The

Chakra

Experience

PATRICIA MERCIER

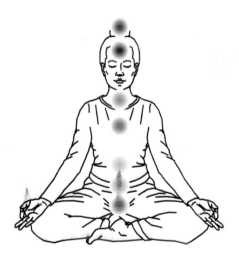

Bounty
Books

An Hachette UK Company
www.hachette.co.uk

First published in Great Britain in 2011 by
Godsfield, a division of Octopus Publishing Group Ltd

This edition published in 2014 by Bounty Books,
a division of Octopus Publishing Group Ltd
Endeavour House
189 Shaftesbury Avenue
London
WC2H 8JY
www.octopusbooks.co.uk

ISBN 978-0-753728-79-6

A CIP catalogue record for this book is
available from the British Library

Printed and bound in China

Note
No medical claims are made for the information in this book and it is
not intended to act as a substitute for medical treatment. In the context
of this book, illness is thought of as a 'dis-ease' – the final
manifestation of spiritual, environmental, psychological, karmic,
emotional ormental imbalance or distress. Wellness and healing mean
bringing mind, body and spirit back into balance and facilitating
evolution for the soul; they do not imply a cure.

CONTENTS

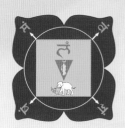

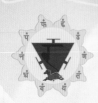

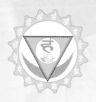

CD tracks

TRACK 1: Colour-Breathing a Rainbow
TRACK 2: Complete Relaxation
TRACK 3: Heart Chakra Visualization
TRACK 4: Sound Experience
TRACK 5: Visualization for my 12 Chakras

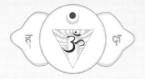

Introduction

Have you ever wondered about chakras, what they could mean for you and how you could understand them? By undertaking this workshop-in-a-book, now you can!

Perhaps you have heard chakras described in a yoga class as something rather mysterious, or have already started to 'tune in' to your own 'subtle body' (unseen, but discernible) energies. In my other books I gave a definitive guide to working with chakras. This book is like coming to one of my chakra workshop courses, because you will benefit from using the tried-and-tested exercises and visualizations, in combination with the CD.

What exactly are chakras?

Around our physical body there is an auric energy field (see page 10). Interacting with our body are spiralling energetic forces known as chakras (both their common and traditional Indian names are given in this book). Teachings originating in yoga refer to seven major chakras or body-power centres as follows, starting from the base of the spine:

1 **Base (Root) Chakra/Muladhara** – colour of influence: red
2 **Sacral Chakra/Svadisthana** – colour of influence: orange
3 **Solar Plexus Chakra/Manipura** – colour of influence: yellow
4 **Heart Chakra/Anahata** – colour of influence: green (or rose-pink)
5 **Throat Chakra/Vishuddha** – colour of influence: turquoise-blue (or sky-blue)
6 **Third Eye (Brow) Chakra/Ajna** – colour of influence: deep blue
7 **Crown Chakra/Sahasrara** – colour of influence: white, violet or gold.

From this sequence you can see how the chakras progress in the light spectrum. Each colour vibrates to its own frequency. We have seven major chakras and 22 interconnected minor and transpersonal chakras that connect us to the wider cosmic field – sometimes called the Quantum Field.

How to use the book and CD

After an explanatory opening section, as you come to each chapter in this book you will learn ways to clear, activate or balance the seven chakras, to facilitate body/mind/spirit harmony and wellness. You will be shown how to use a pendulum and crystals, do colour-breathing and visualizations/meditation and use aromatherapy and sound. Turn to the second part of each chapter for your personal workshop exercises, journal pages and recommendations on when to use the CD.

The CD provides musical tracks to accompany guided instruction for five of the exercises, which you will also find written as scripts in the book. Simply follow the instructions that you hear or, if you prefer, you can record your own.

Journal space is provided in each chapter to record your observations and experiences after the exercises. Remember to write the date. Try using keywords to get your thoughts down quickly. Keep some spare sheets of paper close by, if you prefer to make drawings of your experiences. When you are journaling, record your body's feelings, your thoughts and emotions, how relaxed you feel, whether your energy feels weaker or stronger, whether your sleep patterns are any different, whether your state of wellness is improved and any other information that you wish.

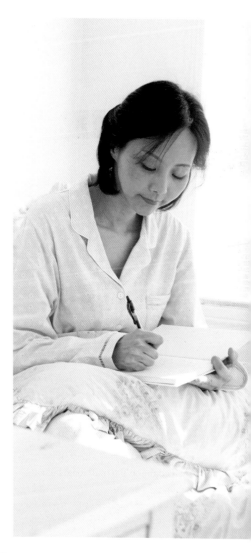

Symbols and recording your insights

Throughout this book you will find symbols to guide you in the next stage of your chakra exploration.

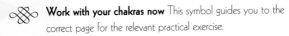

Work with your chakras now This symbol guides you to the correct page for the relevant practical exercise.

I'm not quite there yet If you don't yet feel confident about doing the exercise, this symbol gives suggestions for ways to revise and prepare yourself.

Optional advanced exercise This symbol guides you to the relevant page for more advanced work.

Work with the CD now This symbol tells you when to turn to the CD and which track to select. If you would like to follow the script, turn to the pages indicated.

Subtle energy and the chakras

This workshop-in-a-book experience has been specially designed to lead you step-by-step into a deeper understanding of chakra energy. It is different from an academic course, because you will be asked to familiarize yourself with your own chakras by first reading the written material and then undertaking various exercises. This practical work is essential to appreciate the subtleties of chakras and maintain wellness in a holistic way. You will also be asked to sense the condition and balance of your own chakras and to record this on one of the 'body outline pages' (see page 35 for an example). In addition, each chapter has journal space enabling you to keep notes about your progress. These holistic health teachings will support your realization that you are more than just a physical body. Science can now measure the body's electromagnetic field, which in turn has an even finer, more subtle energy field stretching out as far as 10 m (30 ft), called the aura. This is part of your life-force energy system and is regarded as a 'rainbow of light' – indeed, ancient Indian yogis (dedicated practitioners of yoga) called the chakras 'wheels of light', and this is a very good way to envisage them.

Energy transmission points

Energy is received and transmitted through our chakras. They draw information through a fine network of bio-energy lines called nadis (see page 28). Examples of energy transmission are: a crowd of people in a supermarket feeling stress at the checkout; euphoria at a wedding celebration; or sharing happiness with another person. Where did that energetic feeling come from, and how was it picked up? It is not just something we are hearing or seeing, but *sensing* with all parts of our energy body, comprising the aura and chakras. In Nature, our chakras communicate with all life around, opening us to the natural flow of Creation. Water is affected by our thoughts and emotions, and trees 'talk' to each other, sharing information about soil conditions, predators, rainfall and perhaps even the human beings walking beneath them.!

From the moment we are born, our chakras are concerned with survival and basic instincts, yet simultaneously they remind us that we are Children of Light. All life on this planet is sustained by solar light and spiritual Light (with a capital letter), within the electromagnetic spectrum of colour that is sometimes described as the '49th octave of vibration'.

My aura and luminous body

It is important to understand your aura when studying the chakras. The aura is a fluid, fluctuating, egg-shaped energy field surrounding your physical body with different layers of light energy. Beginning closest to your physical body, these layers are called:

- **Etheric Body:** a holographic energy body that interfaces with the physical body
- **Astral or Emotional Body:** a template of the body, and possibly a place to hold your personality beyond death
- **Lower Mental Body**
- **Higher Mental Body**
- **Spiritual Body:** an energy template for the Etheric Body
- **Causal Body:** a repository for lifetimes of experience
- **Ketheric Body:** your link to superconsciousness and Divine Mind.

These layers coexist because they all have different energetic frequencies. Just as communication signals for cellphones, television and radio don't get mixed up with each other, so the layers of your auric body are separately defined.

Back in 1908–14 a doctor in London, Dr Walter Kilner, developed a chemically coated screen that enabled the aura to be seen by anyone, without the faculty of clairvoyance. We have progressed a great deal since then, with the ability to record energies on very sensitive instruments. We now know that the chakras interpenetrate the auric layers, bringing information energy-flows through our auras – even from deep space – into our bodies. Informational energy also goes back out from our bodies, so we are in two-way communication.

The aura of every human, animal, microbe, plant, tree, stone and crystal vibrates in harmony with the cosmic and elemental energies of Earth, Water, Fire, Air and Spirit. When we are with a crowd of people or walk in a forest of tall trees, our energy fields mingle. We are part of a greater 'field of life', constantly interacting with our surroundings and even extending throughout the cosmos, since biophysicists affirm that all matter is interconnected in the Quantum Field.

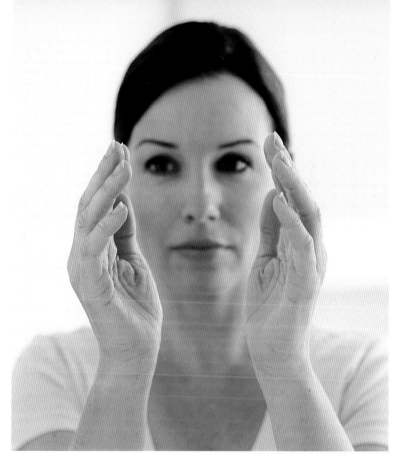

Seeing the aura

You may like to try the following way
of seeing your own aura. Sit in a slightly
darkened room and rub your hands
vigorously together. Then stretch your
arms out in front of you, with your
fingertips curving toward each other,
but not quite touching. Against a dark
background, look to a point *beyond*
your fingertips, without staring and
with a 'soft' gaze. Most people will see
very fine lines of light, or colourless,
luminous auric streamers, moving
from and between their fingers. This
is the first and most visible part of
your aura.

My seven chakras

Chakras focus the energetic forces of life within our bodies. They are situated within the auric field as swirling masses of colour that interact with our physical bodies at the front, as well as at the back through the spine. They relate particularly to the wellness of our endocrine system (the ductless glands), our central nervous system and spinal fluid. These are the seven main chakras, or power centres, with their associated body areas, starting from the base of the spine:

- **Root or Base Chakra/Muladhara** Associated with the most solid parts of the body, such as the bones, teeth and nails; also with the gonads, anus, rectum, colon, prostate gland, blood and blood cells.
- **Sacral Chakra/Svadisthana** Associated with the pelvis, kidneys and the production of adrenaline; also with the bladder and body liquids: blood, lymph, gastric juices and sperm.
- **Solar Plexus Chakra/Manipura** Associated with the lower back, digestive system, liver, spleen, gall bladder, pancreas and the production of insulin.
- **Heart Chakra/Anahata** Associated with the heart, the upper back and general function of the lungs, blood and air circulation. There is another chakra close to the Heart Chakra, which is linked to the thymus gland and lymphatic system, called the Thymus Chakra.
- **Throat Chakra/Vishuddha** Associated with the throat, neck, thyroid and parathyroid glands, ears, windpipe and the upper parts of the lungs.
- **Third Eye (Brow) Chakra/Ajna** – Associated with the face, nose, sinuses, ears, eyes and brain functions (including the pituitary gland, cerebellum and central nervous system).
- **Crown Chakra/Sahasrara** Mainly associated with the cerebrum and pineal gland (which is sensitive to light levels), thus affecting the entire body; linked to the production of cerebral spinal fluid.

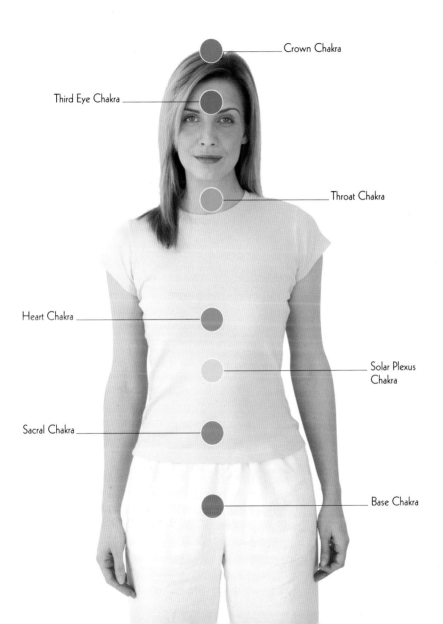

Crown Chakra

Third Eye Chakra

Throat Chakra

Heart Chakra

Solar Plexus
Chakra

Sacral Chakra

Base Chakra

Becoming my own chakra healer

Using the knowledge in this book will help you take responsibility for yourself and understand what is right for you, by listening to the 'inner voice' that comes from your own 'truth'. It is important to be open-minded and to regard this as preventative 'medicine'. Dis-ease will always strike at the weakest part of your physical body. When you get in tune with your chakras, you may also activate spiritual development of a kind that does not normally conflict with religious thinking. The methods described in this book are core to holistic teachings and healing ways developed over the last 100 years, but draw upon ancient truths.

To experience your own chakras and become your own healer, you only need to develop intuition, heeding subtle messages from your body, mind and wider environment around you. There is nothing complicated to learn.

From my own training (first as a teacher of yoga, then as a holistic healer with colour, light, crystals, essential oils and Reiki), I have learned many practical ways to 'nourish' the chakras. You will discover them later in this book. *Give yourself quality time and space to follow them. Avoid being disturbed by people, telephones or excessive noise. Do not undertake the exercises if you are too tired.* If you approach this book in a calm manner, you will settle into a different way of looking at the world, giving yourself permission to relax and explore the mysteries of the chakras. Within these ancient teachings there is enough information for many lifetimes. Central to them is the knowledge gained over centuries through yoga and meditation, which open dimensions beyond your physical body. Understanding your chakra energies will give you command of your life and, most importantly, will bless you with time to be rather than *do*.

 Work with your chakras now Turn to Exercise 1: Sensing and Drawing my Chakra Energies on page 34 and follow the instructions, before you read further.

Understanding the directional spin of chakras

People with auric vision usually describe chakras as having very soft and delicate swirling colours of light merging into one another, and sometimes spinning in a specific direction.

Everyone has a natural direction or spin to their chakra energies – either clockwise or anticlockwise. Whatever others may say, there is no right or wrong direction. This is a fluid situation and many factors can cause the natural spin to reverse temporarily. It may help healers/therapists to know that I use a pendulum to record the directional spin of incoming and outgoing chakra energies – and I do this both before and after a treatment. However, this is an advanced technique and does not feature in this book.

What I have discovered is that when the seven major chakras are harmoniously balanced, they alternate in their direction of spin from the Base Chakra upward. This is an ideal situation to work toward, using the balancing exercises in this book.

All chakras exert an attracting or repelling action, according to their direction. A clockwise chakra attracts an anticlockwise chakra, and vice versa. This is why we sometimes feel repelled by someone for no apparent reason – their subtle energies are just not in synchronization with ours. On the other hand, we are also drawn to some people as if they are an 'energy magnet'. This isn't surprising when we learn more about the chakras, for even our choice of sexual partner is affected by them.

We give off 'vibes' – energy messages – through our chakras to attract a partner. This occurs in both heterosexual and homosexual couples. During lovemaking a chakra ideally aligns with another of the opposite directional spin. So by balancing our chakras we are more likely to attract partners who are destined to enhance our auric energy field. In the future we will realize harmony in relationships and families is intrinsically linked to maintaining vibrant energy fields.

Are my chakras active or passive?

Some people describe chakras as 'open' or 'closed' – but if they were all closed, you would be dead! Better descriptions are 'active', 'underactive', 'passive/balanced' and 'overactive'.

Active means that your chakra is functioning well, maintaining a healthy input and output of the subtle energy known as '*prana*' (see the Glossary of Terms on page 251). When all chakras are active, your whole body and energy field will be vibrant.

Underactive means that your chakra needs help or stimulation – perhaps using the 'Energy Medicine' provided by the exercises in this book and on the CD.

Passive/balanced means that your chakra energies are resting or harmonious. This is the normal state to seek.

Overactive means that one or more of your chakras is functioning excessively to eliminate imbalances in your physical body, such as health issues. Sometimes overactivity aims to eliminate emotional imprints such as addiction, abuse or ancestral karma (see the Glossary).

There are two fundamental ways to influence your chakras and levels of pranic 'life-force', which in itself is usually a measure of well-being.

The first is by exposing your chakras to energy vibrations ('Energy Medicine') in resonance with the frequencies of a naturally balanced chakra. This can be achieved by means of practical exercises, using crystals, colour, light or sound, among other methods. Well-balanced *pranic* energy streaming into your body clears out the chakra like a breath of fresh air, and purification occurs. Sometimes this stimulates a 'healing crisis' (see the Glossary), but soon a deep sense of joy, serenity and clarity will enter.

The second way is to have the courage to just *be*. Take a decision and act upon

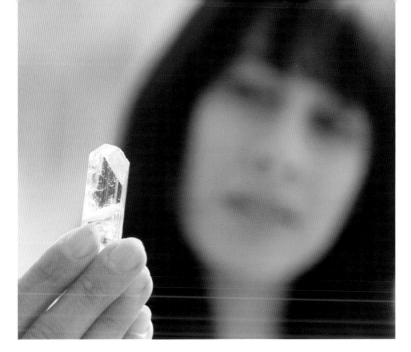

it. Key to this is relaxation, for unless you can relax, the auric mental and emotional bodies hold on to limiting ideas. Many people say they simply can't relax – even in their leisure time and on holiday, they never seem to stop their inner dialogue and never enter into an experience with their entire body/mind/spirit complex. If you recognize yourself in these descriptions, make an extra effort to undertake *all* the exercises more than once.

 Work with your chakras now Turn to Exercise 15: Complete Relaxation on page 110, if you would like to learn a tried-and-tested relaxation technique now.

 Work with the CD now Listen to CD reference Track 2, to hear the same relaxation technique being read out to you.

Using a pendulum

A pendulum is a very useful 'tool' for your work with chakras. Using a pendulum is not a party game – you need to take seriously the energies it shows you. Practise on your own until you develop empathy and get the hang of it. Pendulum 'dowsing', as it is called, gives access to all manner of information that the conscious mind would not have thought possible. The limitation is that you must formulate questions to which there is *only* a 'Yes' or 'No' answer. Please understand the need to disconnect completely from the outcome of the answer, since your mind or ego can influence the swing of the pendulum.

You may use a small jewellery pendant, a natural stone with a hole in it or even a heavy button as a pendulum, although you may prefer to choose a beautiful purpose-made crystal one. Ensure that your pendulum is well balanced and has a pointed tip. It is essential to feel comfortable with whatever you use, for it becomes an extension of your own subtle-energy field, detecting (among other things) slight variations in the surrounding areas that are normally not consciously picked up. If you have a crystal pendulum, wash it and dedicate it to the chakras, keeping it solely for your personal use.

How to hold the pendulum

Hold it between your thumb and first finger, from a chain or cord approximately 15–20 cm (6–8 in) in length. Tuck your elbow tightly into your body, and hold your arm and hand parallel to the floor. This keeps both hand and pendulum in the general area of the Solar Plexus Chakra and enhances the results.

'Yes' or 'No'?

To discover your reactions, relax, take a few calm breaths, then hold the pendulum a little above the palm of your other hand, and ask, 'Is my name...........?' (giving your own name). The pendulum should react immediately, swinging in a circle either clockwise or anticlockwise (occasionally it is a movement from side to side or front to back). This is your 'Yes' response. Run your hand down your pendulum to bring it back to a resting position.

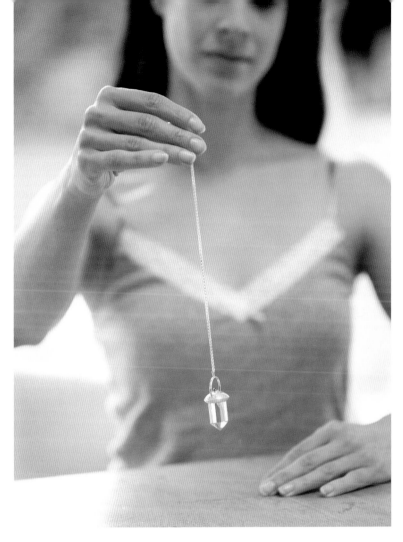

Now check your 'No' reaction. Ask, 'Is my name...........?' (giving a false name). The pendulum should immediately swing in the opposite direction. Practise for a while, asking questions to which you know there is a 'Yes' or 'No' answer.

Setting up my sacred space

Your 'space' – the area your body/mind/spirit complex occupies – is already sacred. Problems with our energies arise when we forget this, and believe that we are separate from our environment or from our connection to the wider influences of the cosmic field of life and light.

To enhance your practice of the exercises in this book, it is helpful either to be in a harmonious natural setting or to create your own special place indoors. In both instances the sacredness within us – actually within our own 'innerscape' – and the 'outerscape' are one and the same, a reflection of each other.

Set aside a space inside where you will not be disturbed, in order to experience your chakras. Turn off the telephone, and every time you use the space, light a candle and some incense to remind you of the sacred Light. Play harmonious music or listen to CD reference Track 2. You may wish to make an altar as a point of focus, because it is a reflection of your connection to 'all that is'. You can create this using:

- Flowers, candles, an aromatherapy oil diffuser/vaporizer;
- Objects you have found in Nature;
- Photographs of your loved ones or the spiritual being/s who guide you;
- Offerings of bread, salt, food, water or other items that respect the traditions in which you were raised or that you embody today;
- Offerings representing the elemental forces of Earth, Water, Fire, Air and Spirit/Ether;
- Items or photographs representing positive aspects of your life;
- Prayers, poems or inspirational words to read out loud and focus upon.

Keep any crystals that you use for the chakra exercises upon your altar. Explain and share your altar with special friends and members of your family who are interested.

The elements

The elements of Earth, Water, Fire and Air resonate with the first four chakras. You can petition the elemental forces to help clear blockages caused by the stress of daily life – an indication of

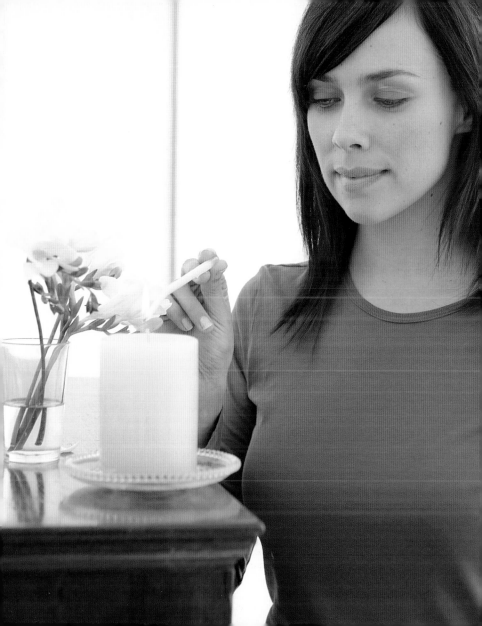

most people's alienation from Nature. Do not think of the elements as abstract ideas, for esoteric teachings have given them form as gods, goddesses or beings: devas/fairies, nymphs, salamanders and sylphs respectively. Above the Heart Chakra, the element of Ether is associated with the Throat Chakra, and Spirit with the Brow and Crown Chakras.

 Work with your chakras now Once you have set up your sacred space, turn to Exercise 27: Candle Meditation on page 197, if you would like to learn a centring and visualization technique leading to meditation.

 I'm not quite there yet Turn to Exercise 15: Complete Relaxation on page 110, if you haven't got time to set up your sacred space.

 Work with the CD now Play CD reference Track 2, to learn how to relax completely.

THE BASE CHAKRA: MULADHARA

 Work with your chakras now Before you read further, turn to Exercise 2: Sensing and Drawing my Base Chakra on page 38.

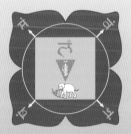

About my Base Chakra

Keypoints: Resonates with the Earth element and the colour red; concerned with sexuality, sensuality, survival and establishing a purpose in living.

The first chakra, the Base, is the source of life – it is from here that the physical body is established and grows. The Sanskrit name, *Muladhara*, means 'root or foundation'. This forms the vital foundation for all the other chakras, so you can understand why it is so important to balance the Base Chakra. This chakra initiates life through procreation and represents our will to live, maintaining existence on planet Earth. Red light, which is the lowest-frequency energy of visible light, stimulates this chakra. At the auric-field level the Base Chakra is linked to the secondary minor chakras in the feet, knees and gonads, and in addition energy flows to the physical body through the lower spinal area. Here are some ways to balance your Base Chakra:

- Relaxing and colour-breathing *red* light (stimulating) (see page 43);
- Relaxing and colour-breathing *pink* light (calming);
- Using crystals or aromatherapy;
- Enjoying healthy, uninhibited sex;
- Eating red-coloured food;
- Wearing red clothes;
- Learning yoga and mantras (see page 152);
- Exercising outside and appreciating Nature.

 Work with your chakras now Turn to Exercise 4: Colour-Breathing Red on page 43.

 Work with your chakras now Turn to pages 152–57 to learn about sound for the chakras.

 Work with the CD now Play CD reference Track 4 for a Sound Experience.

CHART OF THE BASE CHAKRA

Colour of influence	Red
Complementary light colour	Turquoise
Colour to calm	Pink
Physical location	Between anus and genitals, opening downward
Physiological system	Reproductive
Endocrine system	Gonads
Key issues	Sexuality, lust, obsession
Inner teaching	Establishing purpose on Earth
Energy action	Stabilization of Earth energy entering the body through feet and legs
Balancing crystals	Carnelian or 'grounding' stones under feet
Balancing aromatherapy oils	Patchouli, myrrh, cedarwood
Balancing herbal teas	Sage (in moderation), a detox tea containing ginseng or a mix of red clover, raspberry leaf, rosehips and damiana
Balancing yoga position (*asana*)	Virabhadrasana 1 (warrior), Trikonasana (triangle) and Garudasana (eagle)
Mantra/tone	LAM in the note of C (sounds like 'larm')
Helpful musical instruments/music	Organ, drums, double bass
Planet/astrological sign/natural House	Mars/Aries/first: life
Reiki hand position	Hands off the body over the genital area
Power animal (Native American tradition)	Snake/serpent

Body/Base Chakra
connections

Each of the seven major chakras is associated with a point on the spine and with a ductless endocrine gland. For the Base Chakra these are the fourth sacral vertebra and the gonads (testes/ovaries) respectively. Disorders that affect the sacrum, the spine in general, excretion of body waste and the sexual organs are all connected to first-chakra imbalances.

Holistic health practice regards the person as a whole and looks for the underlying causes of disease, rather than the symptoms. It frequently makes a body/mind connection with the more subtle energies of the chakras. For example, chronic constipation could be referred to as a Base Chakra dysfunction caused by holding onto old, unnecessary thoughts and resentments, whereas repeating bouts of diarrhoea could again be a Base Chakra dysfunction, this time a reflection of rejecting ideas without assimilating them, due to deep fear.

Because the Earth element is assigned to this chakra, the best way to keep it in balance is to honour your connection to 'Mother Earth' and Nature. Try to take a walk outside every day and open yourself up to the beauty of your surroundings. Even if you are in a city, enjoy the sky, wind and sun. Seek out a park or some other haven of tranquillity where you might spot some of the creatures or birds that share the planet with us. Walk barefoot on the grass. Because the Base Chakra is your foundation, take a look around your home: is it attractive and safe to live in? Are there ways that you could improve its energy and ambience, for instance by treating yourself to a bunch of flowers or bringing the fragrance of natural aromatherapy oils into it?

❛ We tend the garden of Spirit whenever our chakras begin to open and as we strengthen our resolve to grow toward the Light. Like sunflowers that follow the course of the sun across the sky, we instinctively turn to light and move away from darkness. ❜

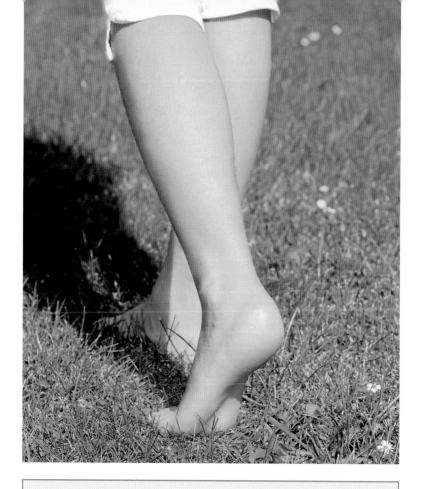

The benefits of grounding energies

When you are relaxing or meditating you might like to have a large stone under each foot, in order to ground what you are experiencing into the Earth Star Chakra beneath (an additional, newly awakened, transpersonal chakra, see page 220). Suitable stones are polished obsidian, iron pyrites or smooth pebbles from a river, garden or beach.

The energy of my Base Chakra

The Base Chakra, opening downward, draws Earth energy upward from the Earth Star Chakra (see page 220) to the feet and legs in order to process and stabilize it. This energy is channelled onward up the spine in a form that the body can handle, as signals that balance the release of endocrine hormones. Unfortunately, the first part of this process is often compromised and we fail to get the full flow of Earth energy. As modern humans, we have become out of touch with Nature by living in cities; by always walking on pavements in shoes and socks made from artificial materials; by buying de-natured food, instead of growing our own and having a relationship with the soil. The most likely and immediate health imbalance caused by alienation from our Earth Star and Base Chakras is persistent tiredness.

Have you noticed that, even in the most polluted, built-up cities, a few large trees manage to survive healthily? They have developed a strong root structure to feed them, which is as wide in its spread as the branches are above ground. Our 'roots', too, are energy connections that need to be strong and expansive.

Kundalini

Kundalini is primal life energy originating at the Base Chakra and normally dormant at the base of the spine. It is likened to a curled-up snake of sexual energy (or a strong *pranic*-type life-force in the Indian traditions). Kundalini is mentioned in the Tantric teachings of Vajrayana Buddhism. Intense sexual practices, such as Tantra, aim to move Kundalini up the spine by way of three major energy channels and the chakras. The central energy channel is called shushumna nadi, whilst the associated ida and pingala nadis intertwine all the way to the Third Eye Chakra. Tantric practitioners aspire to shift a burst of Kundalini energy upward, eventually to the Crown Chakra, where it unites with its opposite polarity, thus achieving enlightenment.

Maintaining the flow of Kundalini during lovemaking produces ecstatic

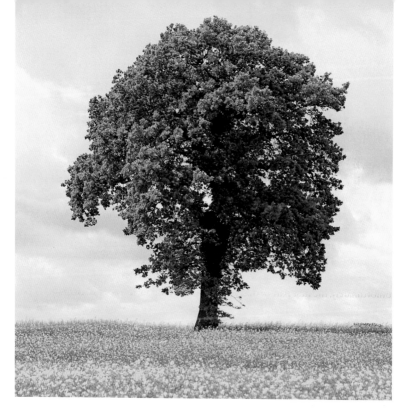

responses, which can be learned through ancient Taoist practices, including intense meditation (which is outside the scope of this book).

Imbalances

If you are unable to fully accept your own sexuality, Base Chakra flow becomes repressed and 'dis-ease' of the sexual organs may result. If you recognize that your fundamental lifestyle is imbalanced, your Base foundation will be imbalanced too. But take heart, for you can rebalance yourself in many different ways. The purpose of this book is to remind you that you can change – you can grow and flourish – simply by learning to be who you really are: ultimately realizing that you are a conscious soul having a physical experience and delighting in your body.

What influences my Base Chakra?

In our technological Western lifestyle, alienated from the world of Nature, we have largely relinquished responsibility for our bodies, in favour of medical intervention and artificial drugs. These are acceptable for supporting specific problems and life-or-death situations, and are administered with tremendous dedication and skill by doctors. But now we are waking up to empowerment through a preventative holistic approach to everyday healthcare. Chakras, body, mind, heart, soul and spirit are irrevocably interrelated. We can therefore choose to approach dis-ease in a different way, whereby a positive attitude of mind is vital. This is how.

Understanding the causes of dis-ease

First, consider what area of your body is affected. What is causing it not to function healthily, and what are the implications of the dis-ease? Explore the physical functions of the associated chakra areas: what is your body telling you?

Second, consider when the illness or dis-ease first manifested – what was happening at that time, and up to two years beforehand?

Third, ask: is this a recurring condition? Has a similar pattern, but a different dis-ease, occurred to me before, to family members or to close friends? Remember, too, that sometimes unwellness is just the process of letting go of old patterns.

Dis-ease may take a long period of time to penetrate the defences of your aura and chakras, before finally resting in your physical body. Natural holistic therapies also take time to clear dis-ease from your body, back out through the aura and chakras. Be prepared to work on yourself, especially on personal emotional issues, which may be the actual 'message'.

More than one chakra may be involved in imbalances in your body. To achieve results, always begin healing practices on the lowest chakra that is implicated.

What emotionally affects this chakra?

We will begin by looking at the message of dis-ease and at body/mind connections to chakras in general. 'Mind' is not just confined to brain functions, because there is an incredible connection between mind and body. With our body we express conscious thoughts and feelings through movement and action. So our body is the mirror of unconscious energies underlying everything we do. On the one hand, complex physical systems convey messages from mind to body; on the other, this is complemented by the intricacies of the chakras. Our bodies are a micro-universe interfacing with vast, converging possibilities. No wonder they sometimes baulk at the immensity of the task and we feel emotionally drained. Yet there is a need to personalize the question and ask: what is the message of this dis-ease in my body?

Every part of your body has a different message to give. You may say, 'I have to shoulder a lot of responsibility' or 'I am fed up to the back teeth'. Take a look at your 'body language' as you say these things. Are your shoulders hunched under too much responsibility, or is your jaw locked, with a habitual grinding of teeth to keep your despair within?

Here are some examples of Base Chakra imbalance:

- Leg tension and circulation problems suggest a holding-on, a lack of security and a disconnection with the Earth. Work on the Base Chakra and feet is needed.
- Imbalanced sexual attitudes may stem from abuse or fear. The key is learning to love ourselves as we are, and accepting that we can grow emotionally and spiritually, even from the direst circumstances.
- Lower-back, hip and pelvic pain all indicate closing down in these areas. We may require more honesty in our relationships, or need to understand that the universe will provide all that we require – but perhaps not all we want!

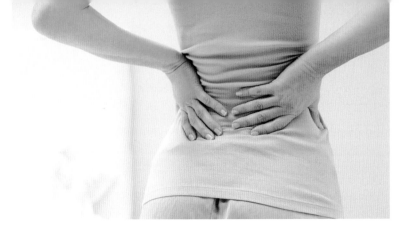

- Our joints are gathering points for energy and can easily block and stiffen – a reflection of our inner attitudes. Knee problems may arise from not accepting a given situation. They may lock with pain, but yoga and t'ai chi ch'uan movements will all work on releasing stubbornness or a fear of progress.
- Ankles and feet move us forward on our life journey. Dis-ease or stiffness in these areas represents conflict about going forward and accepting our direction. This is particularly true in issues to do with the home or with our developing spirituality.

Throughout this workshop-in-a-book you will find many ways to overcome limiting emotional states of mind. Have you ever been to a workshop that was really challenging – it will be the one you remember most, because no one promised you an easy ride? So remember that it is through life's challenges that we all grow. Many years ago my yoga teacher gave me a small piece of paper to study. On it was written: 'I am my own limitation. Without my own limitation I am.' Realizing 'all is perfection', gently accept or gracefully work upon limitations.

 Work with your chakras now Turn to Exercise 3: Swallowing the Inner Smile on page 41.

 I'm not quite there yet Turn to Exercise 1: Sensing and Drawing my Chakra Energies on page 34. (There are additional body outlines at the end of the book.)

BASE CHAKRA EXERCISES

The following exercises develop the Base Chakra or Muladhara, which is the foundation of your being. Like the root system of a large tree, this chakra supports life, giving you your strength and drive. Because it resonates with the frequencies of red light you will learn how to 'colour-breathe' with the help of the CD, learn to smile inwardly, as well as learn to sense and draw the chakra energies.

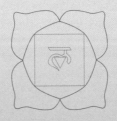

Developing intuition

Do this exercise before reading beyond this page. It will become a record of your subtle energy, to which you can refer back in order to chart your progress. This simple colouring-in of your body outline has been used successfully to train many holistic chakra therapists. It will enhance your intuitive powers.

Exercise 1 SENSING AND DRAWING MY CHAKRA ENERGIES

You will need: a set of coloured pencils or pens (all colours, including magenta, one of the high-frequency colours associated with chakras); keep the book open, ready to colour in the body outline opposite, which represents you (sign and date it before you begin).

- **To begin,** take five minutes sitting in a quiet place, breathing slowly, relaxing and closing your eyes. Now start to sense your body and your aura. Release any emotions that arise. Forget anything you have ever heard or read about chakras and auras. You are simply 'sensing' how your own unique energies are flowing at present. Check from your feet up to your head, to pick up any little clues that your body is giving you. Sense your auric energy field around you as well.

- **When you feel ready,** open your eyes and — immediately and without thinking — quickly colour in any parts of the body outline opposite as you wish. There is no right or wrong place to apply the colour: it is entirely up to you.

- **Once you have completed the exercise,** turn to pages 36–37 to assess your results.

My sensing and drawing my chakra energies experience

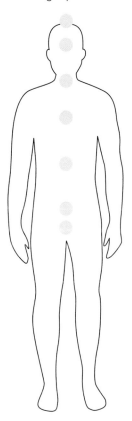

Date _____   Signature _____

Assessing my results for Exercise 1

Remember, there is no right or wrong way to have done this exercise, and there are no right or wrong colours to have used. To help you assess what you have drawn, here are some questions to consider:

- Have you placed colour on or near the chakras?

- Have you mainly used light or dark, heavy shades? What could that mean?

- If you have a pain or an issue with a particular part of your body, what have you drawn there? What colour have you used?

- Can you see areas where there is a concentration or a lack of colour? What could that indicate to you?

- Did you only colour within the body outline? Or did you use the whole page, thus showing your auric field as well?

- Look at your drawing carefully: are some parts of it strong and assertive, while other parts are weak? This is not a judgment, just a reflection.

- Look at the balance of your drawing from top to bottom. Is there more happening above or below your heart level? What could that indicate?

- Look at the balance of your drawing from side to side. Is your left side (feminine influences) or your right side (masculine influences) the strongest?

- Look at the feet — are they 'grounded', or is the body 'floating' and not connected to Earth?

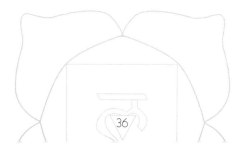

BASIC COLOUR INTERPRETATION OF BODY IMAGE AND THE SURROUNDING AURA

Is there a good balance of colour throughout? If not, ask why this is. Use the following guidelines to interpret your colouring:

Red Strength. Vitality. Or anger. Dull red in the aura = dis-ease or misplaced sexual energy.

Pink Unconditional Love. Excessive pink = ungrounded.

Orange Joyfulness. Balanced sexuality. Excessive orange = imbalance.

Gold/yellow Joy. Intellect. Mental processes. Excessive yellow = imbalance.

Lemon yellow Vitriolic personality/defensive attitudes. In the aura = change.

Leaf-green Balance. Dark green = moodiness, intransigence, unwellness.

Turquoise blue A very positive balanced colour.

Bright blue A very positive balanced colour.

Indigo blue Below heart level = heavy personality. Above heart level = dreamer/thinker/meditator. In the aura = sluggish energy.

Violet and purple Below heart level = ungrounded person. Above heart level or in the aura = spiritual development.

Magenta/ultraviolet A visionary spirit. But if in excess = need to 'ground' and work with the Earth.

Black Small areas of black in the aura or body = unwellness. At the feet = groundedness. Large areas of black = depression/repressed anger/addictions/dominance.

Grey Authority/control/repression. In the aura = unwellness.

Brown Similar to black.

Developing intuition further

Do this exercise before reading beyond this page. It is similar to Exercise 1, but will become a record of your Base Chakra – showing how grounded and realistic or how insecure you are – to which you can refer back in order to chart your progress.

Exercise 2 SENSING AND DRAWING MY BASE CHAKRA

You will need: a set of coloured pencils or pens (all colours, including magenta); keep the book open, ready to colour in the body outline opposite, which represents you (sign and date it before you begin).

- **To begin,** take five minutes sitting in a quiet place, breathing slowly, relaxing and closing your eyes. Now start to sense your body and your aura. Release any emotions that arise. Forget anything you have ever heard or read about chakras and auras. You are simply 'sensing' how your own unique energies are flowing at present. Check from your feet up to your head to pick up any little clues that your body is giving you. Sense your auric energy field around you as well. Now focus upon your Base Chakra area, from the pelvis downward. What is it 'telling' you? What can you sense? Does it feel free, flowing, harmonious? Or is an old pain or trauma held there? Does it feel 'grounded' — or have you shut off all feelings and thoughts of this chakra?

- **When you feel ready,** open your eyes and — immediately and without thinking — quickly colour in the Base Chakra area and any other parts of the body outline opposite as you wish. There is no right or wrong place to apply the colour: it is entirely up to you.

- **Read the interpretation** on page 40 after completing this exercise.

My sensing and drawing my base chakra experience

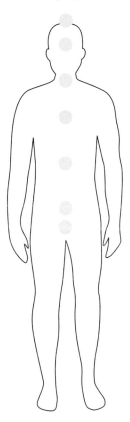

Date _____ Signature _____

Assessing my results for Exercise 2

A balanced Base Chakra will show strong and vibrant colours in the red/orange range. It will reflect trust in the natural flow of life, including your sexuality. It shows the basis of your health, vitality, flexibility, security and love for yourself and all beings. Balance here indicates being centred, grounded, realistic and able to take control of your life.

An unbalanced Base Chakra will show either very weak or very strong colours. These colours may be dark shades — black, brown or grey. It will reflect an attachment to material security, body-weight issues, pessimism and an inability to survive happily. Old childhood traumas are stored here, and weakness/excessive energy indicates low self-esteem, depression, repressed sexuality and fear.

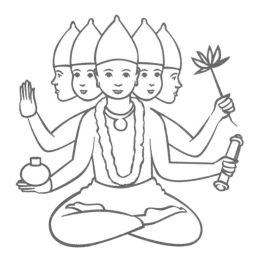

How to 'stress less'

The key to chakra balance is deep relaxation. Listen to CD Track 2 if you feel stressed or before undertaking other exercises. When any of the exercises in this book ask you to sit, use a hard chair with an upright back. Hold your spine straight, chin tucked in, shoulders back and feet firmly on the floor. Rest your hands on your lap, with the right palm on top, clasping the left palm. Breathe deeply through your nose with soft, long, smooth breaths right down to the base of the lungs – both in and out. This takes energy to your belly. Your tongue is a bridge for two channels of energy that flow through your chakras: hold it near the upper teeth over the palate. This prepares you for visualization or meditation.

Sitting as described above, you are now ready for the experience of swallowing your inner smile! This is an ancient Taoist practice and it will give you great inner strength and wellness.

Exercise 3 SWALLOWING THE INNER SMILE

- **The front line:** close your eyes. Allow an inner smile into your eyes, face, neck, heart and blood circulation, lungs, liver, kidneys, adrenal glands, pancreas and spleen.

- **The middle line:** feel saliva collecting in your mouth as your tongue continues to rest over the palate. Collect this saliva with your tongue, then swallow it down with a smile to your stomach, small intestine, large intestine and rectum.

- **The back line:** smile into your eyes, then down the inside of the vertebrae of your spine, from the top downward, one by one.

- **Open your eyes,** be gentle with yourself and with those you meet. Now record your experience in the space provided on page 42.

My swallowing the inner smile experience

Date _____   I saw _____
_____

I felt _____
_____

I learned _____
_____

Date _____   I saw _____
_____

I felt _____
_____

I learned _____
_____

Date _____   I saw _____
_____

I felt _____
_____

I learned _____
_____

Tree visualization

This powerful colour-breathing exercise will connect you to your roots, which draw their sustenance from deep within the Earth, like the roots of a tree. You may record your colour-breathing red experience on the next page and/or make a drawing of your tree on a separate piece of paper.

Exercise 4 COLOUR-BREATHING RED

- **To begin,** sit in an upright chair or a cross-legged yoga posture. Ensure you are fully relaxed. Be in a place where you will not be disturbed for approximately half an hour — indoors is okay, but it would be even better to sit outside with your back against a large tree. Your spine must be as straight as possible and your chin pulled in, to straighten the back of your neck.

- **Close your eyes,** breathe slowly — visualizing your incoming breath as a vibrant red-coloured light — and deeply for a few minutes, focusing on the Base Chakra.

- **Be aware of the ground beneath you** (even if you are in a building) and start to visualize a strong root growing from the bottom of your spine and going into the Earth. Feel you are a seed that has the potential to grow into a huge tree.

- **See roots growing** from the soles of your feet, seeking out flows of water in the Earth. Be aware of tiny rootlets developing from your spinal root, anchoring you in the ground.

- **Now move to your trunk,** sensing that — like the main part of your body — it is a channel through which nourishment from the Earth can flow.

- **Check your body is finely balanced** on either side of your spine. Move on up into your branches. Imagine your neck and head, and perfectly balanced branches going out in the four directions: east, west, north and south.

- **Observe the shape of the leaves** on your tree; maybe there are flowers or fruit, or perhaps the branches are bare. Whatever you see, accept it.

- **Know that you have inner strength,** like a tree, that you can pull into yourself from the Earth. Thank the water and sun for nourishment, and the wind for its cleansing of dead leaves and wood in your branches. Know that you are connected to all other trees and life on this sacred Earth. Really, nothing is separate. All is One.

- **To finish,** start to breathe the red-coloured light more deeply. Reach down to your feet and rub them, then your legs. Finally stand up and stretch 'as tall as a tree'.

- **Now consider** the questions on page 45.

My colour-breathing red experience

Date _____   Signature _____

Circle the relevant answers below:

How well did I relax?   Well / With difficulty / I couldn't relax at all

Did the colour-breathing help me focus on my Base Chakra?   Yes / No / A bit, but then I lost the focus / Don't know

Did you see a tree?   Yes / No

What kind of tree was it? _____

Was it strong / tall / large / small/weak?

Did it have a large trunk / a flexible trunk / a thin trunk?

Did it have leaves?   Yes / No

Did it have buds or flowers?   Yes / No

Describe them _____

_____

Did it have seeds?   Yes / No

How did this exercise affect me? _____

_____

What have I learned from this experience? _____

_____

Does my Base Chakra feel more balanced?   Yes / No / A bit / Don't know

Pendulum dowsing

This exercise in pendulum dowsing builds up empathy and confidence with your pendulum, so that you can use it reliably to determine degrees of activity in your chakras. Avoid holding the pendulum over a chakra, particularly if it is a crystal pendulum; instead, point a finger of the other hand toward and near the chakra – this ensures that the pendulum does not falsify the reading.

Exercise 5 DOWSING MY CHAKRAS

You will need: a pendulum, and a pen to record your results.

- **To begin,** remain focused and silent for a moment. Then work systematically through each chakra, beginning with the Base Chakra and asking: 'Does this .... Chakra require balancing?' It is also relevant to ask: 'Is this .... Chakra overactive?' or 'Is this .... Chakra underactive?'

- **Record your pendulum results** on page 48 (date and sign your record), so that you can begin to see repeating (or varying) patterns of chakra activity. You may dowse just the Base Chakra, or you have space there to record the condition of all your chakras, if you wish. You can also compare the effects that various methods described in this book have upon your chakras, by dowsing before and after any balancing.

- **As an optional method of dowsing,** use a blank 'body outline' as given at the end of this book (see pages 238–49). Sign it (this is your 'witness' or energy imprint). With the understanding that this body outline represents you, rest your index finger on each chakra in turn. Hold the pendulum in the other hand, well away from your physical body. Ask the questions given above. Record your results on the following page, remembering to put the date on it.

- **Don't be concerned** if you can't immediately get reliable results. For some people, dowsing can take a long time to learn — particularly if the mind gets in the way! Continue practising another day, when your energy will be different, and eventually you will succeed. Helpful hint: don't look at the pendulum as you dowse.

Later, when you feel ready to do so, you may also work on the Base Chakra with any of the other balancing methods mentioned on other pages of this book. Consult the chart on page 25 to ascertain which aromatherapy oil to use, which yoga postures, colour breathing, and so on.

I'm not quite there yet Reread pages 18 and 19, for clarity on pendulum dowsing.

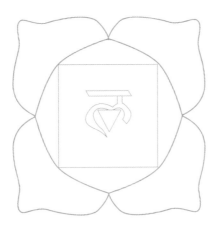

My dowsing my chakras experience

Date _____ Signature _____

- Does this _____ Chakra require balancing?   Yes / No
- Is balance required on a physical level?   Yes / No
- Is balance required on a mental/emotional level?   Yes / No
- Is balance required on an energy level in my auric field?   Yes / No
- Is this _____ Chakra overactive?   Yes / No
- Is colour-breathing required?   Yes / No
- Is crystal balancing required?   Yes / No
- Is a change in my lifestyle required?   Yes / No
- Is this _____ Chakra underactive?   Yes / No
- Is colour-breathing required?   Yes / No
- Is crystal balancing required?
- Is a change in my lifestyle required?   Yes / No
- Ask any other questions that you wish to pose.

Circle the relevant states below:

Base Chakra	Balanced	Underactive	Overactive
Sacral Chakra	Balanced	Underactive	Overactive
Solar Plexus Chakra	Balanced	Underactive	Overactive
Heart Chakra	Balanced	Underactive	Overactive
Throat Chakra	Balanced	Underactive	Overactive
Third Eye Chakra	Balanced	Underactive	Overactive
Crown Chakra	Balanced	Underactive	Overactive

THE SACRAL CHAKRA: SVADISTHANA

 Work with your chakras now Before you read further, turn to
Exercise 6: Sensing and Drawing my Sacral Chakra on page 66.

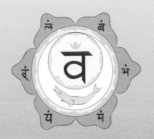

About my Sacral Chakra

Keypoints: Resonates with the Water element and the colour orange; concerned with sexuality, sensuality, emotions, karma and relationships.

The second chakra, the Sacral, is your vitality centre – flexibility here lets you feel content in your own body. The Sanskrit name, *Svadisthana*, means 'one's own abode'.

This chakra comes into play during puberty. It is responsive to the cycles of the moon and balances women's 'moon times'. A harmonious Sacral Chakra moves energy up from the Base Chakra to create sensual sensitivity and joy. It gives us fluidity in our actions, the ability to let go and express ourselves through dance, music and other creative arts.

However, if it is unbalanced, we may deprive ourselves of joy or spontaneity. It's not so much our feelings that will ebb and flow with this chakra, but our response to them. Unpleasant feelings aren't bad – they just need to be worked through and, if severe, may need professional assistance. Our vitality centre is watery by nature and is subject to mood swings, yet it is only by embracing our darker, more difficult side that we grow. And if we do not grow through adversity, then our inner child (see Glossary of Terms, page 251) becomes stuck at second-chakra level and we are unable to move energy up to other levels.

So allow time for recreation, non-competitive sport/exercise, play and laughter. Enjoy playing make-believe with children – they are great teachers because many of them remember who they really are at soul level.

In humanity's present collective incarnation, karma is an outdated attachment to time, causing compliance with archaic control mechanisms that rob us of our true inheritance as beings of Light having a physical experience – not only in this life, but in future lives too.

Orange light stimulates this chakra. At the auric-field level the Sacral Chakra is linked to secondary minor chakras in the groin and behind the knee, which are close to waste-removing lymph nodes. It is also linked to two minor spleen chakras.

CHART OF THE SACRAL CHAKRA

Colour of influence	Orange
Complementary light colour	Blue
Colour to calm	Blue
Physical location	Upper part of sacrum, below navel
Physiological system	Genitourinary
Endocrine system	Adrenals
Key issues	Relationships, emotions, addictions
Inner teaching	Seeking meaningful relationships with all life forms
Energy action	Transmutes sexual energy
Balancing crystals	Moonstone/aquamarine
Balancing aromatherapy oils	Sandalwood/jasmine/rose/ylang-ylang
Balancing herbal teas	Mix of spearmint, chamomile, liquorice, cleavers, corn silk and horsetail
Balancing yoga position (*asana*)	Parivrtta trikonasana (twisting triangle), Utthita parsvakonasana (extended lateral), Natarajasana (pose of Shiva)
Mantra/tone	VAM in note of D (sounds like 'varm')
Helpful musical instruments/music	Viola, lute, chords played on a guitar
Planet/astrological sign/natural House	Mercury and Venus/Gemini and Taurus/third: Education and second: Possessions
Reiki hand position	Two palms over the belly, then lift the hands off and place two palms below the navel
Power animal (Native American tradition)	Dolphins

Body/Sacral Chakra connections

The Sacral Chakra, also called the Navel Centre, is associated with the first lumbar vertebra and with the ductless adrenal endocrine glands above each kidney. Disorders that affect the bladder, kidneys, intestinal complaints and circulatory problems as well as the reproductive organs are all connected to Second Chakra imbalances.

The Sacral Chakra is concerned with assimilation, both in the sense of digestion of food and ideas, which bring about a natural sense of joy. When unrepressed, this produces a strong creative urge. This chakra is where sexuality is transmuted into the creative arts through self-expression.

Holistic health practice makes a body/mind connection with the more subtle energies of the Sacral Chakra. For example, because the adrenals release adrenaline at critical and stressful moments, the 'flight or fight' response is activated: we cannot decide whether to get up and run, or stand our ground and fight, so issues of self-survival are key. Closely linked to this area is the spleen, which supports (among other things) the production of immune cells in the blood. It is known that negative emotions impinge upon our body functions and the spleen is no exception, because anger particularly affects it.

Male and female concerns

Sexual dysfunction, such as sterility, may be concerned with hidden fears about having children, responsibility, financial worries or past traumas from our own childhood. Prostate problems in men are related to the sense of sexual power and performance. So, like women approaching middle age or the 'golden years', men too would be advised to move energy upward creatively through the higher chakras in order to relax in the fullness of older life.

Gynaecological or breast problems may be closely linked to feelings that a mother has when her children leave home. Her life had centred on the family,

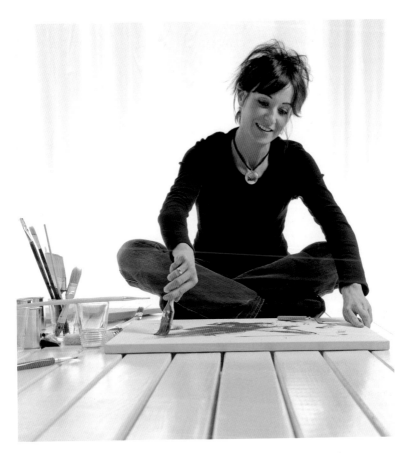

but then alternative interests are needed, which move the emphasis of her energies up from the Sacral and Heart Chakras onto other levels of understanding and into a time of personal spiritual growth.

 Work with the CD now Listen to CD reference Track 2 to help you relax, if you are feeling stressed.

The energy of my Sacral Chakra

The energy of the Sacral Chakra is softer and more 'feminine' than the strongly 'masculine' drive of the Base Chakra. It is the source of vitality for our etheric/auric body and the fountain of our passion for all of life – not just sexuality. It is the centre that leads us on to achieve marvellous things, triumphing over adversity and feeling happy and content in the process.

If your Sacral Chakra energy is imbalanced, you may ignore your feelings, disconnect from your sensuality and simply be too engrossed in your mind, living an ascetic life. Ask yourself the following questions:

- Do I celebrate my life and my accomplishments?
- Do I look after my body?
- Do I eat healthily and get enough sleep?
- Do I express my feelings?
- Do I take the time to look nice?
- Do I smile often?
- Do I sing or dance?
- Do I give and receive gracefully?
- Do I have a fulfilling sex life?
- Do I channel my life-force into creative pursuits?
- Do I regularly give myself a 'day out of time' just to relax?
- Do I exercise enough?

If you answered 'No' to one or two of these questions, then your vitality is weakened. If you answered 'No' to five or more of these questions, then your vitality is imbalanced. And if you answered 'No' to seven or more of these questions, your imbalance needs to be corrected: turn to page 41 immediately and do Exercise 3: Swallowing the Inner Smile.

Later on undertake more than once the exercises that you find particularly helpful in this book, until you feel you are achieving your full potential as a vibrant radiant being.

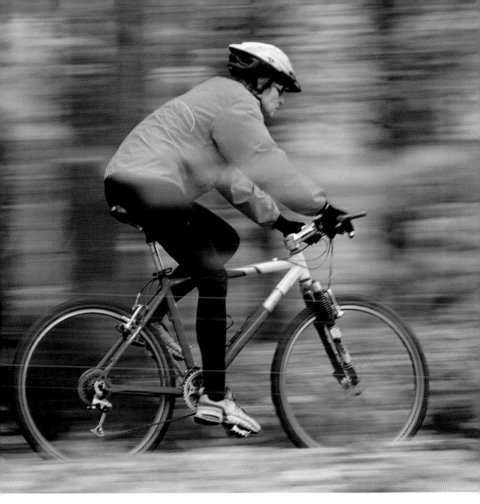

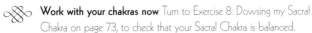 **Work with your chakras now** Turn to Exercise 8: Dowsing my Sacral Chakra on page 73, to check that your Sacral Chakra is balanced.

Work with your chakras now Turn to Exercise 9: Using Crystals on page 75, to balance your Sacral Chakra.

What influences my Sacral Chakra?

The element of Water is associated with the genitourinary system and influences the Sacral Chakra. Our sense of taste is linked to this chakra. It is well known that the moon controls the flow of all liquids on the Earth, and in us! The water we take into our bodies is beneficially encoded with an imprint of cosmic forces transduced through the moon. Even our hormones respond to the flow of tides, the phases of the moon and psychic changes that occur as waves of life experience.

Watery remedies

Because the Water element is assigned to Svadisthana, balance it by enjoying your connection to 'Mother Earth', the moon and Nature. Try to swim often. Drink sufficient pure water; increase your intake of salad foods and orange-coloured fruits and vegetables, because their water and mineral content cleanses the body. Create your own spa by giving yourself a few hours of luxury. Start with a mud or seaweed face-pack, then take a long, hot soak in a bath with mineral salts (or sea salt if you cannot get genuine mineral salts). Finish with a cool shower and pamper yourself with your favourite body lotion.

If this chakra is underactive there will be an urge to overindulge in food or sex as compensation, causing obesity, food intolerances, chronic skin conditions or possibly even impotence, sexual cravings and disease. Overactivity will lead to confused sexuality, unless it is balanced by the influence of the Heart Chakra. These effects are the physical body making its demands known. *Listen to your body;* take notice of any early symptoms it communicates to you. Even talk back to your body, telling it what you are doing to help yourself. Have a conversation with each of your chakras in turn, asking them what they need – unless you ask, you will never know!

 Work with your chakras now Turn to Exercise 10: Colour-Breathing a Rainbow on page 77, to begin to balance all your chakras.

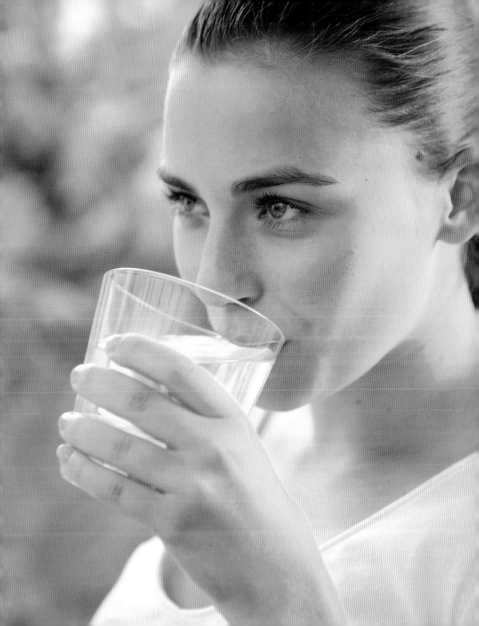

What emotionally affects this chakra?

Clairvoyants say this chakra naturally has an anticlockwise or feminine spin in both men and women. Psychologically it is linked to the Throat Chakra, which – if repressed – will have a detrimental knock-on effect. A healer will therefore often work upon both of these chakras in order to bring about balance.

In Eastern traditions this whole area is called the Hara, and is the centring point for body energies. In the Twelve Chakra System there is a separate Hara Chakra just above the Sacral.

The sacred dwelling place

Two 'serpents' of energy – the nadis called Ida and Pingala, representing dualities – bring energy up from the Base Chakra. They leave the Base where they were united and separate into male and female energies, then meet up once again in the Sacral Chakra in the 'sea of the Moon Goddess'. She symbolizes our sacred womb, the protectress of conception and development of new life. But in both sexes this chakra is also the sacred dwelling place of personal transformation, where we can move beyond the limitations of mind and emotions. When we are centred in this sacred place, we interact with our circumstances through mindfulness and generosity rather than through 'wants'. We can develop discernment, especially where sexuality is concerned, learn how to conserve energy, and what and whom we will allow to perceive our sacred centre.

However, if our own sexuality, mental stress or uncontrolled emotions are the issue, then this chakra requires balance, by looking closely at how we deal with duality in our lives. It requires us to centre an emotional and physical sense of self. Because ancestral and family issues are stored here, past-life regression will often move unhelpful blocks or lingering karmic ties.

On page 50 we explained how karma is closely linked to the Sacral Chakra and gave a modern definition of it. In

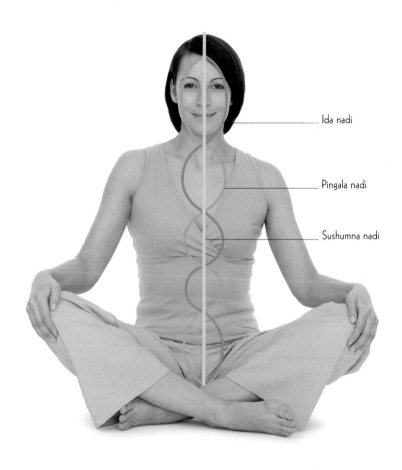

Ida nadi

Pingala nadi

Sushumna nadi

India, karma is considered to be the continual wheel of birth–death–rebirth, the cycle of cause and effect, or 'as ye sow, so shall ye reap'. Another thought-provoking definition is: 'Karma is an expression of the degree to which we have become separate from the Creator/God/Goddess.'

Balancing my Sacral Chakra

To help harmonize this important chakra you can regain equilibrium in a number of ways: through dance, laughter (a good 'belly' laugh), yoga, breathing exercises and visualization of orange-coloured light and even through eating orange-coloured food.

Free expression: dancing with light

As you will see in later chapters, a wonderful way to 'nourish' all your chakras is to feed them with beautiful harmonious music. To release your Sacral Chakra, and indeed balance all your chakras, dance! One evening choose to make a focus of a coloured candle, flowers and objects on a coloured cloth in the centre of a room. For the Sacral Chakra the colours should be predominantly orange, orange-yellow and orange-red. Then begin to play some joyful or perhaps passionate music. Stand very still, getting in touch with your inner energies. Breathe deeply, drawing in and around yourself the colour that you have chosen to work with.

Have a sense of your breath and of the music shifting colour to the place where it is most needed in your body. Begin to move that part of your body. Next, allow the music to flow into the rest of your body. Experience the exhilaration of spinning around, or the point of stillness as you hold a particular position. Be aware of how the music loosens your movements so that you use all the space in your room – lying and moving on the floor, or stretching toward the ceiling. Shiva, Lord of the Cosmic Dance, releases an ecstatic response within our chakras as we dance with joyous abandon.

The piece of music you have chosen will take you to the natural ending of your freely expressed Dance of Light. Lie down for a few minutes after you have finished. Your chakras, now harmonized, will make you feel refreshed and recharged.

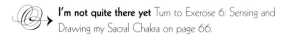 **I'm not quite there yet** Turn to Exercise 6: Sensing and Drawing my Sacral Chakra on page 66.

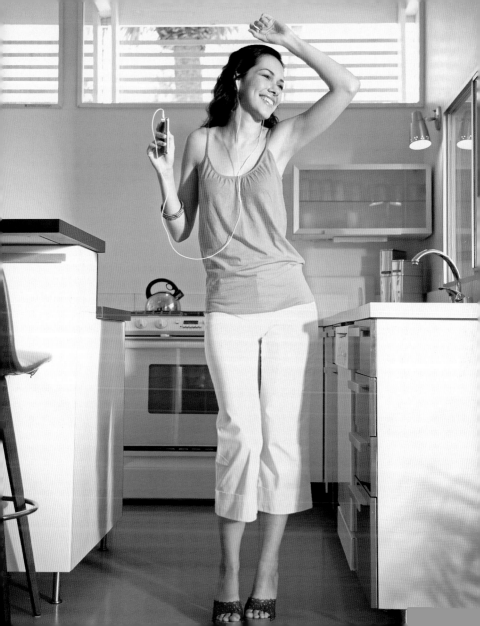

Using crystals to balance my chakras

By the time you have finished this book you may have made a collection of a number of crystals. If possible, this should include:

- Two 'grounding' stones (beach/river pebbles or obsidian)
- Two natural, clear quartz, pointed crystals, any size up to 10 cm (4 in) long
- A set of seven crystals: one in the colour of each major chakra; they may be small, inexpensive 'tumbled' (smooth and rounded) polished crystals
- You may also have a crystal pendulum. Keep your crystals in a special place, such as on your altar or sacred space, or wrap them carefully in red fabric – silk or natural fibre is best.

Cleanse your crystals before and after use. Cleansing methods include soaking the crystals in pure water; wafting them

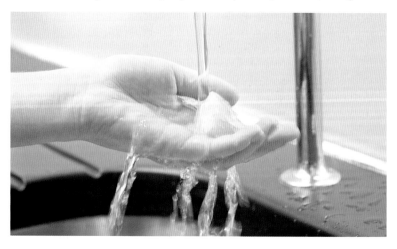

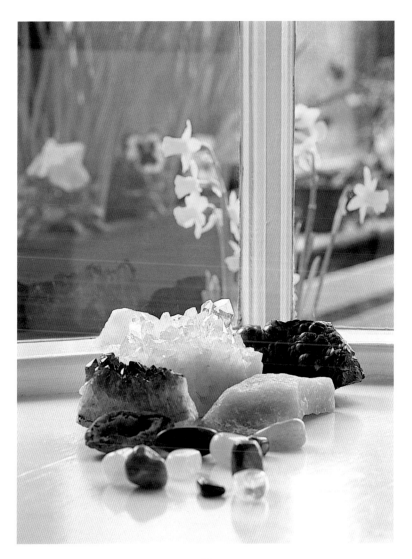

through incense smoke; prayer; flower remedies; or placing them on the earth or on a growing plant. You can also use the power of your mind: visualize them illuminated with clear white light. Occasionally you will need to recharge your crystals in sunlight or moonlight for 12 hours or so.

Before each exercise involving crystals, dedicate them to your chakra work, saying, for example, 'May this crystal draw upon the power of Unconditional Love and Light to balance my chakras and energies, for the highest good.'

Body/chakra boost

It has been proven that our physical and energy bodies respond to the presence of crystals. For this reason it is recommended that you obtain two pointed, clear quartz crystals, as mentioned above. Use the crystals to give a regular body/chakra boost and balance, to yourself or a friend, as follows.

First, find a pleasant place to lie down on your back, such as on a blanket in your sacred space. Then place one quartz crystal at the top of your head, pointing toward your feet, and the other crystal beyond your feet, pointing toward your head. *It is most important that the points of the quartz crystals point inward, because you wish to increase your subtle energy, not drain it away.*

Then just relax and let the crystals exert their influence. Finish by breathing deeply, stretching and sitting up slowly. Visualize the inner strength you could gain by making crystals a natural and intrinsic part of your life.

 Work with your chakras now Turn to Exercise 9: Using Crystals on page 75, to begin to use crystals upon the Sacral Chakra.

SACRAL CHAKRA EXERCISES

The following exercises develop the Sacral Chakra or Svadisthana, which is your vitality centre. This chakra fulfils your life through appreciation of sexuality and creativity, and eventually will bring your feelings into a state of discernment. You will be using a pendulum to ascertain the chakra energies and how to rebalance them using various methods, such as Colour-Breathing a Rainbow (with the help of the CD) and crystals.

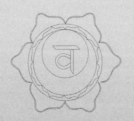

Developing intuition

Do this exercise before reading beyond this page. It will become a record of your Sacral Chakra – reflecting your emotions and your ability to trust others – to which you can refer back in order to chart your progress.

Exercise 6 SENSING AND DRAWING MY SACRAL CHAKRA

You will need: a set of coloured pencils or pens (all colours, including magenta); keep the book open, ready to colour in the body outline opposite, which represents *you* (sign and date it before you begin).

● **To begin,** take five minutes sitting in a quiet place, breathing slowly, relaxing and closing your eyes. Now start to sense your body and aura. Release any emotions that arise. Forget anything you have ever heard or read about chakras and auras. You are simply 'sensing' how your own unique energies are flowing at present. Check from your feet up to your head to pick up any little clues that your body is giving you. Sense your auric energy field around you as well. Now focus upon the Sacral Chakra area of your belly, navel and lower back. What is it 'telling' you? What can you sense? Does it feel free, flowing, harmonious? Or is an old pain or trauma held there? Does this area feel fluid and open, or have you shut off all feelings and thoughts of this chakra?

● **When you feel ready,** open your eyes and — immediately and without thinking — quickly colour in the Sacral Chakra area and any other parts of the body (and surrounding page) as you wish. There is no right or wrong place to apply the colour: it is entirely up to you.

● **Read the interpretation** on page 68 after completing this exercise.

My sensing and drawing my sacral chakra experience

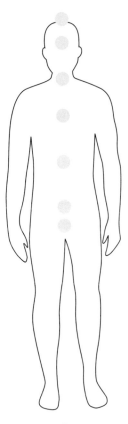

Date _____ Signature _____

Assessing my results for Exercise 6

A balanced Sacral Chakra will show strong and vibrant colours in the light-red/orange range. It will reflect your emotions and your ability to trust others. Like the Base Chakra, it is concerned with sexuality and life's pleasures, the basis of your vitality, your flexibility, security and love for yourself and all beings. Balance here indicates being joyful and able to take control of your own life — feeling happy in your own body.

An unbalanced Sacral Chakra will show either very weak or very strong colours. These colours may be dark shades — black, brown or grey. It will reflect addictions of all kinds, the inability to trust in the abundance of the universe, lack of vitality and sexual perversions and fears.

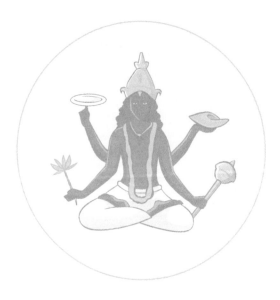

Scanning Sacral Chakra energy

Scanning is a method of using your hands to detect imbalances in the chakras and energy field. Your sensitivity gradually increases with practice. The minor chakras in the palms of your hands will pick up indications in different levels of the auric field, within the chakras and within the body itself. Eventually you will find this a very valuable 'diagnostic' method. Although at present you are using scanning on yourself, many healers who channel healing energy find it invaluable in their work.

 ### Exercise 7 SENSING MY SACRAL ENERGY
CD REFERENCE TRACK 2 (TO FOLLOW THE SCRIPT, TURN TO PAGE 110)

- **To begin**, ensure you will not be disturbed. Sit on your blanket and rub your hands vigorously together to stimulate pranic/ki energy to flow strongly through them. They should feel warm and energized. For this exercise you may use whichever hand you feel most comfortable with.

- **Lie down and relax,** using Track 2 on the CD, or following the instructions for Exercise 15: Complete Relaxation on page 110.

- **Keep your eyes closed** and begin to focus inwardly upon your Sacral Chakra energy. Increase that focus. After a few minutes move your hand slowly around the area of your Sacral Chakra, both within your auric field and on/over your body (this is 'scanning').

- **Notice whether your energy** feels different close into the body or further away. You may feel warmth/cold, lightness/heaviness, vibration/stillness, a colour, dense areas, vibrant areas or other sensations.

- **Remember what you feel,** so that you can record it on the following page.

- **To finish,** take a deep breath, stretch, roll onto one side of your body and sit up slowly.

- **Now consider** the questions on page 71.

- **Note:** You may use this exercise for sensing your Base, Solar Plexus, Heart, Throat, Third Eye and Crown Chakras as well.

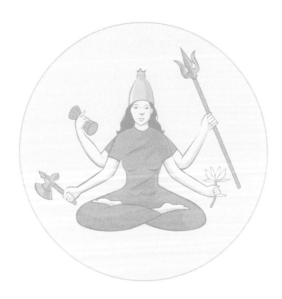

My sensing my Sacral energy experience

Date _____ Signature _____

This exercise was: Easy / Hard / Took a while to get used to it

What did I sense? (tick or expand on what you felt)

Heat _____   Cold _____

Lightness _____   Heaviness _____

Vibration _____   Stillness _____

A colour _____

Dense areas _____

Does this mean my Sacral Chakra energy is clogged/underactive?   Yes / No

Do I need to activate it with colour-breathing orange?   Yes / No
(if your answer is Yes, go to page 77)

Vibrant areas _____

Does this mean my Sacral Chakra energy is balanced?   Yes / No

Did my Sacral Chakra energy seem overactive?   Yes / No

Do I need to calm it with long, slow breaths of the colour peach?   Yes / No
(if your answer is Yes, please do so)

Other sensations? Describe _____

Checking my Sacral Chakra is balanced

This dowsing exercise uses a pendulum to check whether your Sacral Chakra is balanced. As recommended on page 18, try to build up empathy and confidence in your pendulum, so that it can be used reliably to determine degrees of activity in each of your chakras.

Remember to avoid holding the pendulum over a chakra, particularly if it is a crystal one – instead, point a finger of the other hand toward and near the chakra in question. This ensures that the pendulum doesn't falsify the reading.

Below are just some of the questions you may ask. Or how about asking if you need aromatherapy or sound healing exercises? Perhaps you need yoga or other balancing body movements? Any questions that you ask must have only 'Yes' or 'No' answers.

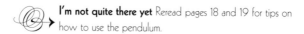 **I'm not quite there yet** Reread pages 18 and 19 for tips on how to use the pendulum.

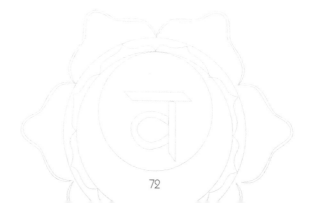

Exercise 8 DOWSING MY SACRAL CHAKRA

You will need: a pendulum, and a pen to record your results.

- **To begin,** remain focused and silent for a moment.

- **Then ask** the following questions:
  'Does this chakra require balancing?'
  'Is balance required on a physical level?'
  'Is balance required on a mental/emotional level?'
  'Is balance required on an energy level in my auric field?'

  It is also relevant to ask:
  'Is this chakra overactive or underactive?'
  'Is colour-breathing required?'
  'Is crystal balancing required?'
  'Is a change in my lifestyle required?'

- **Record your pendulum results** on page 74 (date and sign them), so that you can begin to see repeating (or varying) patterns of chakra activity. You may dowse just the Sacral Chakra, or you have space there to record the condition of all your chakras, if you wish. You can also compare the effects that various methods shown in this book have upon the chakras, by dowsing before and after any balancing work. It becomes very exciting when you do this, because you can start to see positive results.

- **As an optional method of dowsing,** use a blank 'body outline' (see pages 238–49). Sign it (this is your 'witness' or energy imprint). With the understanding that this body outline represents you, rest your index finger on each chakra in turn. Hold the pendulum in the other hand, well away from your physical body. Ask the questions given above. Record and date your results.

My dowsing my sacral chakra experience

Date _____   Signature _____

- Does this _____ Chakra require balancing?   Yes / No
- Is balance required on a physical level?   Yes / No
- Is balance required on a mental/emotional level?   Yes / No
- Is balance required on an energy level in my auric field?   Yes / No
- Is this _____ Chakra overactive?   Yes / No
- Is colour-breathing required?   Yes / No
- Is crystal balancing required?   Yes / No
- Is a change in my lifestyle required?   Yes / No
- Is this _____ Chakra underactive?   Yes / No
- Is colour-breathing required?   Yes / No
- Is crystal balancing required?   Yes / No
- Is a change in my lifestyle required?   Yes / No
- Ask any other questions that you wish to pose.

Circle the relevant states below:

Base Chakra	Balanced	Underactive	Overactive
Sacral Chakra	Balanced	Underactive	Overactive
Solar Plexus Chakra	Balanced	Underactive	Overactive
Heart Chakra	Balanced	Underactive	Overactive
Throat Chakra	Balanced	Underactive	Overactive
Third Eye Chakra	Balanced	Underactive	Overactive
Crown Chakra	Balanced	Underactive	Overactive

Clearing my aura

This exercise uses crystals to clear your aura and balance your Sacral Chakra. Depending on the effect that you require, you can use the following crystals:

- To balance: use moonstone or aquamarine
- To activate: use carnelian or fire opal
- To calm: use emerald, green aventurine or green calcite.

You can use this technique with the recommended crystals for each chakra, but work on just one chakra at a time.

Later, when you feel ready to do so, you may also work on the Sacral Chakra with any of the other balancing methods mentioned in this book. Consult the chart on page 51 to ascertain which aromatherapy oil to use, which yoga postures, colour breathing, and so on.

 ### Exercise 9 USING CRYSTALS
CD REFERENCE TRACK 2 (TO FOLLOW THE SCRIPT, TURN TO PAGE 110)

- **Wear white clothes** or place a white sheet over your naked body. Lie down on a blanket and relax. Have your cleansed and dedicated crystal/s (see page 62) nearby.

- **When it feels right**, gently place your crystal over the Sacral Chakra. Then relax for ten minutes or so, before slowly coming back to everyday awareness. Now record your experience in the space provided on page 76.

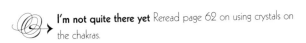 **I'm not quite there yet** Reread page 62 on using crystals on the chakras.

My using crystals experience

Date _____

Chakra and crystal used _____

What I wanted to achieve _____

What I felt _____

_____

What I would like to do next time I try this exercise _____

_____

Does my chakra feel balanced? _____

If not, ask the chakra what it needs. Close your eyes and talk to your chakra.
Record here what it needs _____

_____

Record here what you have done as a result, and the date _____

_____

_____

_____

Breathing colour into all the chakras

This exercise helps you to breathe colour into all of your seven chakras, in a continuation of the relaxation exercise on page 110.

 Exercise 10 COLOUR-BREATHING A RAINBOW
CD REFERENCE TRACK 2 (OPTIONAL) (TO FOLLOW THE SCRIPT, TURN TO PAGE 110) CD REFERENCE TRACK 1 (TO FOLLOW THE SCRIPT, SEE BELOW)

- **To begin,** lie flat on your back with your feet slightly apart. If you have a back problem, bend your knees, but keep your feet flat and about 75 cm (30 in) apart and support your knees with cushions. Close your eyes. Take three deep breaths, and breathe out any feelings of stress when you exhale. Check through your body from your feet to the top of your head to ensure you are relaxed.

- **Focus on your Base Chakra** and legs. Visualize your incoming breath as a bright-red light. 'Pull' and direct it to your Base.

- **Focus on your Sacral Chakra** and abdomen. Visualize your incoming breath as a vibrant orange light. 'Pull' and direct it to your Sacrum.

- **Focus on your Solar Plexus Chakra,** stomach and digestive organs. Visualize your incoming breath as a sunny yellow light. 'Pull' and direct it to your Solar Plexus.

- **Focus on your Heart Chakra** and chest. Visualize your incoming breath as a bright grass-green light. 'Pull' and direct it to your Heart.

- **Focus on your Throat Chakra,** neck, throat, face and back of head. Visualize your incoming breath as a bright turquoise-blue light. 'Pull' and direct it to your Throat.

- **Focus on your Third Eye Chakra,** the centre of your brow, eyes and brain. Visualize your incoming breath as a clear deep-blue light. 'Pull' and direct it to your Third Eye.

- **Focus on your Crown Chakra,** the top of your head and just above your head. Visualize your incoming breath as a clear violet light. 'Pull' and direct it to your Crown.

- **Now visualize clear golden-white light** streaming into the top of your head. Pull the golden-white light into each chakra in turn: Crown, Third Eye, Throat, Heart, Solar Plexus, Sacral, Base. Take the golden-white light right down to your feet, and release it through your soles into the Earth and the Earth Star Chakra beneath you.

- **Return to a normal breathing pattern** and enjoy the feeling of your recharged chakras. Wait a few moments, then stretch and slowly sit up.

- **Now consider** the questions on the opposite page.

My colour-breathing a rainbow experience

Date _____

Is it becoming easier to do colour-breathing?   Yes / No / A bit / Don't know

Base Chakra/red breath
How did my chakra feel? _____
Did it change my mood? _____
Did it bring up a particular emotion or thought? _____
Does my Base Chakra now feel balanced? _____

Sacral Chakra/orange breath
How did my chakra feel? _____
Did it change my mood? _____
Did it bring up a particular emotion or thought? _____
Does my Sacral Chakra now feel balanced? _____

Solar Plexus Chakra/yellow breath
How did my chakra feel? _____
Did it change my mood? _____
Did it bring up a particular emotion or thought? _____
Does my Solar Plexus Chakra now feel balanced? _____

Heart Chakra/grass-green breath
How did my chakra feel? _____
Did it change my mood? _____
Did it bring up a particular emotion or thought? _____
Does my Heart Chakra now feel balanced? _____

Throat Chakra/turquoise-blue breath
How did my chakra feel? _____
Did it change my mood? _____
Did it bring up a particular emotion or thought? _____
Does my Throat Chakra now feel balanced? _____

Third Eye Chakra/clear deep-blue breath
How did my chakra feel? _____
Did it change my mood? _____
Did it bring up a particular emotion or thought? _____
Does my Third Eye Chakra now feel balanced? _____

Crown Chakra/violet breath
How did my chakra feel? _____
Did it change my mood? _____
Did it bring up a particular emotion or thought? _____
Does my Base Chakra now feel balanced? _____

Next time I do this exercise, should I allow myself more time? _____

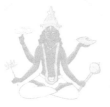
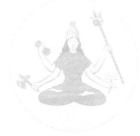

THE SOLAR PLEXUS CHAKRA: MANIPURA

 Work with your chakras now Before you read further, turn to Exercise 11: Sensing and Drawing my Solar Plexus Chakra on page 98.

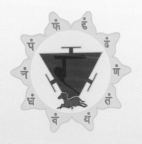

About my Solar Plexus Chakra

Keypoints: Resonates with the Fire element and the colour yellow/gold; concerned with power, empowerment by overcoming our limiting personal ego, becoming non-judgmental and finding our own truth.

The third chakra, the Solar Plexus, is our power base – flexibility here allows us to break away from external control. The Sanskrit name, *Manipura*, means 'the place of jewels', indicating that it is a precious powerful link to our body.

The element of Fire rules the active 'solar power station' of this chakra, and the sun's bio-compatible energies, charged with *prana*, are stored here. In Western esoteric teachings, salamander Fire elementals are interdimensional beings who control, live in and direct the energy of fire. They are keepers of sacred flames. Understanding them aids your appreciation of diverse subtle energies and the secret workings of this chakra.

The seat of the emotions lies within the Solar Plexus Chakra. The more our inappropriate emotions are processed through it, the more the Fire energy there will burn them up. *The ego is closely allied to this chakra* – it is a modern trend to refer persistently to the ego, a psychological construct not recognized until the 20th century. In the past the Devil sat on our shoulder, but now it is our ego that needs to be put in the fire of transformation. Some people consider that ego becomes apparent in childhood due to demands to conform and succeed. If so, then ego is an addiction every bit as powerful as smoking or drinking. Are you using your ego as an excuse? Reflect that you are now an adult, working consciously upon your chakra system to evolve yourself. Every ego eventually has to be released, if humanity is to reach Oneness and Unity.

Golden-yellow light stimulates this chakra. At auric-field level the Solar Plexus Chakra is linked to the secondary minor chakras of the stomach and liver and two minor spleen chakras.

CHART OF THE SOLAR PLEXUS CHAKRA

Colour of influence	Yellow
Complementary light colour	Violet
Colour to calm	Violet
Physical location	Between bottom of sternum and navel
Physiological system	Metabolic/digestive
Endocrine system	Islets of Langerhans (groups of cells in the pancreas)
Key issues	Power, fear, anxiety and introversion
Inner teaching	Honouring the wisdom of others, leading to personal empowerment
Energy action	Transduces incoming solar and *pranic* energy; expels negative body energies
Balancing crystals	Citrine quartz
Balancing aromatherapy oils	Clary sage, juniper, geranium
Balancing herbal teas	Juniper/fennel or detox tea; or a soothing mix of chamomile, marshmallow root, raspberry leaf, fenugreek seed, meadowsweet, slippery elm bark, comfrey and liquorice root
Balancing yoga position (*asana*)	Gomukasana (cow), Ardha matsyendrasana I (sitting spinal twist), Ustrasana (camel)
Mantra/tone	RAM in note of E (sounding like 'rarm')
Helpful musical instruments/music	Loud brass/saxophone to clear 'dead' energy, classical guitar music to calm
Planet/astrological sign/natural House	Sun/Moon/Leo/Cancer/fifth: Love/fourth: Family
Reiki hand position	Lying on back: both palms over the Solar Plexus and stomach; lying on front: both palms on middle back/lungs
Power animal (Native American tradition)	Birds and especially eagles

Body/Solar Plexus connections

The action of the Solar Plexus Chakra on the glandular system occurs through the pancreas, which has small clumps of cells (called the islets of Langerhans), the source of insulin, which is involved in the metabolism of sugar. The physical location of the chakra stretches from the bottom of the breastbone (sternum) to the navel, covering a large area, including the stomach, gall bladder and liver – organs primarily concerned with the digestive system. The coeliac plexus is a network of nerves that meet here. Additionally, the sympathetic nervous system and the health of our muscles are influenced by this chakra.

Links with diabetes and cancer

In the case of diabetes, a holistic practitioner may work with a client to establish why they do not enable sweetness (both of sugars and of personality) to be properly absorbed. From a body/mind perspective, sweetness or love in our lives can become unbalanced. Often love is overprotective or smothering (as from mother to child), and so repetitive patterns of diabetes frequently occur in families. Regular whole-body chakra balancing is required as well as medical treatment.

In cancer and pre-cancerous indications, this chakra can be holding onto unprocessed emotions of anger, fear or hate. Genetic analysis of tumours by the Howard Hughes Medical Institute and Johns Hopkins University in the USA (reported in 2010) suggested that the first cellular mutations may occur 20 years before they develop and become fatal.

Balancing the Solar Plexus may influence your level of wellness. Its natural function is to process energies both from the lower chakras and from the Heart Chakra. Balance may be achieved through healing, meditation, visualization, colour-breathing, using crystals (particularly green emerald or citrine quartz) or simply by consciously breathing in the power of the sun. While these modalities do not replace medical treatment, they do enhance and support medical techniques, through the body's innate desire to return to equilibrium and sustain its own healing, without dependency.

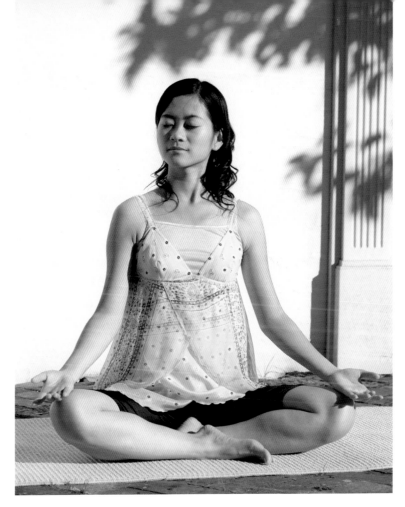

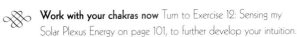 **Work with your chakras now** Turn to Exercise 12: Sensing my Solar Plexus Energy on page 101, to further develop your intuition.

Optional advanced exercises See pages 174, 197, 199 and 206 for more advanced work.

The energy of this chakra

This chakra is where upward-flowing Earth energy meets downward-flowing energy called apana – a specialized type of *prana*.

The expression 'To have a gut feeling' – meaning a sense of feeling something at a very deep level – is actually the Solar Plexus Chakra in action. It enables us to discriminate between good and bad feelings. Maybe you have felt 'butterflies in your stomach' – or a tightening of the whole area – just before an important event. This is the chakra closing down a little, becoming more passive, and pulling in and slightly away from the physical body as a form of protection.

The main action of energy entering the Solar Plexus Chakra assists transmutation and the assimilation of food into a type of coloured light/*pranic* energy that body cells can use. This is why we say it is concerned not only with emotions, but with digestive processes and with nourishing our bodies. One way to harmonize this chakra is by increasing intake of yellow-coloured food, remembering the cleansing properties of lemons, for instance, and the soothing properties of bananas. Other ways are shown on the following pages.

The Solar Plexus is like an inner fire of transmutation, burning up negativity and harmonizing your emotions. If you are going through a period of inner turbulence, allocate some 'me' time. Do something you enjoy and try to relax. Then sit quietly and look at the situation in which you find yourself or which you have drawn toward yourself as a life lesson. Remember that, at soul level, we learn from seemingly the most dire situations and gain inner strength as a result.

Settle down and, as you breathe in, take back all the judgments you have made. Hold them with your breath. Then, as you breathe out, release them one by one. Make sure they have all gone. Maybe you need to expel them with a great sigh. Finally, accept the situation as it is. Be gentle with yourself and with those around you. Perhaps you would like to sit with your partner, or with a friend who is willing to help you, and do the exercises together?

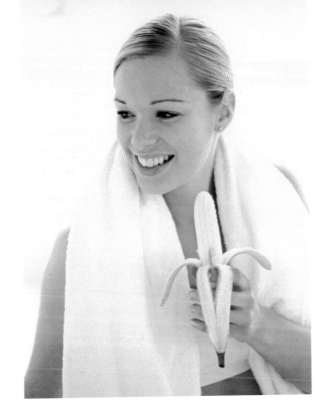

Work with your chakras now Turn to Exercise 13: Dowsing my Solar Plexus Chakra on page 103, to check the balance of this chakra. You can do this both before and after doing any 'remedial' exercises or inner work upon yourself. Remember that it is useful to record your results.

Optional advanced exercise Alternatively, turn to Exercise 28: Releasing Negative Patterns on page 199, for more advanced work, and read page 216.

I'm not quite there yet Go back to Exercise 10: Colour-Breathing a Rainbow on page 77 and CD reference Track 1.

What influences this chakra?

The region of the Solar Plexus Chakra is known in Traditional Chinese Medicine as 'the Triple Warmer' because of the heat generated there during digestion. When this heat is properly regulated through a wholesome and balanced diet, we have health and wellness. However, the nutritive value of junk food and fast food is insufficient to maintain health at many levels. Not only does our body

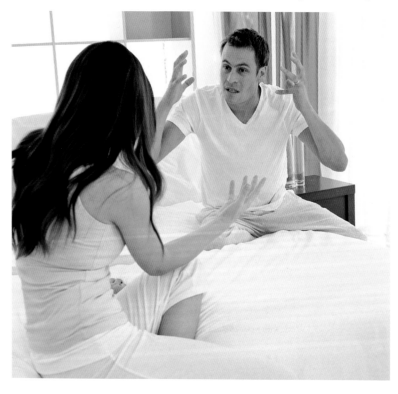

suffer on this type of diet, but our energy reserves also become depleted. If this applies to you, endeavour to correct your diet while simultaneously undertaking the exercises in this book.

Body/mind connections

Sometimes the physical Solar Plexus is referred to as our 'lower mind', because the nerve ganglion there is considered to be a kind of 'visceral brain' where our digestive processes are regulated. Hence this area is subject to various stress-related disorders, such as ulcers. On a body/mind level, people suffering from ulcers may live too much in their mind and be emotionally repressed.

Energy blockages at the Solar Plexus can manifest as domination, anger and abuse. A person exhibiting these qualities of internal conflict becomes stuck at this level, between dominance and submission, where the only escape seems to be aggression or timidity respectively. These body/mind symptoms finally manifest as adrenal-gland weakness, leading to loss of energy and lack of vitality. When considering body/mind connections, do realize that they are often deeply buried in the subconscious and, while it is acceptable to work upon them yourself, it can be damaging to use them as an excuse or as a 'diagnosis' on other people. Most of the inner conflicts or spiritual-growth opportunities within the chakras are not usually recognized consciously, and it would be hurtful to express them about others unless you are in a therapist–client role.

However, this book is about healing yourself, and *the Solar Plexus is a vital chakra centre to take care of*, because a whole range of emotions can cause it to be overstimulated. Through my energy work I have noticed that misuse of personal power is a result of overactivity of the Solar Plexus, while introversion of personality is a result of underactivity. The happy balance is personal empowerment that honours the wisdom and knowledge of others.

 Work with your chakras now Turn to Exercise 14 Breathing in Solar Energies on page 107, for an excellent way to learn how to balance the Solar Plexus Chakra.

Calming my emotions

Has your Solar Plexus Chakra gone into emotional overload? Are you stressed? Does your whole Solar Plexus area feel 'knotted up', or tight and painful, if you prod it with your fingers? This can indicate long-held stress or the kind of tension that builds up before a particularly important event, such as speaking in public.

Firm circular massage in a clockwise direction will usually give relief, using aromatherapy oils such as chamomile to calm the area. You could also try geranium essential oil, because it helps to regulate hormone secretion throughout the whole endocrine system. Also helpful will be a soak in a warm bath containing a few drops of pure chamomile or clary sage essential oil, followed by a cool shower. This releases negativity into the water, leaving you feeling refreshed.

Using a Yantra

In the Indian tradition a Yantra – which means a mapping 'machine' of sacred design in Sanskrit – takes you into a space of relaxation. The Shri Yantra is a traditional design formed by nine interlocking triangles, which surround and radiate out from the central bindu (dot) point, the junction between the physical universe and its unmanifest source. Four of the triangles point upward, representing the Divine Masculine Shiva, and the other five point downward, representing the Divine Feminine Shakti – and hence their union. Together the nine triangles are interlaced to form 43 smaller triangles in a weblike structure that is symbolic of the entire cosmos, or a womb of Creation through the union of Shiva and Shakti.

You may use a Yantra as a focus to still your mind. Look gently at the centre of the Shri Yantra opposite, trying not to blink or close your eyes for some minutes. After a while close your eyes, but keep the image in your 'mind's eye'. Next open your eyes, expanding your focus from the centre of the Shri Yantra to the whole image. Do this repeatedly, looking back at the Yantra when you need to, until your mind is still. This practice reduces stress and develops concentration, leading to relaxation and meditation and eventually to enlightenment.

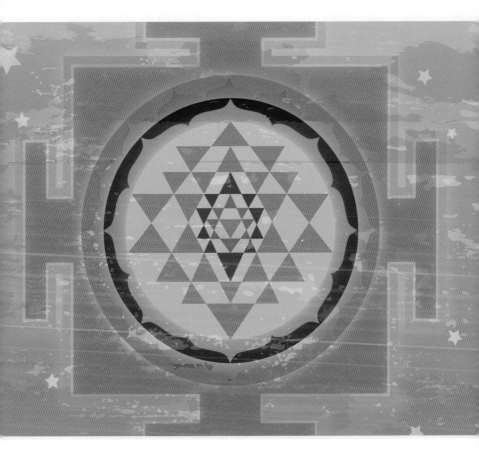

 Work with your chakras now Go to Exercise 14: Breathing in Solar Energies on page 107, to balance this chakra.

 I'm not quite there yet Read pages 92–3 to learn how to balance the Solar Plexus Chakra. Then consider treating yourself to a wonderfully relaxing aromatherapy bath.

Balancing my Solar Plexus Chakra

Relaxation techniques and yoga are both good ways of balancing the Solar Plexus Chakra. 'Your Health is in your own Hands', so make a start on healing yourself using self-taught practices now.

Yoga

You are strongly recommended to take up regular practice of an energy-based discipline that harmonizes the Solar Plexus and all the chakras – t'ai chi ch'uan or yoga are ideal. The development and function of our chakras are of primary importance in yogic tradition, and present-day knowledge of the chakras can be traced to some of the most ancient written texts in the world. These include the *Hathapradipika*, the *Yoga Sutras of Patanjali* and the *Bhagavad Gita*.

For thousands of years Indian mystics knew the nature of chakra energies, and Ayurvedic doctors (traditional healers who restored balance through the 'doshas' or elements of yoga teachings) practised a holistic approach to healthcare. Then at the end of the 19th century meditation arrived in Western esoteric circles. It was like a lotus plant that had lain dormant in Western consciousness. Later many kinds of meditation developed and suddenly blossomed during the late 20th century into a beautiful flower.

Also arising in the East was Shaktism, an organized religious sect dating from the 5th century, and it is their interpretation of the chakras that is most widely used today. In the charts accompanying each of the seven chakras you will find some recommended yoga *asanas* (postures), and there is considerably more about yoga in *The Chakra Bible*.

Relaxation techniques

Stress and tension are necessary for success; but when they become prolonged, or our reaction to them is inappropriate, the body protests in various ways, leading eventually to illness. However, your body has a remarkable ability to heal itself, if you give it the

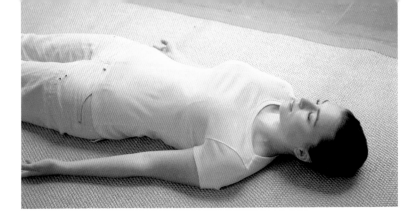

chance. To counter stress, you will find a tried-and-tested relaxation technique on page 110. A technique such as this can be learned by anyone and can then be applied to situations in daily life. It involves no drugs and there are only *pleasant* side-effects. You are asked to participate fully and to practise using the CD supplied with this book. As you begin to lower your stress levels, regular deep relaxation will prove its worth.

During relaxation you remain awake, although afterwards you may feel as if you have had a long, refreshing sleep. When you first learn the technique you will be focusing intently on every part of your body. It is known that whenever you do this, your energy body, chakras and aura receive beneficial activation. Medical

science also demonstrates that if you think about a particular part of your physical body, blood flow there increases and healing can occur more rapidly.

With deep relaxation you:

• Learn how to breathe fully and have a positive attitude to life
• Naturally bring your chakra energies into balance
• Can expect to improve your physical skills and performance
• Are likely to enrich your personal relationships, because it is easier to get on with people when you are relaxed
• Can change your habits, sleep better, feel more fulfilled and perhaps will not need to combat your stress using cigarettes, drink or drugs.

 Work with your chakras now Turn to Exercise 13: Dowsing my Solar Plexus Chakra on page 103, to check whether this chakra is balanced.

Aromatherapy for my chakras

In the evolutionary plan that includes all life on this planet, flowers are the essence and ultimate concentration of a plant's life-force, which is a specialized type of *pranic* energy. They end the cycle of plant growth by providing fertility mechanisms for the reproduction of the species.

Pure essential oils are processed from all parts of plants using different methods, such as steam distillation or maceration. Flowers provide the most fragrant and beneficial oils for the chakras; for example, rose, lavender, linden, ylang-ylang, jasmine, chamomile and neroli. This is because the vibrational level of a flower essential oil is highly charged and compatible with spiritual, mental and emotional dimensions of the human body through a process of resonance. Leaves and the woody parts of aromatic herbs are used to provide slightly larger, less expensive quantities of essential oil; for example, sage, juniper, rosemary, thyme and basil.

These oils, while still working upon the chakra system, offer measurable benefits to the physical body, improving the function of all systems, from relaxing the muscles to balancing hormones. All essential oils are volatile by nature and their small molecular structure easily permeates the skin or is inhaled. Once inside the body, minute aromatized particles circulate through the bloodstream, bringing therapeutic effects to specific organs and body systems. The essential oil that you choose can therefore produce a therapeutic, relaxing, stimulating or sensual effect.

There are many different ways of using essential oils, including the following:

- **Oil diffusers**, sometimes called vaporizers or oil burners (although you should never burn precious essential oil!) give a wonderful boost to the emotions and help respiratory conditions. Simply place a little water in the diffuser's reservoir, add up to five drops of pure essential oil and light a 'tea light' candle underneath.
- **Aromatherapy massage** uses essential oils diluted with a base 'carrier' oil, such as sweet almond, grapeseed or

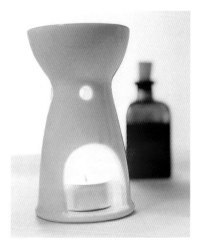

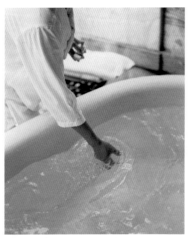

avocado. The dilution rate for adults is: 2.5 per cent essential oil to 97.5 per cent base/carrier oil. To ascertain the correct level, measure your base oil in millilitres and divide by two; the answer gives the number of drops of essential oil required. For example, 20 ml of base oil requires a maximum of ten drops. It is far better to mix your own oil when needed than buy ready-made preparations, because you can assure yourself of the quality of the oils. If you cannot afford a professional massage, ask a friend or treat yourself by massaging the oil into any appropriate parts of your body that you can reach, using firm circular movements.

- **Aromatherapy bathing** is a luxurious way to pamper yourself. Run a warm bath and, just before you get in, add no more than ten drops of your chosen essential oil in the base oil or even in milk. Relax and rebalance your whole chakra system.
- **Steam inhalation** helps the respiratory system. It is excellent for coughs, colds, sore throats and sinus infections – all of which indicate that your Throat, Heart and Thymus Chakras are under stress. Boil 1 litre (1 3/4 pt) of water and pour it into a bowl. Add ten drops of essential oil or a big bunch of a fresh herb (rosemary or thyme are excellent). Put a towel over your head and inhale the vapour for a

few minutes at a time until the water has cooled.

- **Room-spray fragrance** is excellent for cleansing crystals before and after use, as well as for scenting and cleansing your sacred space. Take a glass spray bottle and for each 5 ml of water use up to three drops of essential oil. For example, a 100 ml bottle will take 60 drops of essential oil. Add 10 ml of alcohol (such as vodka) to disperse it.

- **Purification breathing** uses essential oils to assist the release of despair, depression and other negative states of mind. Use an uplifting oil such as juniper, myrrh, basil or frankincense in an oil diffuser/vaporizer and go into a deep-breathing exercise and colour-breathing visualization for your chosen chakra. Continue until you feel purified and as if your mind is clear.

Finally, take a breath of pure white light to recharge your entire body and subtle-energy system.

- **Anointing the chakra area** with essential oil diluted with a carrier oil.

- **Ceremonial cleansing of the auric field** or 'aura brushing', by spraying your auric field (avoid the eyes) to disperse any heavy vibrations trapped there. Use a mix of water, oil and alcohol, as recommended for room sprays.

- **Note:** Never take essential oils orally. Test them first, if your skin is likely to be sensitive. Do not use essential oils at all during pregnancy or on children under the age of 12, except under the supervision of a professional. Some oils, such as clary sage and chamomile, should not be used if you need to drive a car afterwards, for they make you too relaxed.

Seven useful essential oils for the chakras

You will find a number of recommended essential oils for the chakras in the charts that accompany the opening of each chapter, of which the best are:

- Base Chakra — Patchouli
- Sacral Chakra — Sandalwood
- Solar Plexus Chakra — Juniper
- Heart Chakra — Rose
- Throat Chakra — Lavender
- Brow Chakra — Frankincense
- Crown Chakra — Ylang-ylang

SOLAR PLEXUS CHAKRA EXERCISES

The following exercises develop the Solar Plexus Chakra or Manipura, the 'power-centre', where solar energies from food are transformed into light 'nutrients' for your body. You will be shown ways to increase solar light in your energy field, as well as continuing 'colour-breathing', 'scanning', dowsing with a pendulum and relaxing completely with the help of the CD.

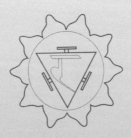

Developing intuition

Do this exercise before reading beyond this page. It will become a record of your Solar Plexus Chakra – showing how much you respect yourself and others and how accurate your 'gut feelings' are – to which you can refer back to chart your progress.

Exercise 11 SENSING AND DRAWING MY SOLAR PLEXUS CHAKRA

You will need: a set of coloured pencils or pens (all colours, including magenta); keep the book open, ready to colour in the body outline opposite, which represents you (sign and date it before you begin).

- **To begin,** take five minutes sitting in a quiet place, breathing slowly, relaxing and closing your eyes. Now start to sense your body and your aura. Release any emotions that arise. Forget anything you have ever heard or read about chakras and auras. You are simply 'sensing' how your own unique energies are flowing at present. Check from your feet up to your head to pick up any little clues that your body is giving you. Sense your auric energy field around you as well. Now focus upon your Solar Plexus Chakra area, which is centred slightly below the ribs. What is it 'telling' you? What can you sense? Does it feel free, flowing, harmonious? Or is an old pain or trauma held there? Does this area feel fluid and open — or have you shut off all feelings and thoughts of this chakra?

- **When you feel ready,** open your eyes and — immediately and without thinking — quickly colour in the Base Chakra area and any other parts of the body (and the surrounding page) as you wish. There is no right or wrong place to apply the colour: it is entirely up to you.

- **Read the interpretation** on page 100 after completing this exercise.

My sensing and drawing my solar plexus chakra experience

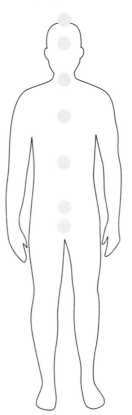

Date _____   Signature _____

Assessing my results for Exercise 11

A balanced Solar Plexus Chakra will show strong and vibrant colours in the light-orange/yellow range. It will reflect your 'gut feelings' and your ability to discriminate between helpful and unhelpful emotions. Balance shows self-respect and respect for others. You will be outgoing, cheerful, relaxed and spontaneous, demonstrating emotional warmth.

An unbalanced Solar Plexus Chakra will show either very weak or very strong colours. These colours may be dark shades — black, brown or grey or a strong, dull red. When weakened, this chakra will reflect depression, insecurity, fear and poor digestion. Overactivity may make you judgmental, a workaholic, a perfectionist and resentful of authority.

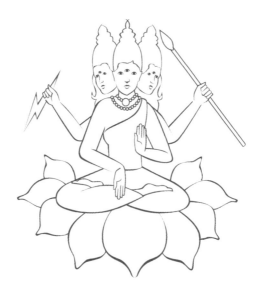

Scanning my Solar Plexus Chakra

Develop your intuition with this exercise. Make a tight fist with one hand – imagine it is your Solar Plexus, all knotted up! Imagine holding that tightness all day, every day. What does it mean to you? Is it fighting, holding on, aggressive acts, defence, anger or self-protection? Now unlock and relax your fist. Shake your hand vigorously. Let both your hands rest openly in your lap. How would your Solar Plexus feel if it was relaxed? Imagine what it would be like if everyone was like this, with open loving, caring hands and Solar Plexus Chakra.

Exercise 12 SENSING MY SOLAR PLEXUS ENERGY

CD REFERENCE TRACK 2 (OPTIONAL) (TO FOLLOW THE SCRIPT, TURN TO PAGE 110)

- **To begin,** lie down and relax. Keeping your eyes closed, push your fingers into your Solar Plexus area. What does it feel like? Relax, placing your hands by your sides.

- **Now begin to focus inwardly** upon this chakra's energy. Increase that focus. After a few minutes move one hand slowly around the area of your Solar Plexus Chakra, both within the auric field and on the body.

- **Notice whether your energy feels different** close into the body or further away. You may feel warmth/cold, lightness/heaviness, vibration/stillness, a colour, dense areas, vibrant areas or other sensations.

- **Remember what you feel,** so that you can record it on the following page.

- **Take a deep breath,** stretch, roll onto one side of your body and sit up slowly.

- **Now consider** the questions on page 102.

My sensing my solar plexus energy experience

Date _____ Signature _____

This exercise was: Easy / Hard / Took a while to get used to it

What did I sense? (tick or expand on what you felt)

Heat _____ Cold _____

Lightness _____ Heaviness _____

Vibration _____ Stillness _____

A colour _____

Dense areas _____

Does this mean my Solar Plexus Chakra energy is clogged/underactive?   Yes / No

Do I need to activate it with colour-breathing golden yellow?   Yes / No
(if your answer is Yes, please do so)

Vibrant areas _____

Does this mean my Solar Plexus Chakra energy is balanced?   Yes / No

Did my Solar Plexus Chakra energy seem overactive?   Yes / No

Do I need to calm it with colour-breathing violet?   Yes / No
(if your answer Yes, go to Colour-Breathing a Rainbow on page 77, exchanging yellow
for violet at the Solar Plexus level)

Other sensations? Describe _____

Checking my Solar Plexus is balanced

This exercise uses a pendulum to check whether your Solar Plexus Chakra is balanced. As recommended on page 18, try to build up empathy and confidence in your pendulum, so that it can be used reliably to determine degrees of activity in each of your chakras.

Remember to avoid holding the pendulum over a chakra, particularly if it is a crystal one – instead, point a finger of the other hand toward and near the chakra in question. This ensures that the pendulum doesn't falsify the reading.

Below are just some of the questions you may ask. Or how about asking if you need aromatherapy or sound healing exercises? Perhaps you need yoga or other balancing body movements? Can you think of more questions to enable you to go deeper? Any questions that you ask must have only 'Yes' or 'No' answers.

Exercise 13 DOWSING MY SOLAR PLEXUS CHAKRA

You will need: a pendulum, and a pen to record your results.

- **To begin,** remain focused and silent for a moment.

- **Then ask** the following questions:
  'Does this chakra require balancing?'
  'Is balance required on a physical level?'
  'Is balance required on a mental/emotional level?'
  'Is balance required on an energy level in my auric field?'

It is also relevant to ask:
'Is this chakra overactive or underactive?'
'Is colour-breathing required?'
'Is crystal balancing required?'
'Is a change in my lifestyle required?'

- **Record your pendulum results on** the opposite page (date and sign them), so that you can begin to see repeating (or varying) patterns of chakra activity. You may dowse just the Solar Plexus Chakra, or you have space there to record the condition of all your chakras, if you wish. You can also compare the effects that various methods shown in this book have upon the chakras, by dowsing before and after any balancing work. It becomes very exciting when you do this, because you can start to see positive results.

- **As an optional method of dowsing,** use a blank 'body outline' (see pages 238–49). Sign it (this is your 'witness' or energy imprint). With the understanding that this body outline represents you, rest your index finger on each chakra in turn. Hold the pendulum in the other hand, well away from your physical body. Ask the questions given above. Record and date your results.

 I'm not quite there yet Don't give up. Pendulum dowsing is a skill that can be very accurate as chakra 'diagnosis' and is a natural ability that many people once had in the past, but which we have now largely lost. Remember, practice makes perfect — but release your attachment to results. Maybe you would like to begin with a relaxation session? If so, Turn to Exercise 15: Complete Relaxation on page 110.

 Work with the CD now Listen to CD reference Track 2 before you next attempt dowsing.

My dowsing my solar plexus chakra experience

Date _____ Signature _____

- Does this _____ Chakra require balancing? Yes / No
- Is balance required on a physical level? Yes / No
- Is balance required on a mental/emotional level? Yes / No
- Is balance required on an energy level in my auric field? Yes / No
- Is this _____ Chakra overactive? Yes / No
- Is colour-breathing required? Yes / No
- Is crystal balancing required? Yes / No
- Is a change in my lifestyle required? Yes / No
- Is this _____ Chakra underactive? Yes / No
- Is colour-breathing required? Yes / No
- Is crystal balancing required? Yes / No
- Is a change in my lifestyle required? Yes / No
- Ask any other questions that you wish to pose.

Circle the relevant states below:

Base Chakra	Balanced	Underactive	Overactive
Sacral Chakra	Balanced	Underactive	Overactive
Solar Plexus Chakra	Balanced	Underactive	Overactive
Heart Chakra	Balanced	Underactive	Overactive
Throat Chakra	Balanced	Underactive	Overactive
Third Eye Chakra	Balanced	Underactive	Overactive
Crown Chakra	Balanced	Underactive	Overactive

Recharging the Solar Plexus

The sun transduces (steps down) energies from outside our solar system and directs them to the planets. Esoterically the sun has been a metaphor for Divinity or Great Spirit – sunlight being 'Divine Light'. Native American traditions, as well as many other cultures, revere their cosmic connections, naming Father Sun, Mother Earth and Sister Moon. People who honour the sun in this way strengthen connections to their Solar Plexus Chakra – finding pleasure in the simple things of life, becoming less troubled by stress and having a tendency to be of a fiery nature, where negative emotions are released quickly. Ceremonies to give prayers and offerings to the sun are an everyday part of their culture. This exercise recharges your Solar Plexus with the power of the sun.

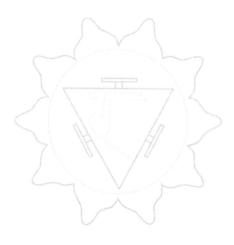

Exercise 14 BREATHING IN SOLAR ENERGIES

For this exercise you ideally need to meditate outside at dawn and watch the sun rise through half-closed eyes. Alternatively, stand before an open window. You may use any form of meditation that you are familiar with, or just go straight into the following visualization and colour-breathing.

- **Standing, breathe deeply** and place your hands on your solar plexus. Then, with each out-breath, extend your arms and hands toward the rising sun. Continue in this way for 13 breaths. Visualize each incoming breath as a beautiful golden yellow, the colour of the rising sun.

- **Then sit down** on a firm chair or in a cross-legged yoga posture and continue focusing upon your breath. Visualize each in-breath charged with a beautiful golden colour that revitalizes your Solar Plexus Chakra and then spreads to the whole of your body.

- **Once you feel your body glowing** with vitality, you will know that the visualization is working and complete.

- **Finish gently,** stretching your body and continuing with your day, recognizing with gracious appreciation that you are a little piece of the sun and that your solar meditation will sustain you.

- **Now consider** the questions on the following page. There is an extra page so that you can do the exercise more than once.

My breathing in solar energies experience

Date _____

How well did I relax?   Well / It was difficult / I couldn't relax at all

Was I outside at sunrise?   Yes / No

Or did I stand before an open window?   Yes / No

Was it easy to breathe in the energy of the sun?   Yes / No

Did the colour-breathing help me focus on my Solar Plexus Chakra?   Yes / No / A bit, but then I lost the focus / Don't know

How did this exercise affect me? _____

_____

_____

_____

_____

_____

_____

Does my Solar Plexus Chakra feel more balanced?   Yes / No / A bit/Don't know

My breathing in solar energies experience

Date _____

How well did I relax?   Well / It was difficult / I couldn't relax at all

Was I outside at sunrise?   Yes / No

Or did I stand before an open window?   Yes / No

Was it easy to breathe in the energy of the sun?   Yes / No

Did the colour-breathing help me focus on my Solar Plexus Chakra?   Yes / No / A bit, but then I lost the focus / Don't know

How did this exercise affect me? _____

_____

_____

_____

_____

_____

_____

Does my Solar Plexus Chakra feel more balanced?   Yes / No / A bit/Don't know

How to relax — fully!

I have taught this relaxation technique for more than 20 years to all my yoga and healer students. You will be lying very still, in order to relax and start 'communicating' with your chakras. Switch off your telephone and arrange not to be disturbed. This is your own quiet time; the CD track allocates 11 minutes, but once you are familiar with the process, you can extend it to 45 minutes or more. However, even relaxing for five minutes during a busy day is useful. You need to move into a state of deep relaxation, but not fall asleep. If you wish, you may place a 'grounding' stone (see page 62) beneath each foot. Wear loose clothing, if possible.

 ## Exercise 15 COMPLETE RELAXATION
CD REFERENCE TRACK 2 (TO FOLLOW THE SCRIPT, SEE BELOW)

- **To begin,** lie on your blanket on your back and place a 'grounding' stone beneath each foot (optional). Close your eyes.

- **Be aware of the floor beneath your back.** Stretch your feet, then let them relax completely, slightly apart. Let your arms rest loosely at your sides, and move your head a little until your head and neck are in a comfortable position. Relax.

- **Take three really deep breaths** — breathe out slowly and relax totally. Your body will feel soft and warm. Your limbs will feel heavy, and it is not unusual to experience a floating sensation as you relax deeper.

- **Feel your arms and hands becoming limp** and heavy. Move your head gently from side to side to release any tension in your neck. Relax all the muscles of your face and scalp, and let the activity in your brain slow down.

- **Now focus inwardly on your Base Chakra** and legs. Let your legs and feet soften and sink down. Let your lower back relax a little more. Feel that through

110

your feet you are closely connected with the Earth, and allow the strength and energy of the Earth element to flow upward to clear any disharmony in your Base Chakra.

- **Focus inwardly on your Sacral Chakra.** Let your hips, buttocks, sexual organs and pelvis relax. Feel that through this chakra you can draw the cleansing power of Water to clear any disharmony.

- **Focus inwardly on your Solar Plexus Chakra.** Relax all your digestive organs, and soften the middle part of your back. Feel that through this chakra you can connect with the positive energies of the sun and draw in the power of Fire to clear any disharmony.

- **Focus inwardly on your Heart Chakra.** Relax and let the activity of your heart and lungs slow down. Experience waves of deep relaxation washing over you. Feel that through this chakra you can draw into your heart the freedom and empowerment of the Air element to clear any disharmony.

- **Allow the elemental quality of Spirit** to flow upward from your Heart Chakra to your throat and neck. Let a clear white light flow to the top of your head, dispelling any disharmony. Then gently let this light flow down and around your body, right to your feet. Wait a while in a lovely relaxed state.

- **To finish your relaxation,** begin to breathe a little deeper for some minutes. Deeper breathing integrates the elements of Earth, Water, Fire, Air and Spirit in your body. Return to everyday consciousness, sit up very slowly and take the rest of the day at an unhurried pace. Now record your experience in the space provided on page 112.

Later, when you feel ready to do so, you may also work on the Solar Plexus Chakra with any of the other balancing methods mentioned on other pages of this book. Consult the chart on page 83 to ascertain which aromatherapy oil to use, which yoga postures, colour breathing, and so on.

My complete relaxation experience

Date _____   Time _____

Before I started this relaxation I felt _____

_____

_____

_____

_____

During the relaxation I experienced _____

_____

_____

_____

_____

_____

After the relaxation I felt _____

_____

_____

_____

_____

_____

_____

THE HEART CHAKRA: ANAHATA

 Work with your chakras now Before you read further, turn to Exercise 16: Sensing and Drawing my Heart Chakra on page 130.

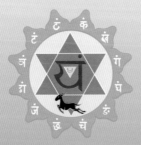

About my Heart Chakra

Keypoints: Resonates with the Air element and the colour crimson red, for the physical heart, and green for the chakra. In a healthy balance of this chakra we give empowerment, empathy and unconditional love to other people, as well as interacting in a caring way for the creatures and environment of our planet.

The fourth chakra, the Heart, is our inner power – harmony here allows us to break away from limiting external control. The Sanskrit name, *Anahata*, means 'the unstruck or unbeaten sound', which is the primordial source of all sound.

When you are on a path of personal growth, unconditional love and compassion develop through the Heart Chakra. You can encourage this within yourself by random acts of kindness. You will never regret making a commitment to work on this chakra. On one level, your dedication to the exercises in this book is designed to realign your state of wellness as preventative medicine. On another level, if you consistently align yourself to the Heart Chakra, you will make a swift discovery of a fundamental change that filters through your entire being. The presence you create will become noticeable to others in your life – a transcendence will occur.

The physical heart may be balanced with the colour of bright grass-green, and you can then bring in a soft pink for the chakra. If you are using crystals, first hold a cleansed aventurine to the Heart Chakra, then a rose quartz.

The Heart Chakra as lotus

Sometimes this chakra is visualized as a beautiful lotus flower: red for energy, pink for love, white for purity. When using a lotus (like a water-lily) as your visualization, consider this is a flower that began its life in the muddy 'waters of emotion' and rose magnificently to blossom above the water in the light. Imagine its petals opening up, as an inner radiance fills your being; remain in this space, immersing yourself in the experience. Then close each petal with love and care as you end your visualization.

CHART OF THE HEART CHAKRA

Colour of influence	Light and bright green
Complementary light colour	Magenta
Colour to calm	Pink
Physical location	Centre of chest on the sternum
Physiological system	Circulatory, lymphatic and immune systems
Endocrine system	Thymus
Key issues	Passion, tenderness, inner child and rejection issues
Inner teaching	Developing unconditional love and compassion
Energy action	Reception and distribution of unconditional love energy
Balancing crystals	Watermelon tourmaline, rose quartz, rhodocrosite, green aventurine
Balancing aromatherapy oils	Rose, melissa, neroli
Balancing herbal teas	Mix of lemon balm (melissa), hawthorn, rose petals and hips and raspberry leaf
Balancing yoga position (*asana*)	Bhujangasana (cobra), Janusirsasana (forward bend), Matsyasana (fish)
Mantra/tone	YAM in note of F (sounds like 'yarm')
Helpful musical instruments/music	Classical violin or piano sonatas, particularly by Mozart
Planet/astrological sign/natural House	Venus/Mercury/Libra/Virgo/seventh: partnerships/sixth: health
Reiki hand position	Two palms on the upper chest, then lift the hands off and place in a T-shape, with upper palm across the Heart Chakra and lower palm beneath it on the centre line
Power animal (Native American tradition)	All mammals

Body/Heart Chakra
connections

The Heart Chakra influences our physical heart and lungs, respiratory system, circulatory and immune systems. At the back it is connected to the fourth thoracic vertebra, and at the front to the centre of the chest. It is common knowledge that our heart works like a pump, oxygenating blood. But the Heart Chakra also pumps energy in and out of our auric body, circulating it through the nadis.

The body/mind connection

The constant action of the physical heart is marvellous, pumping more than 2.5 million litres (4.4 million pints) of blood a year, and coping with regular sport/exercise in normal circumstances. But it does respond adversely to stress and strain. Looking at the body/mind connection, a heart attack is a way for our body to demonstrate that we are overextending ourselves, paying too much attention to material, external and shallow aspects of our lives. Instead, can we express ourselves, and our love to others, and move on from hurtful

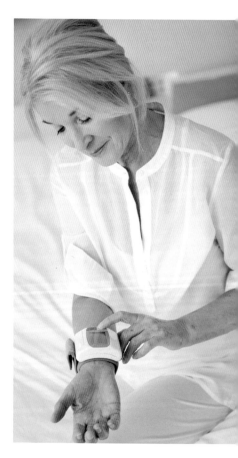

situations to a state of equilibrium? Likewise, high blood pressure (which can be a precursor to a coronary) may be brought about by repressed anger and strong emotions, restricting the natural synchronization of the circulatory system – and cutting us off from letting our 'heart feelings' show. Maybe we feel we want to protect or hide our emotions because they are painful.

Continuing this body/mind connection, there is a logic in exploring the following clinical conditions, fibrositis, arthritis, pain or stiffness of the muscles or joints, because each may indicate rigidity in mental attitudes. There is a consequent stagnation of energy flow through the limbs, so you need to exercise more, balance the Heart Chakra and those chakras nearest the seat of the problem, to encourage self-love. Releasing emotional issues and improving breathing may also help bronchitis, which suggests repressed anger and the need to 'get things off your chest'. Remember that physiological signals are often an indication of something that has been held in your energy field for a long time.

❛ Believe in the impossible — visionary sight is our birthright. ❜

 Work with your chakras now Turn to Exercise 18: Japanese Dō-In Energy Balancing on page 136, and start some simple movement techniques.

 I'm not quite there yet Turn back to Exercise 3: Swallowing the Inner Smile on page 41. Remember, a smile is the cheapest facelift you can get!

The energy of my Heart Chakra

Within the auric field the Heart Chakra is linked to a secondary chakra, the Thymus or Higher Heart, in the centre of the chest. Medical science now accepts that the nearby minor thymus gland plays an important part in our immune system and in helping to regulate growth.

Some yogic teachings also associate the Heart Chakra with an additional spiritual heart centre just below, which develops as we remember our reason for incarnation. It is traditionally called the Kalpatree Chakra, Ananda-Kanda or, in modern terms, the Heart Seed. The associated colours of light to balance these chakras are pink-violet for the Thymus and yellow-gold for the Kalpatree.

It may surprise you to know that your hands are part of the flow of Heart Chakra energies too, for it is through them that we can experience the gift of touch. For example, when we sit or stand in a circle holding hands with a group of people, we move a constant wave of energy around the circle. It comes into one person's left hand, goes across the chest and is passed out via the right hand. This is just another instance of how we are all connected.

Life is an unfolding journey, and we rarely grow if we shut ourselves off from other people, who can reflect so much back to us. It is one of the ways we learn life's lessons. Again, the body/mind connection teaches us. Look at your feet, asking, 'What direction do I want to go in?' Look at your hands, asking, 'What are they really expressing?' Look at your face: what is your smile really saying?

When your heart energy is balanced, you may find yourself in energetic rapport with another person, based on complete understanding of one another. You are 'on the same wavelength' – literally, resonating together. People whom we describe as 'charismatic' have a well-balanced Heart Chakra and draw others toward them like a warming fire.

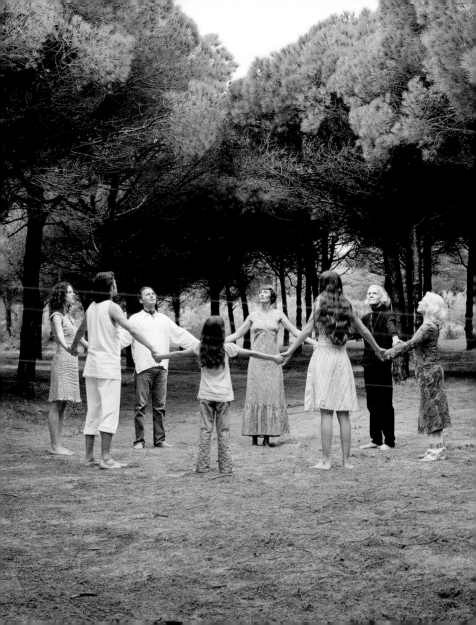

Yogic life lessons

The yogic symbol for the Heart Chakra is a circle surrounded by 12 green petals bearing Sanskrit letters for specific sounds. The 12 traditional lessons of life represented by this chakra are: lustfulness, fraudulence, indecision, repentance, hope, anxiety, longing, impartiality, arrogance, incompetence, discrimination and defiance. These lessons, concentrated at this chakra, have much to teach us about its function. They challenge us to overcome adversity, rising above our lower nature into the vibrations of the higher chakras.

According to these ancient esoteric yoga teachings, the Heart Chakra, in the centre of the Seven-Chakra System, is a 'gateway'. Locked below it are the energies of the first three chakras, which are primarily concerned with establishing our physical presence on Earth. Above it are the chakras more concerned with Spirit. When someone has worked sufficiently with all their challenging aspects, the Heart Chakra unlocks the gate to spiritual development. Energies then flow through an awakened spiritual heart to the higher chakras above it, where the core essence of humanity is destined to evolve and co-create a newly realized superconsciousness.

Love of Nature

In our hurry to fill the day with our 'doings' we have become quite separate from the world of Nature, seeing it as something out there to be enjoyed at weekends. Yet we too are part of the natural world, and every thought, every action we take, has an effect upon it. This occurs particularly through the Heart Chakra – where there is a need to take time to tend our 'inner garden'. When we work enthusiastically with this centre for positive personal growth, we discover that it leads us into 'seeing' that we are part of a greater picture. When we sustain this relationship, the wider cosmic field of life and Light becomes apparent.

What influences my Heart Chakra?

We have seen how, on a physical level, the circulation of air and oxygenated blood through the body are harmonized by the balanced functioning of this chakra, and that energy blockages may manifest as heart or lung disease. The flow of lymph is also closely linked to this area of the physical body. On a subtle-energy level, when the heart and its associated chakras (particularly the Thymus Chakra) are fully balanced, the physical body comes into a state where its basic needs are met. There is nothing more to do, for the heart is a marvellous organ that normally takes care of itself.

But on yet another level, heart care is people care! Now the real work of this chakra begins: the development of hope, forgiveness, peace, acceptance, openness, harmony and contentment.

❛ Smile into your heart. This could prove to be the single most powerful act you can make to assist in self-healing. ❜

All these are aspects of unconditional divine love that we express toward ourselves and others.

The power of positive thinking

Wherever there is pain, ache or discomfort, place your hand upon the area. Medical research has proven that if positive thought is directed to any part of the body, blood flow increases and healing processes are initiated or improved through the enhanced circulation. In addition, circulate unconditional love by drawing it into your body with each breath, from whatever you feel is the source of divine love, within your own spiritual tradition. *Focus intently on your hands.* As they become much warmer, you will know that unconditional love is being transmitted into the area of discomfort. *Smile, and feel the release passing into your physical heart and out through the Heart Chakra.*

Holistic therapies show us that we are not fighting a battle with dis-ease.

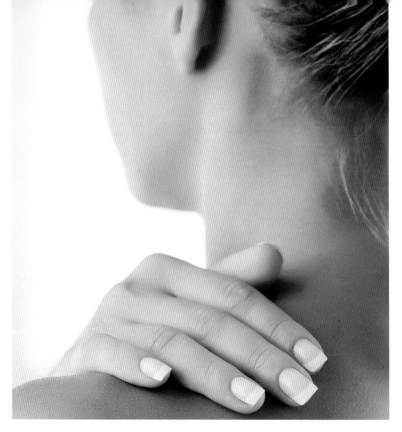

Nor should we become angry or despondent because of what we see as our limitations. When I give workshops, I teach that love is the only emotion that has ever made a positive difference to life. So never think of any part of your body as a nuisance because it is not completely healthy – *always* give praise for its marvellous intricacy, and direct loving thoughts toward it.

Adjust your perception, and be mindful of how you refer to certain body conditions: you don't want to fix dis-ease in your whole body/mind complex. For example, never say, 'I am an asthmatic' (instead, 'At present my physical body has asthma') or 'I am a diabetic' (instead, 'At present my physical body has diabetes'). Attitude of mind is a very important messenger for your body.

Balancing my Heart Chakra

Crystals and aromatherapy using rose essential oil are both excellent ways to balance the Heart Chakra. Rose has a sympathetic resonance with both the female and male reproductive systems, because it may contain plant hormone precursors.

Crystals

Here is a beneficial method that I have used many times with those who respond well to crystal energy. Begin by cleansing and dedicating your crystals, as suggested on page 62. Choose a green crystal to balance the physical heart – aventurine, green calcite or amazonite – and place it over your heart for a short while.

Then make a simple crystal layout of a six-pointed star. Ideally you will need six pink crystals, such as rose quartz or rhodocrosite, or six clear quartz tumbled stones, which will give you an overall boost and balance. Lie supine on your blanket and place a crystal on each side of your knees and one at your head – this forms the triangle of upward-flowing energies. Then place a crystal on each side of your shoulders and one

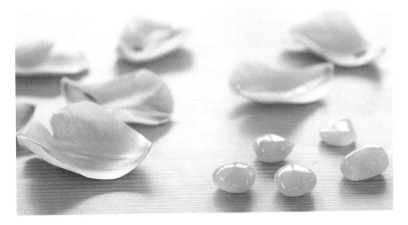

between your feet – this forms the triangle of downward-flowing energies.

Together the two triangles make the Heart Star of Harmonization and attract into your space – if you wish to call upon him/her – your guardian angel or the Archangel Chamuel and the angels of love who bring Christ Consciousness. Relax within the Heart Star of Harmonization crystal layout, and absorb the 'gifts' being brought to you through the crystals.

Aromatherapy using rose essential oil

It is believed that rose was the first-ever essential oil to be distilled by the Arab physician Avicenna in 11th-century Persia. He was probably attempting to produce alchemical gold by heating a combination of red and white rose petals in water – but made an essential oil instead! Rose oil is usually produced today as highly concentrated 'attar of rose'. Rose was traditionally known as an aphrodisiac; rose petals scattered on the nuptial bed have now been replaced by paper petals at weddings. Treatment from a qualified aromatherapist using rose and perhaps other essential oils aids postnatal depression and general anxiety. Rosewater is especially good for skincare.

A lovely way to connect with the natural energies of rose is to place a fragrant real rose (of whatever colour you wish) before you, then meditate upon its beauty. However, the use of rose oil is intended to stimulate the subtle-energy fields that link to the heart, thus bringing balance so that you can find the mystical 'alchemical gold' at the heart-centre. You can do this with aromatherapy, or by showing everyday concern for those nearest and dearest to you, as well as random acts of kindness to strangers. As the heart centre becomes more loving and 'open', you naturally shift your life emphasis away from the lower self to altruistic concerns and development of your spiritual self.

For details of how to use this and other essential oils, see page 94.

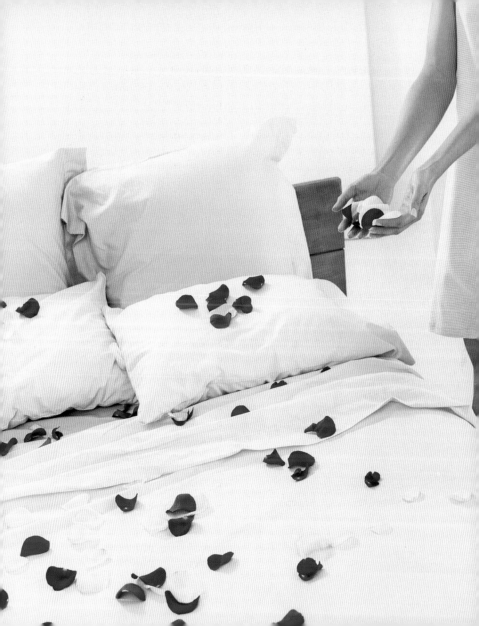

Understanding stress

Despite our best efforts to look after ourselves, the midpoint balance of the Heart Chakra in the Seven-Chakra System is sometimes challenged. Stress is a major contributory factor to any imbalanced chakras that affect our body functions and our state of wellness. So check yourself out from the head down.! Do any of the following manifest themselves in your physical body?

- Headaches, dizziness
- Insomnia
- Panic attacks
- Blurred vision
- Difficulty in swallowing
- Aching neck muscles, stiff jaw
- A susceptibility to infection
- High blood pressure, cardiovascular disorders
- Overbreathing, asthma, palpitations

- Excessive sugar in the blood
- Nervous indigestion, stomach ulcers
- Backache, aching muscles generally
- Nervous rashes and allergies
- Excessive sweating
- Mucous colitis, irritable bowel syndrome, constipation, diarrhoea
- Sexual difficulties, hormonal imbalances, inability to conceive.

Realize that, from a metaphysical point of view, all body dysfunction has first permeated the auric field, entered the chakra and nadi systems and finally come to rest in (usually the weakest part of) the physical body.

A healer will not endeavour to shift physical symptoms, but these will often lessen as the whole body/mind/spirit complex comes into balance.

 Work with your chakras now Turn to Exercise 20: Dowsing my Heart Chakra on page 141, to check that this chakra is balanced.

 I'm not quite there yet Listen to CD reference Track 2 again, for relaxation is the key to harmony.

What can I do about stress?

You need to recognize that too many lifestyle changes at the same time put a major strain upon the body. By 'lifestyle changes' we mean milestones in life, such as divorce, the death of a loved one, personal injury or illness, a change of job, moving house, getting married, having a baby, an abusive relationship or encounters with law-enforcement or other authorities. Try the following steps to reduce your stress levels:

- Take action before you 'crack up' or become ill. Recognize your tiredness and exactly how much of it you can tolerate.
- Change your environment: get away from the situation that causes you stress, if you can. It may save your life.!
- Detox regularly. Avoid alcoholic drink and drugs.
- 'Switch off' for a while during your working day.

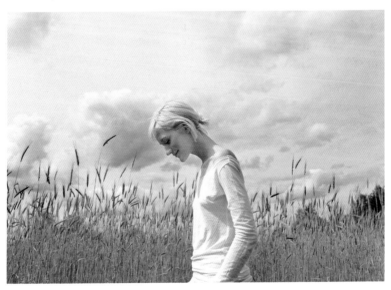

- Keep fit and eat healthily.
- Learn a relaxation technique and how to breathe fully (see Exercise 15: Complete Relaxation on page 110).
- Be aware of your energy field, all your chakras and how to keep them in balance. Use Japanese Dō-In (see Exercise 18 on page 136).
- Treat yourself to a relaxing health treatment, sauna or weekend break.
- Walk outside more often and enjoy Nature.
- Take up hobbies and leisure activities, such as yoga, t'ai chi ch'uan or other energy techniques.
- Gracefully accept whatever good and positive things are around you.
- Examine your feelings of stress, and don't let them alarm you. When you have recovered, use the experience to deepen your understanding of other people.
- Help others, and be an example of how to 'cope with stress *without* distress'.

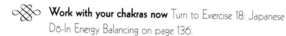 **Work with your chakras now** Turn to Exercise 18: Japanese Dō-In Energy Balancing on page 136.

Work with your chakras now Turn to Exercise 17: Heart Chakra Visualization on page 133, or listen to CD reference Track 3 to meditate.

I'm not quite there yet Turn to Exercise 19: Colour-Breathing the Thymus Chakra on page 139

HEART CHAKRA EXERCISES

The following exercises develop the Heart Chakra or Anahata. It is the centre of your innermost love, which ideally is expressed to others unconditionally. You will use a self-assessment about the power of love, plus 'colour-breathing' and developing intuition and meditation skills with the CD, among other ways of rebalancing this important chakra.

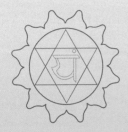

Developing intuition

Do this exercise before reading beyond this page. It will become a record of your Heart Chakra – showing how content or insecure you are – to which you can refer back in order to chart your progress.

Exercise 16 SENSING AND DRAWING MY HEART CHAKRA

You will need: a set of coloured pencils or pens (all colours, including magenta); keep the book open, ready to colour in the body outline opposite, which represents you (sign and date it before you begin).

- **To begin,** take five minutes sitting in a quiet place, breathing slowly, relaxing and closing your eyes. Now start to sense your body and your aura. Release any emotions that arise. Forget anything you have ever heard or read about chakras and auras. You are simply sensing how your own unique energies are flowing at present. Check from your feet up to your head to pick up any little clues that your body is giving you. Sense your auric energy field around you as well. Now focus upon your Heart Chakra area. What is it telling you? What can you sense? Does it feel free, flowing, harmonious? Or is an old pain or trauma held there? Does this area feel fluid and open – or have you shut off all feelings and thoughts of this chakra?

- **When you feel ready,** open your eyes and – immediately and without thinking – quickly colour in the Heart Chakra area and any other parts of the body (and the surrounding page) as you wish. There is no right or wrong place to apply the colour: it is entirely up to you.

- **Read the interpretation** on page 132 after completing this exercise.

  I'm not quite there yet Listen to CD reference Track 2, if you don't feel relaxed enough to do this exercise yet; come back to it later on.

My sensing and drawing my heart chakra experience

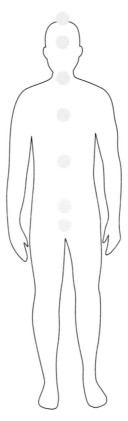

Date _____ Signature _____

Assessing my results for Exercise 16

A balanced Heart Chakra will show strong and vibrant colours of red, green or pink. It will reflect your inner feelings of self-worth, contentment and the ability to give empathy, unconditional love and compassion.

An unbalanced Heart Chakra will show either very weak or very strong colours. These may be dark shades — black, brown or grey or a strong, dull red. When weakened, it will reflect depression, insecurity or 'a broken heart'. Excessive activity may make you overreactive, intolerant and bombastic, or continually seeking loving relationships to balance yourself.

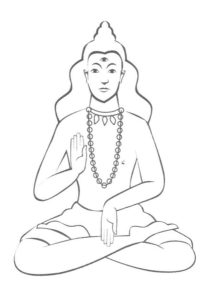

Meditative visualization

This is a meditative visualization to link you to Earth and Sky through the element of Air. If you have an oil vaporizer, use rose or rose geranium oil in it; alternatively, place a pink flower in a vase or hold a rose quartz crystal in your hand, putting you in touch with Heart Chakra energy frequencies.

 ## Exercise 17 HEART CHAKRA VISUALIZATION
CD REFERENCE TRACK 2 (OPTIONAL) (TO FOLLOW THE SCRIPT, TURN TO PAGE 110) CD REFERENCE TRACK 3 (TO FOLLOW THE SCRIPT, SEE BELOW)

You will need: a set of coloured pencils or pens.

- **To begin,** light a candle. Sit and relax, then close your eyes. Remember to keep your spine straight.

- **Breathe slowly and deeply,** feeling the expansion of your lungs. Listen to your beating heart.

- **Notice the expansion of your chest** as you breathe. Breathe in all aspects of the Nature element of Air, ranging from a strong gust of air to a soft breeze. Feel this air rush into your body and energize it with *prana*.

- **Connect to your Heart Chakra,** visualizing it as a beautiful pink lotus flower. Observe the flower closely. Notice whether it is a tightly shut bud or fully open. If it is open, what do you see inside?

- **Now visualize the place** where the lotus is growing. It needs water to grow and flower. So see the water, sky and whatever else is around. Are there more lotus flowers?

- **Focus on your own lotus,** the one you first visualized, as a single bloom. Notice whether it has changed, and whether you can now see its centre of golden stamens.

- **To finish,** ask the lotus to close its petals. Then put a circle of clear bright emerald-green light around it. As you do so, ask for the protection of your Heart Chakra with another circle of clear bright emerald-green light.

- **Finally,** put your right hand crosswise across your chest, followed by the left in the same manner.

- **Open your eyes** and blow out the candle.

- **As with all meditative visualizations,** it is a good idea to record your experiences on the next page, and to draw your lotus, if you wish.

- **Now consider** the questions on page 135.

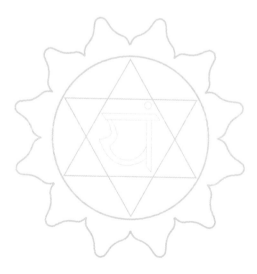

My heart chakra visualization experience

Date _____

Was this exercise difficult ?: Yes / No / A little

How well did I visualize the lotus flower? _____
_____
_____

What did it look like? _____
_____
_____

What (if anything) could I see inside the lotus? _____
_____
_____

What did I feel about this exercise? _____
_____
_____

What did I learn from it? _____
_____
_____

Daily exercise for total balance

This once-daily exercise is based on teachings stemming from the Tao of Shin Sen, an ancient collection of Dō-In exercises and the practice of them as a spiritual path. It was originally used by Zen monks over a wide area of China, Japan, Korea and Vietnam.

Exercise 18 JAPANESE DŌ-IN ENERGY BALANCING

- **To begin,** kneel on a mat with your hands resting lightly on your lap. Aim to keep your consciousness in the unlimited ocean of tranquillity of Oneness. Clap your hands together twice to purify your space. Rub your face all over with the palms of your hands. Then tap your face all over with your fingertips.

- **With lightly gripped fists,** tap your entire head lightly, as if they are bouncing off it. Use the side of the fist at the little finger. This stimulates all its physical and mental activities and the coordination of various physical and energy systems.

- **Pound the opposite shoulder** with one fist about 30 times. Repeat on the other side and at the back of your neck.

- **Kneel up and vigorously pound** with both fists as much of your back, buttocks and the backs of your legs as you can reach. Gently pound the centre of your chest to stimulate the thymus region.

- **Kneel down again.** Open your arms in front of you and vigorously tap with the fingertips of one hand up the inside of the other arm from fingers to shoulder, then round and down the outside of the arm, right to the fingertips. Repeat seven times on each arm.

- **With one palm over the other,** slowly and deeply massage the whole of the soft abdominal area in a clockwise action about 20 times.

- **Sit, stretching out your legs.** Vigorously tap with your fingertips from the toes up the inside of the leg to your groin, then round and down the side and back of the leg to the toes. Repeat seven times on each leg.

- **With the soles of your feet together,** hold them with your hands and breathe deeply seven times, harmonizing the energy flow.

- **Now consider** the questions on page 138.

Optional advanced exercise If you enjoyed this exercise, how about following it with Exercise 23: Sound Experience on page 168.

Work with the CD now Play CD reference Track 4 to hear the same Sound Experience.

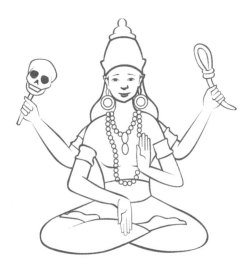

My Japanese dō-in energy balancing experience

Date _____   Time of day _____

What was my physical energy level before the exercise? _____
_____

What was my physical energy level after the exercise? _____
_____

What was my mental/emotional energy level before the exercise? _____
_____

What was my mental/emotional energy level after the exercise? _____
_____

What else did I feel? _____
_____

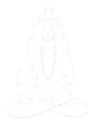

Recharging the Thymus Chakra

This exercise continues your colour-breathing visualization practice, improving the depth and quality of your breathing and bringing a particular emphasis upon the Heart Chakra region.

You need to be in a place where you will not be disturbed for between ten minutes and half an hour – indoors is okay, but it would be even better to be sitting outside in Nature.

 ### Exercise 19 **COLOUR-BREATHING MY THYMUS CHAKRA**

CD REFERENCE TRACK 2 (OPTIONAL) (TO FOLLOW THE SCRIPT, TURN TO PAGE 110)

- **To begin,** sit in an upright chair or a cross-legged yoga posture. Ensure that you are fully relaxed. Your spine must be as straight as possible and your chin pulled in, to straighten the back of your neck.

- **Close your eyes** and breathe slowly, visualizing your incoming breath as a clear, bright grass-green light. Breathe deeply for a few minutes, focusing on the Heart Chakra. Feel this coloured breath suffusing the area of your physical and subtle heart with beneficial new energy, helping to clear and balance it.

- **Now change the colour** of your breath to a pink/violet light, focusing on your Heart Chakra and the Thymus Chakra, just above it, for a few minutes. Feel this coloured breath suffusing the area of your physical and subtle heart with more energy, bringing wellness and inner peace.

- **Return to normal breathing** and, after some minutes, open your eyes.

- **Now consider** the questions on page 140.

My colour-breathing my thymus chakra experience

Date _____

How well did I relax?   Well / It was difficult / I couldn't relax at all

Did the colour breathing help me focus on my Heart Chakra?
Yes / No / A bit, but then I lost focus / Don't know

Did the colour-breathing help me focus on my Thymus Chakra?
Yes / No / A bit, but then I lost focus / Don't know

How did this exercise affect me?_____
_____
_____
_____
_____
_____
_____

Does my Heart Chakra feel more balanced?   Yes / No / A bit / Don't know

Checking my Heart Chakra is balanced

This exercise uses a pendulum to check whether your Heart Chakra is balanced. As recommended on page 18, try to build up empathy and confidence in your pendulum, so that it can be used reliably to determine degrees of activity in each of your chakras.

Remember to avoid holding the pendulum over a chakra, particularly if it is a crystal one – instead, point a finger of the other hand toward and near the chakra in question. This ensures that the pendulum doesn't falsify the reading.

Below are just some of the questions you may ask. Or how about asking if you need aromatherapy or sound healing exercises? Perhaps you need yoga or other balancing body movements? Any questions that you ask must have only 'Yes' or 'No' answers.

Exercise 20 DOWSING MY HEART CHAKRA

You will need: a pendulum, and a pen to record your results.

- To begin, remain focused and silent for a moment.

- Then ask the following questions:
  'Does this chakra require balancing?'
  'Is balance required on a physical level?'
  'Is balance required on a mental/emotional level?'
  'Is balance required on an energy level in my auric field?'

  It is also relevant to ask:
  'Is this chakra overactive or underactive?'

'Is colour-breathing required?'
'Is crystal balancing required?'
'Is a change in my lifestyle required?'

• **Record your pendulum results** on the opposite page (date and sign them), so that you can begin to see repeating (or varying) patterns of chakra activity. You may dowse just the Heart Chakra, or you have space there to record the condition of all your chakras, if you wish. You can also compare the effects that various methods shown in this book have upon the chakras, by dowsing before and after any balancing work. It becomes very exciting when you do this, because you can start to see positive results. There is an extra page overleaf so that you can do the exercise more than once.

• **As an optional method of dowsing,** use a blank 'body outline' (see pages 238–49). Sign it (this is your 'witness' or energy imprint). With the understanding that this body outline represents you, rest your index finger on each chakra in turn. Hold the pendulum in the other hand, well away from your physical body. Ask the questions given above. Record and date your results.

Later, when you feel ready to do so, you may also work on the Heart Chakra with any of the other balancing methods mentioned on other pages of this book. Consult the chart on page 115 to ascertain which aromatherapy oil to use, which yoga postures, colour breathing, and so on.

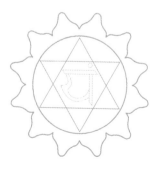

My dowsing my heart chakra experience

Date _____   Signature _____

- Does this _____ Chakra require balancing?   Yes / No
- Is balance required on a physical level?   Yes / No
- Is balance required on a mental/emotional level?   Yes / No
- Is balance required on an energy level in my auric field?   Yes / No
- Is this _____ Chakra overactive?   Yes / No
- Is colour-breathing required?   Yes / No
- Is crystal balancing required?   Yes / No
- Is a change in my lifestyle required?   Yes / No
- Is this _____ Chakra underactive?   Yes / No
- Is colour-breathing required?   Yes / No
- Is crystal balancing required?   Yes / No
- Is a change in my lifestyle required?   Yes / No
- Ask any other questions that you wish to pose.

Circle the relevant states below:

Base Chakra	Balanced	Underactive	Overactive
Sacral Chakra	Balanced	Underactive	Overactive
Solar Plexus Chakra	Balanced	Underactive	Overactive
Heart Chakra	Balanced	Underactive	Overactive
Throat Chakra	Balanced	Underactive	Overactive
Third Eye Chakra	Balanced	Underactive	Overactive
Crown Chakra	Balanced	Underactive	Overactive

My dowsing my heart chakra experience

Date _____ Signature _____

- Does this _____ Chakra require balancing?   Yes / No
- Is balance required on a physical level?   Yes / No
- Is balance required on a mental/emotional level?   Yes / No
- Is balance required on an energy level in my auric field?   Yes / No
- Is this _____ Chakra overactive?   Yes / No
- Is colour-breathing required?   Yes / No
- Is crystal balancing required?   Yes / No
- Is a change in my lifestyle required?   Yes / No
- Is this _____ Chakra underactive?   Yes / No
- Is colour-breathing required?   Yes / No
- Is crystal balancing required?   Yes / No
- Is a change in my lifestyle required?   Yes / No
- Ask any other questions that you wish to pose.

Circle the relevant states below:

Base Chakra	Balanced	Underactive	Overactive
Sacral Chakra	Balanced	Underactive	Overactive
Solar Plexus Chakra	Balanced	Underactive	Overactive
Heart Chakra	Balanced	Underactive	Overactive
Throat Chakra	Balanced	Underactive	Overactive
Third Eye Chakra	Balanced	Underactive	Overactive
Crown Chakra	Balanced	Underactive	Overactive

THE THROAT CHAKRA: VISHUDDHA

 Work with your chakras now Before you read further, turn to Exercise 21: Sensing and Drawing my Throat Chakra on page 162.

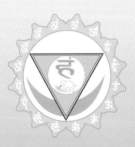

About my Throat Chakra

Keypoints: Resonates with the Ether element (akasha in Sanskrit) and the colour turquoise-blue; concerned with developing our self-expression, communication and will.

The fifth chakra, the Throat, is the centre of our personal expression and flexibility, enabling us to break away from limiting external control. The Sanskrit name, Vishuddha, means 'to purify'. At the fifth chakra we have the opportunity to purify the energies of all the lower chakras, so that they may pass through the narrow channel of the neck into the head.

This chakra develops speech, communication, song, telepathy and channelled information. Sound is the sense held within it, brought about by the Earth element at the Base Chakra dissolving in Water at the Sacral Chakra, leaving a sense of smell. The Water is then vaporized by Fire at the Solar Plexus, leaving a sense of taste. As Fire enters the Heart Chakra, the Air moves, leaving a sense of touch. When the Air enters the Throat, it becomes sound.

The crystal of choice to activate the Throat Chakra is blue topaz for spiritual insights and yellow topaz for physical energy. You do not need expensive gem-quality topaz; natural, uncut topaz, which is just as beneficial, can be obtained. Excellent balancing crystals are chrysocolla and turquoise; always try to get natural turquoise, not a reconstituted or a dyed stone. One way to use crystals is to place a small one in the notch of the collarbone, or two on either side of the neck, for 10–20 minutes for best effect.

To calm the Throat Chakra, consider sipping turquoise solarized water (see page 187 for its preparation). Using the resonant frequencies of light, the water becomes intentionally aligned with a minute homeopathic quantity of the turquoise frequency required by this chakra.

 Work with your chakras now Turn to Exercise 22: Throat Chakra Visualization on page 165, to enjoy a relaxing meditation visualization.

CHART OF THE THROAT CHAKRA

Colour of influence	Turquoise-blue
Complementary light colour	Red
Colour to calm	Turquoise-blue, pale blue or pale green
Physical location	Between collarbone and larynx on the neck
Physiological system	Respiratory
Endocrine system	Thyroid and parathyroid
Key issues	Self-expression, communication and will
Inner teaching	To develop compassion and caring self-expression
Energy action	A bridge between the physical and spiritual
Balancing crystals	Turquoise, gem silica, chrysocolla
Balancing aromatherapy oils	Lavender, Roman chamomile (and rosemary, thyme, sage, unless pregnant)
Balancing herbal teas	Mix of echinacea, lobelia, elderberry, marshmallow, red sage, cleavers and honey
Balancing yoga position (*asana*)	Dhanurasana (bow), Simhasana (lion), Paschimottanasana (sitting forward bend)
Mantra/tone	HAM in the note of G (sounds like 'harm')
Helpful musical instruments/music	Flute
Planet/astrological sign/natural House	Jupiter/Mars/Sagittarius/Scorpio/ninth: intellect, eighth: death
Reiki hand position	Two palms gently over the throat
Power animal (Native American tradition)	All humanity

Body/Throat Chakra
connections

The Throat Chakra is located on the front of the neck and at the corresponding part of the spine – the third cervical vertebra – at the back. This is where the body is narrowing and concentrating all its energies, to enable information to pass up through the neck to the brain. It is a major body 'highway' that can become overburdened and blocked; repeated physical infections of the throat may be an indicator of this.

This chakra is primarily linked to the thyroid, a large endocrine gland lying at the base of the neck, affecting cellular metabolism and growth stimulation. It also encourages the onset of puberty and sexual maturity, as well as acting as protection against infection. In addition it is linked to two parathyroid glands in the physical body, through the two secondary parathyroid chakras and two clavicle chakras. The hormones secreted by the parathyroids aid normal growth and the vital metabolism of calcium for our bone structure.

The whole of the ear/nose/throat connection, dealing with hearing and speech, and to some extent the respiratory system are also connected to this chakra. So for imbalances in these areas, which show up as dis-ease or discomfort, the Throat Chakra needs to receive healing. Additionally this is the region of your physical body where pollution – such as smoke, inappropriate food or drink – is ingested, and where words/sound/song are emitted.

Neck rotations Japanese-style

The following simple exercise releases tension that builds up in the 'bottleneck' of the body. Sit down, relax your shoulders and then rotate your head *slowly*. If you feel any tightness or pain, stop and massage the area with your fingertips. Then resume the rotations. If you feel dizzy, slow down the speed of rotation. Ensure that you rotate in each direction an equal number of times. Also consider practising Dō-In exercises, to keep your body and chakras balanced.

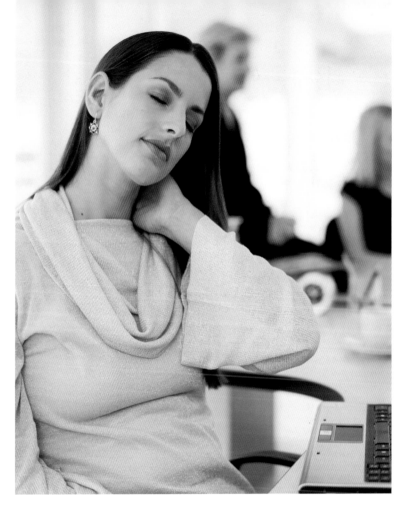

Work with your chakras now Turn to Exercise 18: Japanese Dō-In Energy Balancing on page 136, and remember to spend a little while on these exercises each day, and especially on the neck rotations given above, if you sit in front of a computer for long periods of time.

The energy of my Throat Chakra

The Throat is one of the most important chakras, for not only does it act as a vital 'bridge' on the highway between the physical body and the neck, as I have explained, but also as a bridge between different realities.

Generally the chakras are believed to become most energized or developed sequentially from Base to Crown. In this model of the development of the inner aspects of chakra energies, once the Throat Chakra is receptive, this highway takes us to a different land, another side of the 'River of Life', where access through the dimensions to spiritual realms is achievable.

Mysteriously supporting these other dimensions of soul and spirit is the nebulous Nature element of Ether. In the associated yoga symbol there are petals that are sometimes a smoky-blue, representative of Ether, together with an unyoked elephant, indicating the inherent strength and power that can be developed from this chakra.

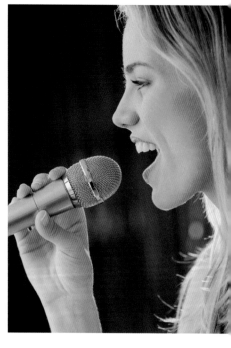

Connections between the Throat and Heart Chakras

The most obvious examples of positive Throat Chakra balance are singing, public speaking and acting. Singers usually have a well-developed Throat Chakra. When this chakra comes into balance, we are able to express ourselves and our love for others through our words.

The Throat Chakra is closely linked with the Heart Chakra, because there is a natural tendency arising in the Heart Chakra for loving words and song. Our intentions are imprinted upon the emanations from our voice, and analysis can confirm that we either have a good range of tones and harmonies or our voice is dull and boring. A voice therapist can improve your public-speaking voice, but Throat Chakra balancing will improve your subtle communication skills, by drawing heart energies into your everyday speech.

For people such as monks who follow a specific spiritual path, these two chakras are where inner light forms, ready to be released through the voice as prayer, hymn, chant or song. This changes their relationship to the mundane world of matter, using the vibrational frequencies of pure spirit.

Throat imbalances are concerned with self-expression. Clearly we all need to speak our truth; this becomes easier once you overcome initial barriers of shyness or social or religious control. Because of the inherent strength of this chakra, a useful affirmation to make is along the lines of 'At every appropriate opportunity I will express my higher wisdom to others.'

 Work with your chakras now Turn to Exercise 22: Throat Chakra Visualization on page 165, if you did not do so previously.

Chakras and sound

Sound is commonly understood as a vibration that travels through a medium, usually air. However, sound also travels through water and blood, as well as through denser materials such as flesh and bone. The all-encompassing word 'sound', for these purposes, includes the speaking voice, singing voice and musical instruments.

Using the voice with or without accompanying instruments, I now want to introduce you to the benefits of mantras (including Bija mantras for the chakras), as well as to voice toning and overtoning. *You don't need to be a good singer to do this!*

Mantras

A mantra is repetitive vocalization of sacred words, syllables or prayer, using voice intonations. Used personally or ceremonially in a group, it produces altered states of consciousness by reducing brainwave levels. Profound realizations are achievable through pure concentrated focus of mind, body and spirit to connect with the core level of our Being.

Bija mantras

These are one-word mantras specific to the chakras, with their origins deep within ancient Hindu and Buddhist teachings. See page 156 for full details.

Voice toning

The express purpose of using the music in your voice for toning is to cause resonation within your physical body and/or etheric fields. Toning involves no melody, no words, no rhythm and no harmony – just the sound of the vibrating breath: re-sonance.

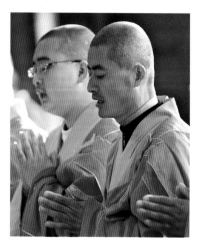

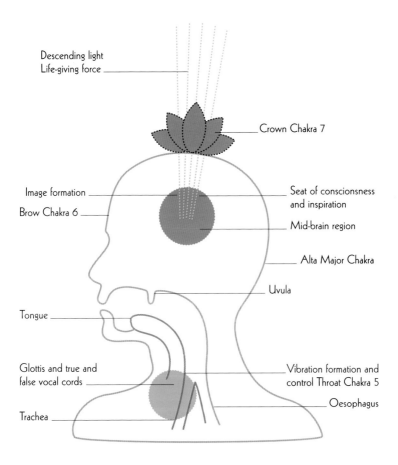

Descending light
Life-giving force

Crown Chakra 7

Image formation

Brow Chakra 6

Seat of consciousness
and inspiration

Mid-brain region

Alta Major Chakra

Uvula

Tongue

Glottis and true and
false vocal cords

Vibration formation and
control Throat Chakra 5

Oesophagus

Trachea

Voice toning can:

- Restore balance and harmony to your mind, emotions and body;
- Awaken and deepen your sense of self;
- Align you to the deepest vibration of soul and spirit;
- Synchronize your brainwaves and help relieve tension;
- Develop your voice–ear connection;
- Improve stamina and concentration;
- Expand your body's ability to breathe deeply.

On the path of toning, you move toward the source of your own inner balance, creativity, well-being and freedom.

When doing any of the sound exercises at the end of this section, begin by feeling calm and centred; drink a little pure water, blow your nose and clear your throat. Correct posture and breathing are important. Breath should be inhaled through the nostrils and out through the mouth – a steady breathing rhythm indicates that you are relaxed. Make your inhaled breath long, slow and as deep as possible. Do not allow your mind to wander or weaken, through thoughts such as 'I can't do it'. Instead, resonate with the frequency of what is forming within you. Enjoy the moment of bliss as you pause before releasing the sound; then focus on the chakra or place to which you wish the sound energy to go. When releasing the sound, do so as slowly as you can by allowing your tones to last for as long as possible. During inhalation, check your posture so that your lungs are fully but comfortably expanded, and each time try to breathe a little deeper and slower.

Keep repeating the appropriate sounds until you have focused your intention on each chakra. Always finish toning with grateful acceptance of what you have achieved at the physical, emotional, mental and spiritual levels. You will find suggestions concerning which tones to use on page 155.

Overtoning

In many references to the use of the voice for toning, mention is made of 'overtoning'. In Bija mantras, for example, you may discover a dot over the letter M; you may also see it written as 'ang' or 'ung' – the 'n' and/or the 'g' give the vital clue to expressing an overtone above the tone, and are an indicator that an overtone sound should be aimed for, by consciously strengthening the muscles surrounding the glottis in conjunction with the appropriate controlled release of breath. Simply begin by exploring different positions of the tongue, glottis and nasal passages while sounding the tone. Overtoning becomes a valuable exercise in muscle control and creates a magical effect, capable of relaxing you into deep alpha and theta brainwave levels. There is a whole beautiful world to explore if you are so inclined, but don't think you've failed if you are unable to produce 'overtones'.

Nada yoga: toning vowels

Nada yoga is the ancient yogic practice of using mantras and sounds in order to elevate consciousness. In ancient times, within Sanskrit, Hebrew and Chinese cultures, vowels were considered sacred. They are an expression of subtle energy. Consonants articulate that subtle energy into shapes. This is why vowels are toned for the chakra centres. To speak or tone the vowel sounds requires breath (ether) to pass out through an open mouth.

Try softly repeating the separate vowels A, E, I, O, U, and notice the effect this has upon you. Let go of any left-brain logical deductions as you do this exercise. As you learn to apply these vowels to the chakra centres, remember that it is always important to ascend through the chakras and then descend, so as to ground the energies. Ascending tones suggest movement toward the transcendence of matter into cosmic reality. Descending tones suggest movement from cosmic refinement into the denseness of matter.

There is a tremendous difference between listening to someone else toning or chanting and doing it yourself.

TONING VOWELS FOR THE CHAKRA CENTRES

Chakra (Sanskrit name)	Element	Keyword	Note	Vowel (as in)	Chakra (English name)
Muladhara	Earth	Depth	Note of C	U (UH)	Base/Kanda
Svadisthana	Water	Flowing	Note of D	OO (TOO)	Sacral
Manipura	Fire	Opening	Note of E	O (GO)	Solar plexus
Anahata	Air	Fullness	Note of F	A (PA)	Heart
Vishuddha	Ether	Balance	Note of G	I (EYE)	Throat
Ajna	Mind	Intensity	Note of A	A (AYE)	Third Eye
Sahasrara	Pure consciousness	Wisdom	Note of B	E (EEE)	Crown

Nada yoga: Bija mantras

Through the use of Bija mantras – one-word mantras specific to the chakras – the chakra system is brought alive. Traditionally they are intoned silently, although since sound is an all-over body experience, you may like to vocalize them out loud using the following scale. Remember to breathe correctly and deeply, so that the sound resonates within your whole body. With focused consciousness and by learning through practice, you will increase your overall state of wellness.

Bija literally means 'seed'. Through intention, correct breathing and vocalization, the seed will germinate and flourish within your awareness as well as in your physical body.

Repeated use of the Bija mantras creates the possibility of transformation, simply because vibration directed with powerfully focused intention aligns the body's physical structure at a molecular level. An Indian 'mala' or 108-bead necklace is used as a method of

THE SAPTAK SCALE AND ASSOCIATED BIJA MANTRAS

SAPTAK SCALE	NATURE SOUND	DIATONIC SCALE	CHAKRA	BIJA MANTRA/ OVERTONE SYMBOL (G)
Sadja/Sa	Peacock's cry	C	Muladhara/Base/Kanda	LAM(g)
Risabha/Re	Cow calling her calf	D	Svadisthana/Sacral	VAM(g)
Gandhara/Ga	Goat bleating	E	Manipura/Navel	RAM(g)
Madhyama/Ma	Heron's cry	F#	Anahata/Heart	YAM(g)
Panchame/Pa	Cuckoo's song	G	Vishuddha/Throat	HAM(g)
Dhaivata/Da	Horse's neigh	A	Ajna/Third Eye	OM(g)
Nishada/Ni	Elephant trumpeting	B♭	Sahasrara/Crown	OM(g)

counting the repetitions, so that the mind can concentrate upon the mantras.

The seven notes of the Indian musical scale associated with Bija mantras, called the Saptak, were established in India by the 2nd century BCE and related humans to the sounds of Nature. The Western musical scale below is only an approximation of this Saptak scale. All traditional mantras are internalized in five stages:

- Likhita: through writing;
- Vaikhari: through speaking and sounding;
- Upamshu: through whispering;
- Manasa: through thinking;
- Ajapa: through uninterrupted inner repetition.

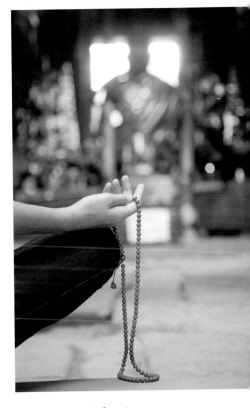

 Work with your chakras now Turn to Exercise 23: Sound Experience on page 168.

 Work with the CD now Play CD reference Track 4, to hear the same Sound Experience.

Energy Medicine

Energy Medicine (sometimes called Vibrational Healing) is a wide-ranging, diverse, holistic type of healthcare and healing that provides treatment by balancing the human energy system. Most importantly, Energy Medicine harmonizes with the natural healing abilities of the body, because it has an innate drive to function at its highest possible state of health. Dis-ease (deliberately hyphenated) is your body demonstrating that you need to start listening to it because something is out of balance.

While doctors are excellent at treating emergencies, they are not so adept at treating dis-ease. Simply addressing the symptoms does not usually get to the original energetic cause. Often symptoms are masked by prescribed drugs, and the imbalance will continue. However, in serious conditions, always heed your doctor's advice.

In many instances Energy Medicine, which focuses upon the chakras, will enable a return to a state of wellness and ease. This is aided by slowing down and, most importantly, learning how to relax and taking numerous stops along the way, to restore optimum balance by developing a harmonious relationship within ourselves.

Scientific discoveries show that our energy system (chakras, meridians, subtle-energy field, and so on) vibrates at many subtle levels. Usually it lies beyond the point where most people can hear or perceive it, but with some practice it can be sensed by any dedicated person.

A healer or practitioner in Energy Medicine uses finely tuned energy-sensing skills to assess and then balance the subtle-energy system, aiming to access and guide a person's subtle energy and assist in its transformation; sometimes it needs to be increased, and at other times decreased. A healer will use crystals, sound, light, colour and numerous other methods, or will channel healing energy through their hands. This workshop-in-a-book enables you to develop these skills to use upon yourself.

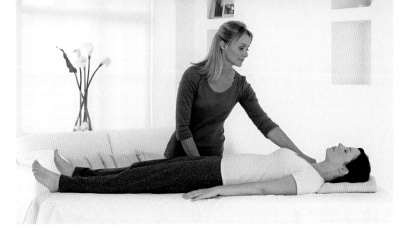

How does it work?

Physicists tell us that everything is simply energy. Energy has a range of low to high frequencies. Lower frequencies are more dense, so they are the ones we can see in our physical world – everything from our pet cat to the table at which we sit. Higher frequencies are much less dense – they are the subtle energies that we refer to when we talk of auras and chakras. Physicists describe how energies interpenetrate one another, from the microscopic cellular and DNA level to the movement of planets and stars in the cosmos.

As we have already discussed, the seven main chakras are specialized energy centres working to regulate the flow of pranic life-force within the body. It enters the body field at a chakra and travels through the network of nadis to particular cells, organs and tissues. These reciprocate by resonating with that chakra's unique frequency. This subtle-energy system is complementary to physical body systems such as the nervous, digestive and circulatory systems. When we interact *consciously* with the energy system, we get to the root cause of dis-ease.

The adverse effects of EMF and noise

This book would be incomplete without mentioning the potential effects upon our chakras of the external electromagnetic fields (EMFs) that we are subjected to in our daily lives. Domestic electrical appliances give out a measurable force field, which may particularly affect the Base and Sacral Chakras if we are exposed to the source for a continuous length of time. So check to ensure that these electrical force fields (and the pulsed micro-waves from cellphones, TVs and other electrical units) are at a safe distance from where you and your family sleep. Any EMF force fields near the head are particularly dangerous to the higher chakras.

Noise is legally defined as a pollutant in a number of countries. Medical studies confirm the adverse effects of noise on the hearing, heart rate, blood pressure, sleep and mental health, as well as on physical performance, measured by inappropriate levels of adrenaline, noradrenaline and melatonin, which have implications for chakra energies.

The effect of sound upon an unborn child in a mother's womb is particularly important. The pineal centre appears at the fifth week in the developing human embryo. By the 18th week the sense of hearing has become active, and its first function is to give 'food' to the brain. It is wise to protect your unborn child from excessively loud noise and music by placing a cushion over your lower chakra areas, because metaphysical teachings regard the foetus's chakras and subtle-energy system as the 'template' upon which life builds from the moment of conception.

For the first seven years of a child's life close contact with the mother is vital, to ensure that the child's etheric body maintains vital interdependence with its mother's energies. Therefore a mother's attention to maintaining wellness through chakra balancing also has implications for the child.

The adverse effects of chemicals

A whole range of chemical vibrational frequencies severely affects chakra functioning. So examine the many ways in which you can bring your life more into tune with Nature, challenging disease and balancing your chakras. Try to choose natural fibres for clothing and bedding, such as cotton, hemp, wool, silk or linen, because they permit the healthy functioning of the auric field. Avoid chemicals and additives in your food – stay natural and read the labels. Especially avoid chemical cleaners such as bleach; a natural alternative for all home cleaning applications is vinegar.

 Optional advanced exercise Turn to Exercise 25: Cutting Emotional 'Cords' on page 174 for an optional advanced exercise.

THROAT CHAKRA EXERCISES

The following exercises develop the Throat Chakra or Vishuddha, which expresses where you are on your path of life through speech, song or devotional words such as hymns, mantras and chants. It reflects how you treat others and whether you speak your truth. You will learn how to rebalance it by practising 'Bija mantras' with the help of the CD, as well as other more advanced methods.

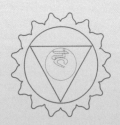

Developing intuition

Do this exercise before reading beyond this page. It will become a record of your Throat Chakra – showing your ability to express yourself – to which you can refer back in order to chart your progress.

Exercise 21 SENSING AND DRAWING MY THROAT CHAKRA

You will need: a set of coloured pencils or pens (all colours, including magenta); keep the book open, ready to colour in the body outline opposite, which represents you (sign and date it before you begin).

- **To begin,** take five minutes sitting in a quiet place, breathing slowly, relaxing and closing your eyes. Now start to sense your body and your aura. Release any emotions that arise. Forget anything you have ever heard or read about chakras and auras. You are simply 'sensing' how your own unique energies are flowing at present. Check from your feet up to your head to pick up any little clues that your body is giving you. Sense your auric energy field around you as well. Now focus upon your Throat Chakra area. What is it 'telling' you? What can you sense? Does it feel free, flowing, harmonious? Or is an old pain or trauma held there? Does this area feel fluid and open – or have you shut off all feelings and thoughts of this chakra?

- **When you feel ready,** open your eyes and – immediately and without thinking – quickly colour in the Throat Chakra area and any other parts of the body (and the surrounding page) as you wish. There is no right or wrong place to apply the colour: it is entirely up to you.

- **Read the interpretation** on page 164 after completing this exercise.

162

My sensing and drawing my throat chakra experience

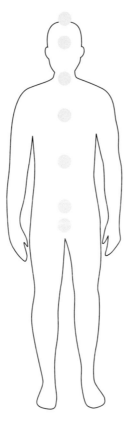

Date _____ Signature _____

Assessing my results for Exercise 21

A balanced Throat Chakra will show strong and vibrant colours of turquoise, blue or green. It will reflect your inner will, self-expression and ability to communicate in a caring way. It may also reflect the ability to speak your own truth without hurting others, and a developed singing skill.

An unbalanced Throat Chakra will show either very weak or very strong colours. These colours may be dark shades — black, brown or grey or a strong, dull red. When weakened, it will reflect depression, dependence and an inability to express yourself. Overactivity may make you overreactive, intolerant and hurtful to others, especially in an uncaring choice of words. Frustration held in the Throat Chakra may manifest as strong anger or violence.

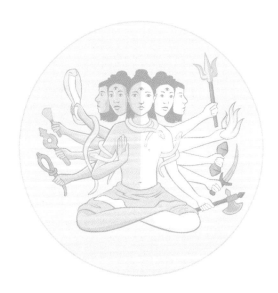

Meditative visualization

This visualization exercise will increase your energy, help to lift depression and boost your immune system. Ideally it should be done outside, while lying on your back looking up at a pure blue sky. If this is not possible, make yourself comfortable inside and imagine that you are gazing into the sky.

 ## Exercise 22 THROAT CHAKRA VISUALIZATION

CD REFERENCE TRACK 2 (OPTIONAL) (TO FOLLOW THE SCRIPT, TURN TO PAGE 110)

- **To begin,** do Exercise 15: Complete Relaxation on page 110, using CD reference Track 2 (optional).

- **Then visualize a pure sky-blue colour** all around you. Imagine you are gazing across a very calm sea that merges with the sky into a shimmering pale turquoise in the far distance.

- **Feel that you can breathe in** pure sky-blue colour into your body. Imagine that you are immersed in a sea of tranquillity and can hear the sounds of the sea blending with the rhythmic sounds of your own body.

- **Know that this colour cleanses** and refreshes your physical body. It brings a spiritual dimension to your whole energy field and chakras. It especially boosts your energy levels by clearing unwanted elements from your Throat Chakra region.

- **Now imagine a bridge of Light** spanning the sea, which it is possible to cross. On arriving at the other side, you meet a beautiful glowing 'Light being'. It may be your guardian angel or Archangel Michael, who brings the qualities of communication and self-expression. Whoever it is, allow them to place their healing hands upon you and transmit Light throughout your whole mind/body/spirit complex.

- **Feel the warmth** from the Light being's hands removing any pain or disharmony from your body. Feel their hands removing any stress and tension from your mind. See them dispersing into the vast Ocean of Life. When they have finished their healing work, they remove their hands, but the warmth and sense of well-being remains with you.

- **Realize that we are each a tiny drop** in the vast Ocean of Life, but as each drop is important in the great universal plan, so you too are unique and important.

- **Thank the Light being** and return the way you came, across the bridge of Light.

- **On reaching your starting point again,** breathe in pure sky-blue colour, reconnect with your physical body, and finally open your eyes.

- **Now consider** the questions on page 167.

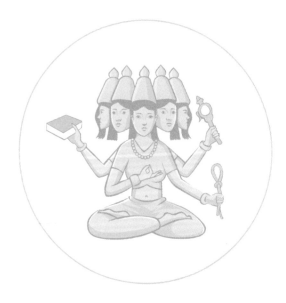

166

My throat chakra visualization experience

Date _____

Where I did my visualization _____
_____
_____
_____
_____

What I experienced _____
_____
_____
_____
_____

What I can learn from this visualization _____
_____
_____
_____
_____

Sounding the Bija mantras

This Sound Experience exercise introduces you to sounding the Bija mantras (see page 156). As a regular practice it is helpful to repeat the Bija mantra at least three times with each chakra. Sit comfortably on cushion or upright chair. Ensure you will not be interrupted. It is best not to have eaten for at least an hour, but do have water to hand. Begin with lighting a candle.

Toning the Bija mantras is not a diagnostic tool; it is about creating transformation so avoid any expectations during toning. Don't be surprised, or think you have failed, if you have sensed nothing – sometimes seeds take time to germinate! Repeat the exercise as many times as you can manage, simply enjoy being a human being instead of a human doing.

 Exercise 23 SOUND EXPERIENCE
CD REFERENCE TRACK 4 (TO FOLLOW THE SCRIPT, SEE BELOW)

- **To begin,** relax your shoulders, keeping your spine straight. Clear your nose and throat. Sit in an upright position, with your palms facing upward and your index fingers touching the thumbs (this is called the 'Chin or Jnana Mudra').

- **Focus on the candle flame,** the rhythms of your heart and breathing.

- **Remain silently focused** for a minute, carefully avoiding any external thought intrusion.

- **Place your left hand** on the perineum (the region surrounding the urogenital and anal openings) for the Base Chakra (if you wish) and focus on your Base Chakra.

- *** Draw a full breath into your lungs,** continuing to concentrate and letting your voice make a sound expressing the Bija LAM (sounds like 'laarmm').

- **Allow your lungs to empty slowly** while maintaining your inner focus.

- **Then begin to focus on the next chakra**, placing your left hand (if you so wish) below the navel.

- **Repeat from * above**, but with the Bija VAM (sounds like 'vaarmm').

- **Repeat from * above**, placing your hand on your solar plexus, sounding the Bija RAM (sounds like 'raarmm').

- **Repeat from * above**, placing your hand on heart, sounding the Bija YAM (sounds like 'yaarmm').

- **Repeat from * above**, placing your hand on the throat, sounding the Bija HAM (sounds like 'haarmm').

- **Repeat from * above**, placing your hand on the forehead, sounding the Bija OM (sounds like 'aumm').

- **Repeat from * above**, placing the palm of your hand downward on top of your head, sounding the Bija OM (sounds like 'aumm').

- **Finish by breathing slowly** and deeply, allowing anything that you wish to release to pass from you with each exhalation.

- **Give silent thanks** for this precious time that you have been able to keep with yourself.

- **Record any notes** that you wish to make on pages 170–71.

I'm not quite there yet Read page 184 about sounding OM, if you found this exercise difficult.

My sound experience

Date _____

● What, if anything, did I experience at a physical, emotional, mental and spiritual level when I toned LAM? _____

_____

_____

_____

_____

_____

● What, if anything, did I experience at a physical, emotional, mental and spiritual level when I toned VAM? _____

_____

_____

_____

_____

_____

● What, if anything, did I experience at a physical, emotional, mental and spiritual level when I toned RAM? _____

_____

_____

_____

_____

_____

• What, if anything, did I experience at a physical, emotional, mental and spiritual level when I toned YAM? _____

_____

_____

_____

_____

• What, if anything, did I experience at a physical, emotional, mental and spiritual level when I toned HAM? _____

_____

_____

_____

_____

• What, if anything, did I experience at a physical, emotional, mental and spiritual level when I toned OM (for the Third Eye)? _____

_____

_____

_____

_____

• What, if anything, did I experience at a physical, emotional, mental and spiritual level when I toned OM (for the Crown)? _____

_____

_____

_____

Recharging the Throat Chakra

For this exercise you need to be in a place where you will not be disturbed for approximately half an hour – indoors is okay, but it would be even better to be sitting outside. Wherever you choose, your spine must be as straight as possible and your chin pulled in, to straighten the back of your neck.

Choose two cleansed and dedicated small pieces of natural turquoise (if you choose to use crystals) and hold one in each hand. Place 'grounding' stones, such as heavy beach pebbles under your feet (see page 27 for more about 'grounding' stones). Light a special candle if you wish.

Exercise 24 COLOUR-BREATHING WITH CRYSTALS

CD REFERENCE TRACK 2 (OPTIONAL) (TO FOLLOW THE SCRIPT, SEE PAGE 110)

- **To begin,** sit in an upright chair or a cross-legged yoga posture. Ensure that you are fully relaxed.

- **Close your eyes** and breathe slowly, visualizing your incoming breath as a clear, bright turquoise-blue light. Breathe deeply for a few minutes, focusing on the Throat Chakra. Feel this coloured breath suffusing the area of your physical throat and neck and its chakra with energy.

- **Now feel this coloured light** spreading across your shoulders, balancing the minor chakras there.

- **'Wrap' a cloak of turquoise light** around your whole body and auric field for protection.

- **Return to normal breathing** and, when you feel ready, slowly open your eyes.

- **Now consider** the questions on page 173.

My colour-breathing with crystals experience

Date _____

How well did I relax?   Well / It was difficult / I couldn't relax at all

Did the colour-breathing help me to focus on my Throat Chakra?
Yes / No / A bit, but then I lost the focus / Don't know

How did this exercise affect me? _____

_____

_____

_____

_____

_____

_____

_____

_____

_____

_____

Does my Throat Chakra feel more balanced?   Yes / No / A bit / Don't know

Releasing emotional suffering

Today, in an advanced exercise, you are going to release – cut the 'cords' – that tie you to outdated emotional suffering. You will cut them *once only* and it will be *for ever*. This is a symbolic act and 'rite of passage'. You will be calling upon the Force of Grace, which, if invoked by your superconsciousness (your higher self), cannot fail to respond.

Ideally you should be outside in a quiet, natural place; alternatively place a chair before an open window. This release is most powerful when done in the presence of two friends: one to witness, the other (the 'reader') to read the words, slowly, for you to repeat. However, it can be done on your own, but the words *must always be read slowly out loud* and with conviction. You do not need to tell your friends any details of the emotional suffering that you are about to release – in fact, it is much better not to transfer any of it to them. So don't chat; just make time and space for this special act.

 Exercise 25 CUTTING EMOTIONAL 'CORDS'
CD REFERENCE TRACK 2 (OPTIONAL) (TO FOLLOW THE SCRIPT, TURN TO PAGE 110)

- **To begin,** play CD Track 2 (optional) to ensure that you are fully relaxed, then sit up.

- **Get your friends to stand** one on each side of you and slightly behind you. (The release that liberates you from emotional 'cords' works through your physical, emotional, mental and spiritual bodies; it is cathartic, so you don't want someone standing in front of you to take on any negativity.)

- **The 'reader' begins,** saying the following words, line by line, which you then speak clearly out loud:

Superconsciousness, by the Force of Grace,

I formally rescind all ties and attachments

to outdated emotional suffering

entered into in this or any other lifetime.

I cut these 'cords' that have bound and limited me

And replace them with light that suffuses my

Energy body with joy.

May the power of that release

be fully manifest in my consciousness. [deep, releasing out-breath]

And so it is.

- **Now record** your experience on page 176.

- **Note** 'Energy Medicine' such as this does not normally conflict with medication, although those with mental health issues should consult their healthcare provider.

Later, when you feel ready to do so, you may also work on the Throat Chakra with any of the other balancing methods mentioned on other pages of this book. Consult the chart on page 147 to ascertain which aromatherapy oil to use, which yoga postures, colour breathing, and so on.

My cutting emotional 'cords' experience

Date of release of emotional suffering _____

Do not discuss what you experienced with those friends who helped you. Instead, write below any positive thoughts or feelings that you wish to record. _____

_____

_____

_____

_____

_____

_____

_____

_____

_____

Use a separate piece of paper to draw anything positive that you experienced (optional)

Should you have experienced any negative emotions, use a separate piece of paper to write them down or draw them and burn it immediately.

Remember that this is a once-only release of energy. It does not need to be repeated. If, at some future date, your mind begins to dwell on similar emotional issues, look back to this day, remember that you released all past and future emotional suffering, congratulate yourself and celebrate.

THE THIRD EYE CHAKRA: AJNA

Work with your chakras now Before you read further, turn to Exercise 26: Sensing and Drawing my Third Eye Chakra on page 194.

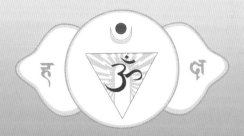

About my Third Eye Chakra

Keypoints: Resonates with the subtle element of Spirit and the colour deep blue; concerned with extra-sensory perception (ESP), clarity, intuition (inner teaching) and balancing our higher and lower selves.

The sixth chakra, the Third Eye or Brow Chakra, is the centre where we control the power of our mind. The Sanskrit name, *Ajna*, means 'to know' or 'to command' and it is traditionally regarded as the place where conflict takes place between ego and Spirit. It is also where we can release the limitations imposed upon us by the psychological construct of ego, which by rights should have already been dealt with at the Solar Plexus Chakra. Once this is achieved, we become open to 'inner sight' through the symbolic celestial marriage of sun and moon, mind and body.

This chakra is depicted with two petals in indigo or white, bearing Sanskrit letters. These petals symbolize the right and left sides of the brain, and represent the combination of the two polarities of human existence. The left side of the brain is our rational, analytical side, while the right is our intuitive, creative and experiential side. Traditionally a downward-pointing triangle is shown at Ajna, signifying the importance of integrating masculine and feminine energies at this stage of human spiritual evolution. This means that we will each become complete within ourselves, no longer depending upon others for our security or nurture. In fact the goddess of Ajna, Shakti Hakini, also illustrates this point, because her many minds are divinely pure – achieved by drinking the divine 'nectar' that constantly flows toward the Base Chakra.

All the ancient texts recommend 'awakening' the Third Eye Chakra slowly. Deep-blue light stimulates this chakra, which is sometimes symbolized by a blue sapphire.

 Optional advanced exercise Turn to Exercise 27: Candle Meditation on page 197, to deepen your experience of meditation using a candle.

CHART OF THE THIRD EYE CHAKRA

Colour of influence	Blue
Complementary light colour	Orange
Colour to calm	Blue and pale blue
Physical location	Centre of brow
Physiological system	Endocrine and nervous systems
Endocrine system	Pituitary
Key issues	Balancing higher and lower self and trusting inner guidance
Inner teaching	Completing and clearing karmic lessons
Energy action	Merging masculine and feminine energies
Balancing crystals	Lapis lazuli and any deep-blue crystal
Balancing aromatherapy oils	Frankincense, basil (in moderation)
Balancing herbal teas	Juniper/lemon balm/chamomile, or a mix (for the brain) of ginkgo, peppermint, nettle, rosehip, basil and anise
Balancing yoga position (*asana*)	Adho Mukha Avanasana (dog face down), yoga mudra in Padmasana (advanced pose), Halasana (Plough), Matsyasana (Fish).
Mantra/tone	OM in the note of A
Helpful musical instruments/music	Harp
Planet/astrological sign/natural House	Uranus/Saturn/Aquarius/Capricorn/eleventh: objectives/tenth: protection
Reiki hand position	Palms covering the face, then lift off to sides of head on the temples
Power animal (Native American tradition)	Spirit guides and ancestors

Body/Third Eye Chakra
connections

This chakra's action on the body's glandular system occurs through the pituitary gland, which lies behind the eyes and is known as the 'leader of the endocrine orchestra'. Our physiological balance and growth are maintained and monitored by the pituitary gland. It is more active at puberty and is concerned with female fertility and pregnancy. The physical location of the Third Eye Chakra is in the centre of the brow, just above the eyebrows, and it is related to the brain, eyes, ears, nose and nervous system.

When this chakra is imbalanced you may experience headaches, migraines, eye and sinus problems, catarrh, hayfever and hormonal fluctuations. Sleeplessness and disturbing dreams may be encountered if you overstimulate this chakra. Relaxation is key to its balance, coupled with many types of 'Energy Medicine' (which was introduced on page 158).

Ajna is particularly receptive to Energy Medicine in the form of visualization,

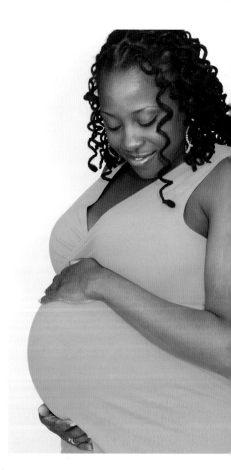

meditation, crystals, colour, coloured light, essential oils and the high vibration of flower essences. You may awaken this chakra by tapping it a number of times with the middle finger of your right hand, then massaging it with a circular clockwise movement. Visualize your Third Eye Chakra – your inner eye, the 'Eye of Shiva' – being cleaned, cleared and balanced.

Associated chakras

The Third Eye Chakra is connected to a smaller chakra called the Soma Chakra, meaning nectar or 'amrita'. This is depicted as a lotus with 12 petals with a silver crescent moon at the centre, said to be the source of the nectar. It is positioned at the centre of the hairline. Lavender-blue light stimulates this chakra. Tantric yoga describes how priests traditionally maintained celibacy to transmute their sexual energies in the Soma Chakra in order to gain enlightenment. It is considered to contain the combined energies of the godhead: Brahma the creator, Vishnu the preserver and Shiva the destroyer.

Two other minor paired chakras are also associated with the Third Eye, and particularly with developing healing abilities; they are the small Temple Chakras at either side of our head.

 All strength, all healing of every nature is the changing of the vibrations from within – the attuning of the Divine within the living tissue of a body to creative energies. This alone is healing.
Edgar Cayce, American healer and visionary

 Work with your chakras now Turn to Exercise 30: Colour-Breathing for my Third Eye Chakra on page 206.

Third Eye energy and imbalances

Energetically this chakra helps us to understand the world around us intellectually, honing our ability to accurately remember the past and helping us to envision the future, while remaining firmly anchored in the present *now* moment. The Third Eye, our inner perceptive faculty, opens our physical eyes to the beauty of the natural world that is all around us, if we take the trouble to look – even if we live in a city. This chakra, in its own way, energetically 'channels' beauty, art and positive vision as vital soul 'food'. It shows us the beauty in others, and in the simplest things in life.

If it is energetically blocked, the Third Eye may make us over-intellectualize, become egotistical or deluded, suffer from memory loss, show paranoia, negativity or deeply engrained sarcasm, or be drawn into controlling types of religion or causes such as conspiracy theories. We might come across to others as controlling perfectionists, putting on a mask for the sake of appearances, instead of displaying honest self-expression.

Physical manifestations

Physiologically, migraine headaches may result from a reduced supply of oxygen to the brain (although they can be food-related). From a body/mind perspective, migraines suggest that deeply held needs are being thwarted. Sometimes they are caused by an overload of responsibility that denies fulfilment in a given area. Look at your lifestyle choices, and whether you need to look deeper into your soul through your inner eye.

Do you have frequent headaches, sinus/ear problems or endocrine imbalances? At an energetic level, this is caused by not wanting to see or hear something that is important to your inner growth and soul's journey. One suggestion to remedy this is to follow the proverb 'Do not put off until tomorrow something that can be done today.' Working with visualization exercises, particularly on the Third Eye, will help to open up new possibilities for you that, if absorbed at deep inner levels, may improve your well-being.

A stiff neck may indicate that you are limiting yourself by only wanting to look in one direction. Work on the Throat and Third Eye Chakras, together with the Base Chakra, to give yourself increased energy levels and to repattern the effects of limitation.

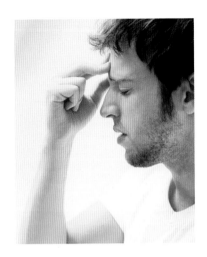

Balancing the whole chakra system – together with focus upon the Heart (self-worth), Throat (self-expression) and Third Eye (Brow) Chakras (visualization of a goal) – will help many symptoms of dis-ease. Chakra balancing through the methods described in this workshop-in-a-book generally brings peaceful acceptance of physical ailments, which may sometimes be ameliorated by adjusting the energy flow through appropriate chakras. Do remember, though, that this is a type of Energy Medicine that is primarily intended to balance energy. The effects are sometimes immediately beneficial to the physical body, but sometimes a 'healing crisis' results, which releases long-held, deeply entrenched dis-ease. If this occurs, know that the body, in its wisdom, is using its own method to restore equilibrium.

 Work with your chakras now Turn to Exercise 29: Dowsing the Third Eye on page 203, to check the balance of your Third Eye with a pendulum.

 I'm not quite there yet. Turn to Exercise 28: Releasing Negative Patterns on page 199.

The sacred OM/AUM

OM/AUM is an ancient Sanskrit word, thought to be the primordial creative sound from which the universe and all of Creation first manifested. Originally it was set forth as the object of profound religious meditation, with the highest spiritual efficacy being attributed not only to the whole word, but also to the three sounds within it.

The two written words OM and AUM describe the same sound. A-U-M represents divine energy (Shakti) and unites the major trinity of Hindu gods: Brahma, Vishnu and Shiva in their three elementary aspects: Brahma Shakti (creation), Vishnu Shakti (preservation) and Shiva Shakti (liberation and/or destruction).

Going deeper in the act of voicing OM/AUM, we find that it consists of three phonemes (units of sound): a, u and m. It symbolizes the Three Vedas, the Hindu Trimurti or the three stages of birth, life and death respectively.

In Tibetan Buddhist tradition, OM ('AUM') represents different aspects of the trinity of the Body (A), Speech (U) and Mind (M) of the Buddha, or an enlightened being. Sounding the AUM in this manner puts one in resonance with these qualities of consciousness. Yet another esoteric teaching of OM ('AUM') reminds us that the 'A' represents the physical plane, the 'U' the mental and astral planes and the 'M' all that is beyond the reach of the intellect. OM ('AUM') is the initial syllable at the commencement of many mantras.

Mantrically repeating OM/AUM will help you connect with the still point within, which may be described as the 'Source' of who you really are. OM is not just a sound or vibration; it is not just a symbol. It enables us to touch the entire cosmos – whatever we can see, touch, hear and feel. It is all that is within our perception and all that is beyond our perception. It is the core of our very existence. If you think of OM only as a sound, a technique or a symbol of the divine, you will miss a profound opportunity to change your whole life and understand who you really are.

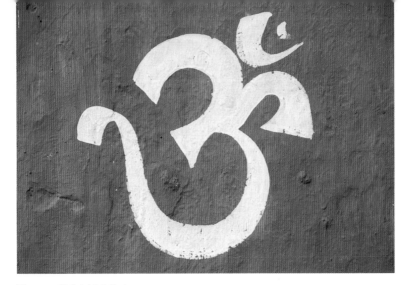

Toning OM/AUM

OM/AUM may be repeatedly toned as a mantra, but to achieve a path of deeper realization requires preparation. The following are guidelines for the beginner:

- Prepare to spend time somewhere you can be quiet and uninterrupted.
- Sit comfortably in an upright chair or in an appropriate yoga position.
- Become aware of your gentle, relaxed breathing.
- Reflect upon the meaning of OM/AUM and integrate these thoughts with your intention to sound the sacred word.
- *Breathe in deeply and, as you do so, visualize a fine strand of light entering through your Crown Chakra from somewhere way above. Feel that connection to the Light in your pineal gland/Crown Chakra area as you form a sound.
- Open your mouth, gently and slowly releasing your breath as you utter in equal length of time A... U... M..., taking care to pronounce the letters clearly and softly. (Enhance your facial muscular movements and give equal weight to each letter.)
- Take care not to force, strain or create tension.
- Enjoy the space after the out-breath and then repeat from *.
- Continue for a minimum of 5 to 10 minutes. When you have finished, be still, and in the silence absorb the vibration and, in turn, the deep realization of what you have created.

Using a crystal on my Third Eye

Having trained as a crystal healer, I recommend that you only *activate* the Third Eye Chakra with a crystal if you:

- Have already worked extensively with the chakras beneath it;
- Are prepared for a deep awakening;
- Are willing to enter other dimensional realities.

If so, use a cleansed clear quartz that is dedicated to your inner spiritual growth. Lie down and place the quartz on your brow for no more than ten minutes on the first occasion.

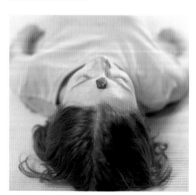

Other Third Eye actions

If you wish to *balance* the Third Eye Chakra, then ideally use lapis lazuli – a deep-blue stone with little golden veins in it – again for no more than ten minutes on the first occasion.

If you wish to *calm* the Third Eye Chakra, then ideally use emerald or sapphire. Although these may sound like expensive precious stones, they can be obtained very cheaply as uncut stones. Again use them for no more than ten minutes on the first occasion.

As you become more used to working with crystals, you can tape a small piece of emerald or sapphire to your Third Eye Chakra before you go to sleep, in order to have a calm night's sleep, untroubled by disturbing dreams. It may cause you to have wonderfully vivid and helpful dreams instead!

Making solarized water

Every chakra takes on and resonates with a specific energetic colour of light. It is a kind of 'food', which the chakra is drawing into the physical body as though it is liquid being poured through a funnel.

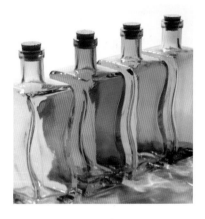

In this book, for ease of visualization, the predominant chakra colour is given, although these colours are never static or solely one shade of colour, because healers realize that there is continual movement in the energy body. Those who can see auric fields and chakras refer to the colours as swirling mist in constant motion. Detection work on the condition of auric fields and chakras can often lead to a perception of disease before it manifests in the body.

Colour healers develop the ability to channel a specific colour or to use instruments to give coloured light. There is also a simple colour-healing vehicle called 'solarized water', which passes sunshine through high-quality translucent coloured glass into water, and this can easily be prepared at home. It should be made with pure spring water, because water has the ability to take on different energetic encodings.

Select small, clean glass bottles or containers in a range of vibrant single colours (of course you may choose the appropriate chakra colour). Add the water and leave in the sun or strong daylight for up to 12 hours. The resulting coloured solarized water should be sipped slowly throughout the day between meals. This is a type of Energy Medicine that gives you a particular frequency of light-encoded water.

The meaning of colours

Different colours have different meanings when it comes to balancing the chakras.

Red ranges from very deep to a very pale red and has the slowest, longest wavelength of any colour. It is a powerful energizer and stimulant. Red increases blood supply to an area and improves circulation, of both physical and subtle energies. It should not be used where there is anger, anxiety or emotional issues.

Orange is more gentle in action than red and lies midway between the red and the yellow rays, therefore influencing physical vitality and intellect. Orange brings about changes in our biochemical structure, making it useful in conditions that require the dispersal or removal of inappropriate energetic imprints in the chakras.

Yellow rays carry positive energies to stimulate mental activity and the power of our mind. Yellow is used when there is a lack of physical or subtle-energy vitality.

Green, being midpoint in the colour spectrum, is neither a 'hot' nor a 'cold' colour. It brings balance, harmony and wholeness. However, do not use green if you are pregnant or have an issue with depression or cancer – in these instances, consult a qualified colour therapist.

Turquoise-blue has a strengthening and protective effect upon the physical body. It is an excellent colour ray to 'cool' any overactive chakras or to visualize as a means of protection around the whole body and auric field.

Blue is the colour ray that symbolizes inspiration, peace and devotion. It is used to slow down any body system or overactive chakra. Blue makes an excellent colour to visualize during meditation or to use in your healing sacred space.

Indigo is not generally used in colour healing, but it is the frequency with which the Third Eye Chakra resonates and takes one into deep levels of expansive, enhanced consciousness.

Violet rays enhance spirituality and self-respect. Its use with the Heart Chakra, or any chakras above it, uplifts the chakra in question and takes one into a realm of pure spiritual awareness.

Magenta is a colour really only seen as light – sometimes visible at sunset. The magenta ray used with the Heart Chakra, or any chakras above it, releases old ideas and conditioning in the chakra in question. It clears and uplifts it, dissolving rigidity and leading to personal spiritual evolution. Magenta is particularly appropriate to use with the higher chakras, such as the cosmic and transpersonal ones. You can read more about these chakras on page 219.

Developing my ESP abilities

Extra-sensory perception (ESP) originates at the Third Eye Chakra, assisted by the two minor chakras at the temples. Taking your time to work through all the exercises in this book, at least twice for each one, will gradually and naturally open your ESP abilities. Regular deep and complete relaxation (such as that taught in this workshop-in-a-book – see page 110), visualization and meditation are key to this process.

Different types of ESP

- The skill to see beyond the physical world is known as 'clairvoyance' – clear seeing.
- Hearing sounds or voices not in the physical world is 'clairaudience' – clear hearing.
- Sensing smells and perfumes not of this world is 'clairsentience' – clear feeling.

Some people appear to be born with these skills, and if these are recognized and allowed to develop, they may work as clairvoyants, mediums or healers. Others have the ability to see fairies or angels, but were told from an early age, 'Don't be silly – they are not really there.' Children frequently perceive auras around people, believing it is the natural way to see things – and, of course, it is – but unthinking adults may take them to have their eyes tested!

In the future, many babies will be born to enlightened parents who will recognize the importance of encouraging, rather than discouraging, ESP. This will create a resurgence of it, linking mysticism, science and spirituality. Just viewing the range of books now available on these subjects, compared to 25 years ago, shows the fundamental changes that are taking place in human consciousness.

A word of caution

Opening up your ESP can make you vulnerable to people who do not understand these energies. At many levels of your being, you will be reflecting an inner Light. Within your social group, ESP may not be a skill that you should talk about unless you are prepared to stand your ground, come out of your shell and reflect this inner

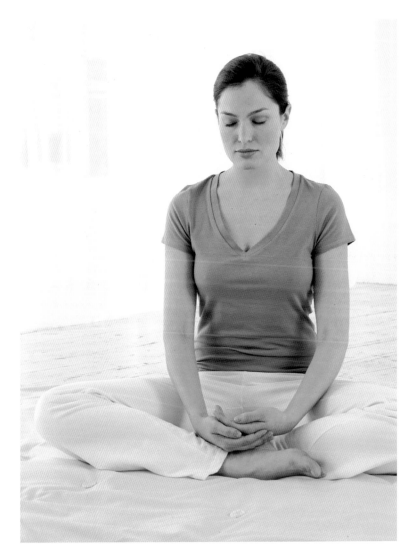

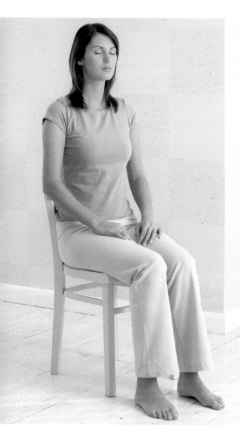

Light, which has gifted you with these abilities. When you really shine strongly as a beacon, it will attract all kinds of people and energies to you. Sometime these people actually prey upon your light energies, sucking into, drawing upon and trying to destroy your inner Light. While they may not be aware that they are doing this, you certainly need to be aware!

Protect yourself

Therefore consistently invoke a strong personal psychic protection. Visualize a cloak of deep-blue light that you can wrap securely around yourself. Or place a circle of clear white light around your body, 'drawing it' with a fingertip and then closing it up into a protective sphere/shell or egg shape of white radiance, which only positive energy can permeate.

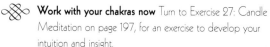

Work with your chakras now Turn to Exercise 27: Candle Meditation on page 197, for an exercise to develop your intuition and insight.

THIRD EYE CHAKRA EXERCISES

The following exercises develop the Third Eye Chakra or Ajna, which shows you other ways of perceiving the world, going beyond what you see with your physical eyes. They are intended to deepen your inner seeing, through visualization leading to meditation. They include a self-assessment that helps the release of negative patterns, a candle meditation and ways to protect your chakras.

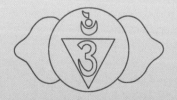

Developing intuition

Do this exercise before reading beyond this page. It will become a record of your Third Eye Chakra – showing your ability to engage with ESP — to which you can refer back in order to chart your progress.

Exercise 26 SENSING AND DRAWING MY THIRD EYE CHAKRA

You will need: a set of coloured pencils or pens (all colours, including magenta); keep the book open, ready to colour in the body outline opposite, which represents you (sign and date it before you begin).

- **To begin,** take five minutes sitting in a quiet place, breathing slowly, relaxing and closing your eyes. Now start to sense your body and your aura. Release any emotions that arise. Forget anything you have ever heard or read about chakras and auras. You are simply 'sensing' how your own unique energies are flowing at present. Check from your feet up to your head to pick up any little clues that your body is giving you. Sense your auric energy field around you as well. Now focus upon your Third Eye Chakra area, in the centre of your brow. What is it 'telling' you? What can you sense? Does it feel free, flowing, harmonious? Or is an old pain or trauma held there? Does it feel 'grounded' — or have you shut off all feelings and thoughts of this chakra?

- **When you feel ready,** open your eyes and — immediately and without thinking — quickly colour in the Third Eye Chakra area and any other parts of the body (and the surrounding page) as you wish. There is no right or wrong place to apply the colour: it is entirely up to you.

- **Read the interpretation** on page 196 after completing this exercise.

My sensing and drawing my third eye chakra experience

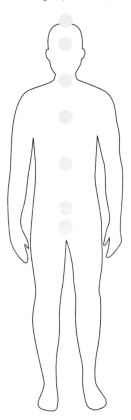

Date _____   Signature _____

195

Assessing my results for Exercise 26

A balanced Third Eye Chakra will show strong and vibrant colours in the blue to violet range. It will reflect your 'inner eye', your ability to engage with ESP, visions and deep transformative meditation. Balance shows your personal empowerment and respect for the life and spiritual paths of others. You will be outgoing, cheerful, relaxed, intuitive, demonstrating natural ESP such as telepathy or the ability to meditate easily. You may be a natural healer or spiritual teacher. You will be drawn to deepen your interest in metaphysical teachings.

An unbalanced Third Eye Chakra will show few or no colours, or possibly very strong and disjointed colours and patterns. These colours may be dark shades — black, brown or grey or a strong, dull red. When weakened, it will reflect depression, insecurity, dubious occult tendencies, fear of other situations or other dimensional realities. Overactivity of this chakra may make you egotistical, controlling, judgmental, sarcastic and a petty perfectionist.

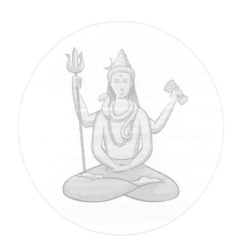

Developing insight

This is an ancient yogic technique called Tratakam, which helps to develop visualization techniques and brings great inner peace. You should do this exercise regularly to develop ESP and Third Eye Chakra sensitivity, but for no longer than 30 minutes at a time.

Exercise 27 CANDLE MEDITATION

You will need: a candle and a pen to record your results.

- To begin, sit in a dark room in front of a candle, placed about 1 m (3 ft) away from you at eye level. Ensure that you are sitting comfortably and upright.

- Close your eyes and take three deep, relaxing breaths.

- Open your eyes and look straight at the candle flame without blinking.

- Close your eyes when they become tired and, with your eyelids closed, look upward to your Third Eye Chakra.

- There you will see an inner image of the candle flame, and probably many colours. Hold this image for as long as you can.

- Eventually all images will disappear and then you can reopen your eyes. Be ready to record your experience on the next page.

- Now consider the questions on page 198.

My candle meditation experience

Date _____

What did I experience when I closed my eyes?_____
_____

What does this teach me?_____
_____

Was this exercise easy/difficult (indicate which)_____
_____

Date _____

What did I experience when I closed my eyes?_____
_____

What does this teach me?_____
_____

Was this exercise easy/difficult (indicate which)_____
_____

Overlaying a pattern of perfection

We all occasionally need some help to see clearly what is limiting us. Our physical and energy bodies – comprising the chakras and aura – accumulate all of life's experiences, both those that we consider good and those we consider bad. They may be held in rigid horizontal banding that prevents upward flow through the whole body field.

Sometimes they linger as negative patterns that need to be identified and then released, through the methods explained in this book. In place of negative patterns we can choose to consciously overlay a pattern of perfection, comprising light-encoded frequencies for the well-being of our mind, body and spirit.

Exercise 28 RELEASING NEGATIVE PATTERNS

You will need: a pen to record your results.

- To begin, remain focused and silent for a moment.

- Assess the simple statements on pages 200–201. Be honest with yourself and circle the statement that reflects your answer.

- Once you have considered all the statements, count the number of nos you scored and read what that means.

- Think about how you can remedy any negative patterns and turn those answers into positive statements. Record those statements on the form on page 202.

My releasing negative patterns experience

Date _____

Take a while to assess the following simple statements. Be honest with yourself.

Circle the relevant answers below:

- I can relax easily   Yes / No / Sometimes
- I feel comfortable in my body   Yes / No / Sometimes
- I can use my mind creatively   Yes / No / Sometimes
- I feel comfortable with spiritual concepts   Yes / No / Sometimes
- I enjoy my own company   Yes / No / Sometimes
- I enjoy the company of other people   Yes / No / Sometimes
- I try not to judge other people by appearances   Yes / No / Sometimes
- I have an open mind   Yes / No / Sometimes
- I have a good and accurate memory   Yes / No / Sometimes
- I can concentrate well   Yes / No / Sometimes
- I look after my body   Yes / No / Sometimes
- I appreciate my home/family/friends   Yes / No / Sometimes
- I like to help other people   Yes / No / Sometimes
- I have a positive self-image   Yes / No / Sometimes
- I see the best in all situations   Yes / No / Sometimes

- I have useful premonitions   Yes / No / Sometimes

- I go to sleep easily   Yes / No / Sometimes

- I have colourful and exciting dreams   Yes / No / Sometimes

- I can visualize something easily   Yes / No / Sometimes

- I enjoy being in Nature   Yes / No / Sometimes

- I often meditate   Yes / No / Sometimes

How many 'Nos' did you score? Record your score here _____

- If you answered 'No' to any of these statements, you are holding some unhelpful patterns in your energy body (chakras and aura).

- If you answered 'No' to five to ten of these statements, you need to work upon these aspects.

- If you answered 'No' to ten or more of these statements, you are holding some seriously unhelpful patterns in your energy body that will ultimately affect your physical body. It means that your personal vision is compromised and you would be wise to open yourself to the wonder of life – and make an extra effort to undertake the exercises in this workshop-in-a-book at least twice each, until you feel you have learned the lessons that you need at soul level.

- Think about how you can remedy the situation and record your thoughts on page 202.

Write here what you intend to do to remedy the situation, by making positive statements. (For example, 'I will be open to the ideas of other people and constructive in my responses'.)

Checking my Third Eye is balanced

This exercise uses a pendulum to check whether your Third Eye is balanced. As recommended on page 18, try to build up empathy and confidence in your pendulum, so that it can be used reliably to determine degrees of activity in each of your chakras. *Remember to avoid holding the pendulum over a chakra*, particularly if it is a crystal one – instead, point a finger of the other hand toward and near the chakra in question. This ensures that the pendulum doesn't falsify the reading.

Below are just some of the questions you may ask. Or how about asking if you need aromatherapy or sound healing exercises? Any questions that you ask must have only 'Yes' or 'No' answers.

Exercise 29 DOWSING THE THIRD EYE

You will need: a pendulum, and a pen to record your results

- To begin, remain focused and silent for a moment.

- Then ask the following questions:
  'Does this chakra require balancing?'
  'Is balance required on a physical level?'
  'Is balance required on a mental/emotional level?'
  'Is balance required on an energy level in my auric field?'

  It is also relevant to ask:
  'Is this chakra overactive or underactive?'
  'Is colour-breathing required?'
  'Is crystal balancing required?'
  'Is a change in my lifestyle required?'

- **Record your pendulum results** on the following page (date and sign them), so that you can begin to see repeating (or varying) patterns of chakra activity. You may dowse just the Third Eye Chakra, or you have space there to record the condition of all your chakras, if you wish. You can also compare the effects that various methods shown in this book have upon the chakras, by dowsing before and after any balancing work. It becomes very exciting when you do this, because you can start to see positive results.

- **As an optional method of dowsing**, use a blank 'body outline' (see pages 238–49). Sign it (this is your 'witness' or energy imprint). With the understanding that this body outline represents you, rest your index finger on each chakra in turn. Hold the pendulum in the other hand, well away from your physical body. Ask the questions given above. Record and date your results.

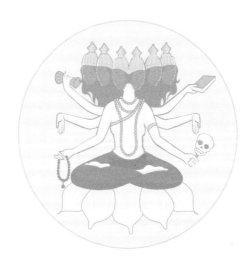

My dowsing the third eye experience

Date _____   Signature _____

- Does this _____ Chakra require balancing?   Yes / No
- Is balance required on a physical level?   Yes / No
- Is balance required on a mental/emotional level?   Yes / No
- Is balance required on an energy level in my auric field?   Yes / No
- Is this _____ Chakra overactive?   Yes / No
- Is colour-breathing required?   Yes / No
- Is crystal balancing required?   Yes / No
- Is a change in my lifestyle required?   Yes / No
- Is this _____ Chakra underactive?   Yes / No
- Is colour-breathing required?   Yes / No
- Is crystal balancing required?   Yes / No
- Is a change in my lifestyle required?   Yes / No
- Ask any other questions that you wish to pose.

Circle the relevant states below:

Base Chakra	Balanced	Underactive	Overactive
Sacral Chakra	Balanced	Underactive	Overactive
Solar Plexus Chakra	Balanced	Underactive	Overactive
Heart Chakra	Balanced	Underactive	Overactive
Throat Chakra	Balanced	Underactive	Overactive
Third Eye Chakra	Balanced	Underactive	Overactive
Crown Chakra	Balanced	Underactive	Overactive

Recharging my Third Eye

Using crystals with this exercise is optional, but if you use them they will increase the energetic frequencies for your Third Eye Chakra as you experience the colour-breathing. You need to be in a place where you will not be disturbed for approximately half an hour – indoors is okay, but it would be even better to be outside in Nature. Protecting the energy of your chakras is vital for well-being, especially as your spiritual journey unfolds. Here it is suggested you use turquoise light since it is the principal protective colour.

 Exercise 30 COLOUR-BREATHING MY THIRD EYE CHAKRA

CD REFERENCE TRACK 2 (OPTIONAL) (TO FOLLOW THE SCRIPT, TURN TO PAGE 110)

You will need: one small clear quartz crystal with a point or five small, tumbled clear quartz crystals (optional), plus a meditation blanket to lie on.

- **To begin,** arrange the five tumbled quartz crystals (if you are using them) in a semicircle on the blanket around your head, or hold the quartz point (if you are using it) in the palm of your left hand, with the point directed up your arm.

- **Lie on your back** on your blanket and ensure that you are fully relaxed.

- **Close your eyes** and breathe slowly, visualizing your incoming breath as a clear, deep-blue light. Breathe deeply for a few minutes, focusing on your Third Eye Chakra. Experience the sensation of this coloured breath suffusing the area of your brow, head, eyes, ears, brain and Third Eye Chakra with energy.

- **Pause for a while**, then feel this coloured light spreading down your neck to your shoulders, relaxing them and bringing a feeling of total well-being. Again pause to let the deep-blue light-encoded frequencies permeate your physical body, energy body and consciousness.

- **Finally 'wrap' a cloak** of turquoise light around your whole body and auric field for protection.

- **Return to normal breathing** and, when you feel ready, slowly open your eyes.

- **Now consider** the questions on page 208.

Later, when you feel ready to do so, you may also work on the Third Eye Chakra with any of the other balancing methods mentioned on other pages of this book. Consult the chart on page 179 to ascertain which aromatherapy oil to use, which yoga postures, colour breathing, and so on.

My colour-breathing my third eye chakra experience

Date _____

How well did I relax?   Well / It was difficult / I couldn't relax at all

Does my Third Eye Chakra feel more balanced?
Yes / No / A bit, but then I lost the focus / Don't know

How did this exercise affect me? _____

_____

_____

_____

_____

_____

_____

_____

_____

_____

_____

_____

_____

THE CROWN CHAKRA: SAHASRARA

 Work with your chakras now Before you read further, turn to
Exercise 31: Sensing and Drawing my Crown Chakra on page 226.

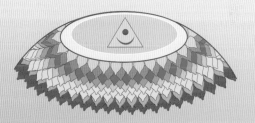

About my Crown Chakra

Keypoints: Resonates with Spirit and with pure white light flecked with gold and violet; has a connection to higher consciousness and inner wisdom.

The seventh chakra, the Crown, has Sanskrit name Sahasrara, 'the thousand-petalled lotus'. Here we finally reach a state of enlightenment when we choose to be released from the karmic 'wheel of life and rebirth'. In accordance with the traditional interpretation of karma, having recognized our divine self, there is no longer any reason to reincarnate.

It is written in the *Dhammapada*, a Buddhist collection of aphorisms or wise words:

'The traveller has reached the end of his journey. In the freedom of the infinite he is free from all sorrows, fetters that bound him are thrown away, and the burning fever of life is no more. He is calm like the earth that endures; he is steady like a column that is firm; he is pure like a lake that is clear; he is free from Samsara, the ever-returning life-in-death. In the light of his vision he has found his freedom; his thoughts are peace, his words are peace and his work is peace.'

The Crown Chakra activates and opens us up to higher consciousness, literally 'crowning' us with Great Spirit/Creator/Goddess/God. In yogic tradition, its many petals represent the spiritual work needed to perceive the source of manifest and unmanifest Spirit through the union of Shiva and Shakti at the Brahman Gate. In practice, this means that energies of duality, masculine and feminine, unite. Here lies the gate where the 'I' – the centre of our being – can transcend, creating superconsciousness beyond Time and Space. A process of unification occurs between human personality and a Higher Self containing tiny jewels of 'all that is, all that has been and all that ever will be', carried as soul seeds from one lifetime to another.

When we begin to glimpse what these yoga-inspired words mean, an enormous power is lit up in our minds. It may happen to you if you are serious about your spiritual practice. Once experienced, there is no going back – life is changed for ever, and everything is a play of subtle energies. In Tantric Buddhism, it is called the Rainbow of Liberated Energies.

CHART OF THE CROWN CHAKRA

Colour of influence	Intense violet/gold/white
Complementary light colour	Magenta
Colour to calm	Green
Physical location	Top of head
Physiological system	Central nervous system and brain
Endocrine system	Pineal
Key issues	Inner wisdom and ageing gracefully
Inner teaching	Releasing attachments to transcend Earth-bound karma
Energy action	Achieving Unity and Oneness
Balancing crystals	Amethyst and clear quartz
Balancing aromatherapy oils	Ylang-ylang, rosewood, linden
Balancing herbal teas	Chamomile or valerian (for sleep), a mix of wood betony, skullcap, chamomile, meadowsweet, hops and peppermint (for headaches), echinacea (for the lymph)
Balancing yoga position (*asana*)	Salamba sirhasana 1 (headstand) – advanced, Bakasana (crane) – beginners, Salamba sarvangasana 1 (shoulderstand)
Mantra/tone	OM in the note of B
Helpful musical instruments/music	Tibetan and crystal bowls
Planet/astrological sign/natural House	Jupiter/Neptune/Pisces/twelfth: challenges
Reiki hand position	Hold the back of the head
Power animal (Native American tradition)	Kachina Universal Spirit

Body/Crown Chakra connections

The Crown Chakra is biologically linked to the whole endocrine system and to one of our most important rhythms of waking and sleeping. Unlike all the other six major chakras, this chakra opens upward like a funnel of energy and connects deep within the brain to the pineal gland, our biological clock. Among its functions are:

• Balancing the action between the pineal gland and the gonads (prostate/testes or ovaries/uterus at the Base Chakra), which work closely together to regulate sexual growth at puberty.

• Producing the hormone melatonin, which peaks during the 28-day menstrual cycle and is stimulated by light levels and particular wavelengths of light, although production of this hormone decreases in continuous light. It also regulates light photo-receptors in the retina of our eye and calms us down at night. During the hours of natural light, serotonin production in the pineal gland is at its peak, urging us into activity, so these two hormones work in a continuous circadian cycle.

More on melatonin

A modern disorder, SAD (seasonally affected disorder) is a type of depression reflecting unnatural cycles of sleep (natural rhythms take us to sleep at dusk and waken us at dawn). It is caused by melatonin/seratonin-cycle imbalance through the artificiality of street lighting, sleeping with the curtains closed or working at night. It can be improved by increasing the light levels in winter, preferably of sunlight, although a special daylight-simulation lamp can also be obtained.

As we begin to work with new awareness, cutting-edge medical research continues to throw more 'light' upon pineal-gland functions, validating chakra wisdom teachings – for example, the efficacy of meditating at night, or ideally at 3 a.m., when biologists confirm that melatonin production is at its peak and the Crown Chakra is active.

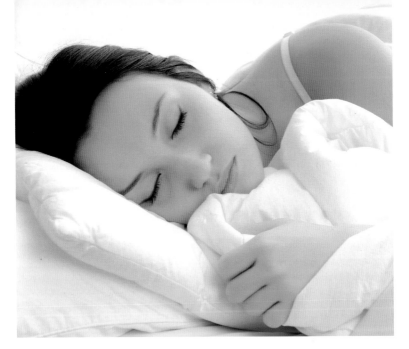

It is interesting to note that various hormones released by the pineal gland, including pinoline, are similar to LSD, producing natural hallucinations and heightened states of awareness. The pineal and adrenals also have a complex biological link that may influence stress levels, through the kidneys and abdominal organs, connected with the Solar Plexus and Sacral Chakras.

At both auric-field level and within our skulls, the Crown Chakra is linked to the pyramid shape of energy formed by the Brow Chakra and the Alta Major Chakra (see page 230 for more on this).

Did you know?
It is the pineal gland of some mammals that causes them to hibernate in winter in response to reduced daylight.

My Crown Chakra in balance

At the Crown, the 'Diamond Lotus', we ask, 'Am I committed to a daily spiritual practice?' If so, it is likely that the harmoniously balanced energies of all the chakras will flow upward to illuminate the Crown. In the past the aura of a saint was shown as a golden halo around the head, indicating development of their Crown Chakra.

The Crown is where we finally liberate consciousness that was previously attached to our physical body. We open up an ability to come into a state of 'superconsciousness' that is both personal and interpersonal, of this world and of other worlds, of this dimension and other dimensions. To achieve this we choose to release ego-driven self-created identity and liberate our wisdom inheritance. On an everyday level this means great challenges. If we let go of something, do we immediately replace it with something else? Or can we let go in order to find ourselves? Letting go of attachment requires us to see life simply as it is – not to embellish it with what is outside our control, but to be open to the many possibilities and energies that stream into our planet from all parts of the cosmos.

Using symbolic language

At the Crown, of necessity, we must turn to metaphysical, deeply esoteric language. Such specialized language was developed thousands of years ago in the Indian subcontinent by practitioners of yoga and related disciplines. It was written in the form of Sanskrit and is still used today for sacred texts that require complex spiritual concepts to be expressed. Using this symbolic language, we visualize our chakras as the lotus, whose roots are in the mud and whose flowers (similar to water lilies in appearance) reach skyward. Ask yourself these questions:

- Do I have a daily spiritual practice?
- Have I learned the lessons of the Base Chakra? Am I well rooted?
- Have I grown through the emotional 'mud' of the Sacral Chakra? Is the

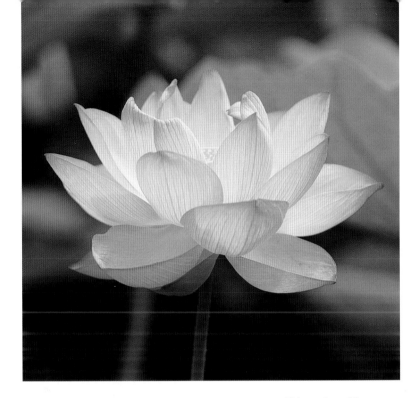

growing shoot of my life strong, straight and well intentioned as I reach for the next chakra?

- Have I allowed the physical and spiritual sun to shine upon my growth as I reached for the light at my Solar Plexus?
- Have I nurtured a precious flower bud with love in my Heart Chakra? Is that love given unconditionally to all beings?
- Can I authentically and honestly express myself through my Throat Chakra?
- When I visualize the lotus flower bud opening at my Third Eye, what does this look like?
- Can I stand fully receptive, vulnerable as an open flower, reflecting my inner and outer light at the Crown Chakra?
- Am I prepared to transcend ecstasy to reach Divine Bliss?

⁶ Believe in miracles. ⁹

Ancestral imprints

Do you think you know your ancestors? How far back in your mother or father's line can you go: can you recall the full names of your grandmothers, great-grandmothers, great-great-grandmothers and grandfathers? Probably not. This probably reflects how, in our modern world, we give them very little significance. But many indigenous peoples can recall names stretching back for generations.

So who do we mean by 'ancestors'? Seven categories of ancestor are listed below. Their energetic imprints are embedded deeply in our auric field and seven chakras. It is up to us whether we are in harmony with this situation, or whether we wish to clear any negative imprints from our chakras.

Personal family bloodlines

The personal bloodlines of our mothers and fathers go right back to the start of time. We carry elements of these ancestors' DNA. We may well still have a living connection with some of them, or they had a strong guiding influence on our present lives. These may be held as inherited imprints of particular

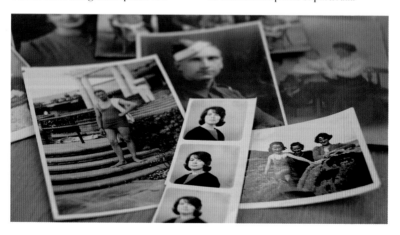

personality traits or dis-ease that we can eradicate at an energetic level. We associate them with red light at the Base Chakra.

National or tribal ancestors

Many of us are of mixed racial descent. Each of our ancestors made us who we are and brings with him or her the folk heroes and national leaders who have led their peoples over the ages. We may bless and release these ancestors, if we wish. We associate them with orange light at the Sacral Chakra.

Earth Spirit ancestors

These are essences of the land/s that have formed us: the elves, fairies, devas, sylphs, undines, salamanders, little people, the Tolilahqui (in Native American tradition) and so on. We may bless and release these ancestors, if we wish. We associate them with yellow/gold light at the Solar Plexus Chakra.

Mythic ancestors

These are supernatural beings in different world creation myths, which created Earth and the first human beings. These ancestors were usually born of both Earth and the stars. In Celtic tradition they are 'the Shining Ones'; but also consider: Athene/Apollo, Isis/Ra, Shakti/Shiva, Quetzalcoatl/Ixchel, plus aspects of the Great Mother Goddess – for example, Celtic: Brigit, Indian: Kali-ma, Egyptian: Hathor, Norse: Freya, Native American: Buffalo Calf Woman.

Our mythic ancestors may influence us strongly. Since some energies associated with them seem to us today to have been violent or war-like, you should only ever invoke the presence of those who will come to you in a peaceful, good way to guide your present life. We associate them with green light at the Heart Chakra.

Personal spirit ancestors

They are the beings that we once were in our karmic memories, our past lives. Included in this category are our parallel lives (past, present and future), the angelic influences that guided (and continue to guide) us, as well as spiritual masters or females to whose lineages we have been aligned. From a shamanic perspective, they are also spirit animals or clan spirits that guided our past lives. We may bless and release these ancestors, if we wish. We associate turquoise light with spirit ancestors at the Throat Chakra.

Star-people ancestors

These ancestors guided and mated with humans, seeded or in other ways influenced our DNA, our bodies and spiritual direction. They are star people with whom we feel a particular resonance – for example, those from the Pleiades or Sirius. Remember to ask for any extra-terrestrial ancestors to come 'in a good way, with good intent'. We associate them with blue light at the Third Eye Chakra.

Ascended-being ancestors

These are profound guiding influences, including Krishna, the Buddha, Mohammed and Jesus, as well as the Archangels. Their positive influences continue to guide many millions of people. Their aim? Unification with the Source! Our present life direction is subtly guided by them. We associate them with violet light, and within our luminous field the energetic imprints of beneficial ancestors merge into white light.

Clearing imprints

If you sense that you are in any way influenced by ancestral blockages, probably generated by deep trauma, then clear each chakra in turn, beginning with the Base Chakra. In your sacred space, light a candle and say out loud: 'I ask the ancestors to come to me in a good way.'

Focus upon flooding the chakra with the appropriate coloured light, as mentioned above. Say, 'I ask those ancestors who carry negative imprints in my energy field to leave me now.' Then seal each chakra in turn with an equal-armed cross of light and say, 'I ask the ancestors who come to me in a good way to remind me of the wisdom of the Ages that is within me, and to seal it within this chakra.'

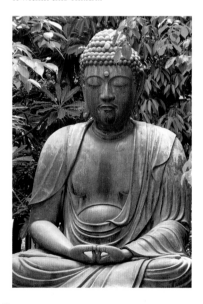

Reaching beyond the seven chakras

Applying a visionary perspective to the Indian chakra tradition, we can see how it has been a great and wise teaching for the past 2,000 years – but today humanity is rapidly evolving. Time appears to be speeding up. We are in the last few years of a great cycle of time spanning 26,000 years and a shorter 5,125-year period within it, which began during the Neolithic era and will end, according to the Maya wisdom teachers of Central America, in December 2012. They do not predict an apocalyptic end to our planet at that time, but rather a period of preparation, of clearing out the old, while humanity is confronted with difficult choices. A new cycle of time will then begin, when fresh patterns of life on Earth will be established. What they are depends upon the choices we make concerning the values by which we live.

Whether we listen to the Maya, Hopi and other indigenous peoples of the Americas, to the wise Hawaiian Kahuna, to elders and spiritual messengers from other aboriginal and tribal peoples or to visionary spiritual teachers within a Western context, we are hearing the same message. The cry is that everyone needs to wake up! We humans are being urged to take responsibility for ourselves and our beautiful planet. Our opportunity to evolve as a human race is *now*, and the outcome of this great 'experiment' in human consciousness depends upon you and me. There are two basic options – two spiralling timelines for us to pursue collectively at this critical time. Will we stay on the same timeline as our forebears and continue with our materialistic goals and destruction of Earth's resources? Or will we, with full awareness of the pulse of life that comes from the cosmos and regulates our chakras and subtle energies, choose to use the skills that we have learned in our lives to care for people and our planet?

At this decisive time in the development – indeed, evolution – of humanity, our spiritual skills take us beyond the Seven Chakra System and deeply into the significance of 12 chakras. One of these,

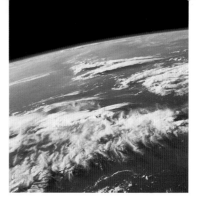

the Earth Star, has only opened in very recent years, with the advent of environmental awareness. These additional chakras (particularly the Earth Star Chakra and three located above the head) link us to the whole planet, the galaxy and the cosmos. Developing awareness of them takes us on a positive timeline that ultimately stretches beyond Time itself, deep into an exploration of other quantum realities.

There is a natural limiting factor within these additional chakras – if you have not completed both practical and spiritual activations upon the traditional seven chakras, in accordance with your soul path, and are not living a good intentioned life from a heart-centred level, you are unlikely to find yourself open or receptive to these energetic gateways.

Conscious intention and meditation vertically align our supreme power as enlightened beings. Light enters through the Stellar Gateway, Soul Star and Causal Chakra (see opposite) into the Crown Chakra. You may visualize it as sparkling golden light with a special quality of Divine Love, opening the heart to activate and ground energies at the Earth Star below. The response is for Earth energies to rise and meld at the Heart Chakra, sending out a strong vibrational signal, so that restructuring of our DNA and the journey to what we, as humans, have always intended to be can continue.

❛ Look with the opened inner eye. You will see everything you need, waiting to be shared. ❜

 Optional advanced exercise Turn to Exercise 32: 'Be in the Flow' Meditation on page 228, for an advanced meditation.

 Optional advanced exercise Or turn to Exercise 33: The Pyramid of Light on page 231, for another advanced meditation.

My 12 chakras

The five newly recognized chakras are transpersonal in nature. When awakened, we are taken beyond limited body/mind perceptions to interact with our wider environment and cosmic inheritance.

Earth Star Chakra

This was introduced on page 27. It is located just below our feet and is connected to the physical body by nerve endings, reflexology points and acupuncture meridians in the soles. It becomes activated when we allow our inner light to interact consciously with our environment and combine people care with planet care. This chakra is black and is not visible in the aura, unless we have strengthened and regained our intrinsic connection to the Earth, when it becomes a beautiful glowing magenta colour that 'walks' below our feet wherever we tread. Its purpose is the recreation of our bodies in preparation for restructuring DNA and, ultimately, luminous light-body ascension.

The Hara

This is closely linked to the Sacral Chakra, but in many people working with Eastern energy techniques it has

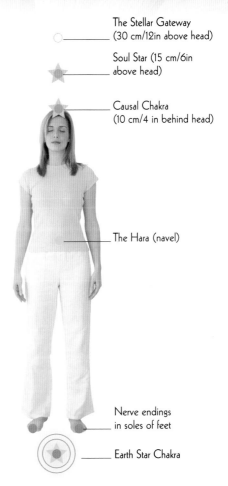

The Stellar Gateway
(30 cm/12in above head)

Soul Star (15 cm/6in above head)

Causal Chakra
(10 cm/4 in behind head)

The Hara (navel)

Nerve endings in soles of feet

Earth Star Chakra

become dominant and is regarded as a separate chakra. It resonates with a strong orange-red colour of light. This chakra is balanced using tiger's eye or carnelian crystals.

Causal Chakra

This is located 10 cm (4 in) back from the Crown Chakra, lying just above the head and aligning with the spinal column. It helps development of the 'higher self' – an aspect of us beyond conscience. Conscience is conditioned, moulded and, at extremes, manipulated by the society in which we live. But the higher self knows, at core level, the right action to take in any circumstances because it is an expression of our soul. When we follow a path of unconditional love and repeatedly act selflessly, we are linked to our higher self in daily action.

The Causal Chakra guides our present lives, if we have released ego and opened up to Spirit – at which point it becomes a purifying filter through which we perceive life on Earth. It enables us to make good decisions and right choices for the benefit of the many, within an 'ocean' of inner peace and tranquillity. You will know when your Causal is balanced because your life will be a reflection of the peace that you feel in your physical and spiritual Heart Chakra. Crystals to enhance awareness of the Causal Chakra are celestite and moonstone, while kyanite directs positive energy and 'cuts' unwanted energy.

Soul Star

This is located 15–30 cm (6–12 in) above the head. Through energy impulses coming from the Crown Chakra, it transmits light-encoded information upward and outward to the Source. Reciprocally it filters incoming galactic information in order that it may be comprehended and acted upon at an awakened human level. It is believed that the Soul Star is where the soul rests immediately after death, before transition to other realities. Crystals to enhance awareness of the Soul Star are selenite, pink petalite or phenacite.

The Stellar Gateway

This is located a little above the Soul Star or is expanded an infinite distance into space. Full activation of this gateway will only occur when humanity is collectively ready to receive the inconceivably high vibrational energy of the cosmos. Crystals to enhance awareness of the Stellar Gateway are dark-green moldavite and Brandenburg crystal.

CHART OF THE 12 CHAKRAS

NAME OF CHAKRA	LIGHT COLOUR	PROPERTIES	LIFE LESSON
Earth Star	Black/magenta	Spiritual grounding point	Transmutation of fears
Base Chakra	Red	Physical grounding point	Establishing purpose on Earth
Sacral Chakra	Orange-red	Generative creative energy	Seeking balance with all life forms
Hara	Orange-yellow	Physical sustenance and strength	Balancing energy and Spirit
Solar Plexus Chakra	Yellow	Development of mental/physical movement	Honouring wisdom in others
Heart Chakra	Green	Unconditional Love/compassion	Honouring Divine Love
Throat Chakra	Turquoise blue	Verbal/artistic expression	Resonating with compassion
Third Eye Chakra	Deep intense blue	Inner sight, purification of thought	Completing karmic lessons
Crown Chakra	Purple/gold/white	Expansion of consciousness	Transcending physicality
Causal Chakra	Aqua	Conscious reprogramming	At-oneness with the solar system
Soul Star	Peach	Abode of soul after death	At-oneness with the galaxy
Stellar Gateway	Silver	Oneness, universal consciousness	At-oneness with the universe

 Work with your chakras now Turn to Exercise 34: Visualization for My 12 Chakras on page 233.

 Work with the CD now Play CD reference Track 5 for the same visualization.

Death and transition

Death is a transition from one reality to another. Our lives in the energy field of Earth Mother. Finally a time comes when we have to release and seek independence in another dimensional experience and so some prefer to call death a transition – of energy, spirit, soul and consciousness. We're born through the Base Chakra and transit out through the Crown. At that point all bio-energy and body functions are released and we are declared 'dead'. Metaphysically the soul rests awhile in the Soul Star Chakra before moving on. This is why a tunnel and intense light are described by those who have had a near-death experience – they are seeing the light of the Crown and the three chakras aligned vertically above it, beckoning them into this other dimension.

A peaceful transition

Knowing this, we can assist in the transition of those we love, or in our own transition. At the appropriate time, consciously move energy up through the chakras and, finally, fully open the thousand-petalled lotus at the Crown. Infinite peace will result, which releases the soul into a great flow, like an enormous river, that carries it toward the Divine Light. A peaceful transition is greatly aided by playing soft music and talking to a loved one even if they appear to be unconscious. Sometimes we are at a loss to know how to use meaningful ceremony, so light candles and make the room comfortable for everyone present. Sometimes in our modern culture we are at a loss to know how to perform a meaningful ceremony that aids transition, particularly when the emotions are in full flow. If it is acceptable, place a quartz crystal pointing upward on the Third Eye Chakra of the dying person; position another just above their head, again pointing upward. This will encourage the upward movement of energy.

Use the ideas and teachings in this book with lightness and love in your Heart Chakra, expanding the wisdom acquired through insights at the Third Eye. Wisdom – different from knowledge – dawns through visionary consciousness. So look at life with an open inner eye. You will see everything you need, waiting to be shared.

CROWN CHAKRA EXERCISES

The following exercises develop the Crown Chakra or Sahasrara, taking you into the dimensions of Spirit whilst remaining on Earth. You may expand deep personal insights of an uplifting, transformative nature. plus the ability to meditate and identify with your life-path through numerous exercises. A guided Visualization for My 12 Chakras follows, complete with CD instructions, and drawing a record of your complete energy field.

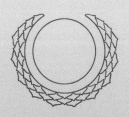

Developing intuition

Do this exercise before reading beyond this page.
It will become a record of your Crown
Chakra and your higher chakras, to which
you can refer back in order to chart your
progress. Your developing ESP may take
you into deep perceptions.

 **Exercise 31 SENSING AND DRAWING MY
CROWN CHAKRA**

You will need: a set of coloured pencils or pens (all colours, including magenta);
keep the book open, ready to colour in the body outline opposite, which
represents you (sign and date it before you begin).

- **To begin,** take five minutes sitting in a quiet place, breathing slowly, relaxing and
closing your eyes. Now start to sense your body and your aura. Release any emotions
that arise. Forget anything you have ever heard or read about chakras and auras. You
are simply 'sensing' how your own unique energies are flowing at present. Check from
your feet up to your head to pick up any little clues that your body is giving you.
Sense your auric energy field around you as well. Now focus upon your Crown
Chakra area, from the pelvis downward. What is it 'telling' you? What can you
sense? Does it feel free, flowing, harmonious? Or is an old pain or trauma held there?
Does it feel 'grounded' — or have you shut off all feelings and thoughts of this chakra?

- **When you feel ready,** open your eyes and — immediately and without thinking —
quickly colour in the Crown Chakra area and any other parts of the body (and the
surrounding page) as you wish. There is no right or wrong place to apply the colour:
it is entirely up to you.

- **There is no need** to interpret the Crown and higher chakras. Their energy is so
personal to you that you will probably require some considerable time to fully
appreciate their subtleties.

My sensing and drawing my crown chakra experience

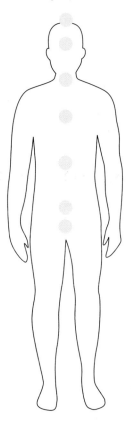

Date _____ Signature _____

Creating a bridge of energy

Our individual spiritual development brings a responsibility to contribute to the spiritual development of the planet. This meditation is termed light-bridging because it sends positive energies from your chakras to the four directions of the Earth in the form of cleansing light. It is best undertaken outdoors in a standing position. The purpose is to generate a bridge of energy between your Earth Star Chakra connection to the Earth and your Stellar Gateway to the cosmos. Only do this meditation for a short time, until you get used to it.

Exercise 32 'BE IN THE FLOW' MEDITATION

- **To begin,** face east. Stand outside with bare feet on the grass or earth. Activate all seven major chakras by visualizing your spine as a luminous column.

- **Send a strong 'root' down** from your feet through your Earth Star Chakra to the centre of the Earth.

- **Raise your arms** and ask to be filled with golden-white light. Imagine that your energy body has become so large that you can touch the stars. You are now 'in the flow' and bridging realities. Breathe deeply.

- **Lower your arms,** with the palms facing outward at shoulder level. Breathe golden-white light into your Heart Chakra, feeling it expand.

- **From your Heart Chakra,** visualize sending out light to the four compass directions of the Earth, turning around clockwise to do this. Start in the east; turn to the south, then west, then north. Imagine the light clearing all the places on Earth where there is pollution, despair or fear.

- **Feel joy** as you know that this work has been done, and gradually release the bridge of light.

My 'be in the flow' meditation experience

Date _____

Place _____

I felt _____

_____

_____

Date _____

Place _____

I felt _____

_____

_____

Date _____

Place _____

I felt _____

_____

_____

Alta Major Chakra

The Alta Major is located at the back of the neck, on the base of the skull. It is one of our 'oldest' chakras because it holds distant memories and links to the rudimentary part of the brain. Yet it is of vital importance when we come to balancing a triad of chakras that comprise a sacred pyramid in the skull, because through the Alta Major we have inherited our ancestral survival patterns, our race memories and past lives. On the one hand, the energy here can be strong, heavy and dense, if our life-path has not enabled us to deal with these inherited traits. On the other hand, if we have cleared negative imprints here and filled the chakra with light, it takes its place in the pyramid, ready to transmute the alchemical gold at the centre. Try this advanced exercise to see the pyramid of light. Note that spiritual evolution – ultimately a spiritual rebirth – takes place through the Crown Chakra, while physical birth takes place through the Base.

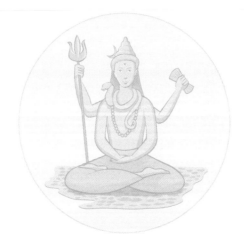

Exercise 33 THE PYRAMID OF LIGHT

- **To begin**, sit in a quiet place, feeling very relaxed.

- **Close your eyes** and begin to activate your head chakras by tapping your fingertips all over your skull for a few minutes in the following sequence: a line from Third Eye to Crown to Alta Major. Then in a circle horizontally from Third Eye to right temple, around the back of the skull to the left temple and return to the Third Eye.

- **Sit quietly** for a few minutes.

- **Concentrate on your Third Eye** and take a line of golden light from it right through your head to the Alta Major. Focus on the Alta Major.

- **Take a line of golden light** from your Alta Major right through your head to your Crown Chakra. Focus on the Crown Chakra.

- **Take a line of golden light** from your Crown Chakra right through your head to your Third Eye. Focus on the Third Eye.

- **Shift your focus** to the sacred golden pyramid now activated in your skull.

- **See the centre of the pyramid** being filled with sparkling golden light. It is the source of 'radiant ether' released through activation of the chakra system. Let this etheric light fill your head.

- **Release the golden light**, closing your Crown and Alta Major Chakras to an acceptable level of activity. Do the same in turn with the Third Eye, Throat, Heart, Solar Plexus, Sacral and Base Chakras.

- **Open your eyes** and be gentle with yourself for the rest of the day.

My pyramid of light experience

Date _____

Fingertip-tapping helped awaken my head chakras.   Yes / No

I was relaxed.   Yes / No

I experienced _____

_____

_____

_____

_____

Date _____

Fingertip-tapping helped awaken my head chakras.   Yes / No

I was relaxed.   Yes / No

I experienced _____

_____

_____

_____

_____

Guided visualization

Blue is the colour that brings peace. In the following visualization it is combined with golden light to balance your 12 chakras with your auric field.

 Exercise 34 VISUALIZATION FOR MY 12 CHAKRAS

CD REFERENCE TRACK 2 (OPTIONAL) (TO FOLLOW THE SCRIPT, SEE PAGE 110)
CD REFERENCE TRACK 4 (TO FOLLOW THE SCRIPT, SEE BELOW)

- **To begin,** lie down, preferably outdoors, but otherwise find a comfortable place indoors.

- **Imagine you are climbing** up the stone steps of a tall pyramid. You observe that it has 12 levels and a flat top with a small temple upon it. You reach the top and enter the temple.

- **Recline within the temple,** where an open circular window enables you to look directly up into the sky. See the vastness of the cloudless sky.

- **Wonder at the magnitude** of this atmosphere, which surrounds our Earth and stretches out beyond. Consider whether space is infinite or has a beginning and an end.

- **Consider how little** we really know about the galaxies and life beyond our own, and how small we are in this huge cosmic field.

- **Now concentrate on the sun,** taking a moment to appreciate its importance in sustaining life. Without it, all would be barren, lifeless and dark. Visualize a shaft of golden light pouring from the sun into the deep mysterious blueness of space. Let yourself travel within this golden light out into the universe. While you are doing so, a dark-blue light protects and holds you in its peaceful cloak.

- **In the immensity of space** you are just floating and moving gently. Without gravity you can effortlessly turn and look at the stars and planets. Each has its own colour of light and its own sound that blends with the whole, to create a 'symphony of the spheres'.

- **Let the colours and sounds** permeate your energy body, surging through your 12 chakras. They cause your physical body — each organ, muscle and bone — to resonate with its own perfect frequency of sound, creating wholeness within you.

- **Remember** that you came from the stars — and to the stars you will return.

- **Focus again** upon the dark blueness of space and consider your own spiritual path: is there a message for you?

- **When you feel ready**, travel within the shaft of golden light through the sun, then back to Earth. Become aware of your body lying within the temple. Descend the 12 levels carefully, step by step, and become once again fully present in your physical body, noting any changes to your chakras.

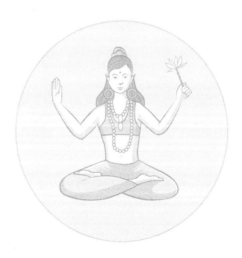

My visualization for my 12 chakras experience

Date _____

I relaxed   Well / not very well

I could visualize the temple easily   Yes / No

I could visualize travelling in the shaft of golden light   Yes / No

Check out each chakra and make appropriate notes _____

_____

_____

_____

_____

_____

I also experienced _____

_____

_____

_____

_____

_____

_____

_____

Developing intuition

This final exercise will become a record of your complete subtle-energy system, chakras and aura, to which you can refer back in order to see the extent to which you have progressed. You may compare it with the very first body outline that you intuitively coloured in on page 35.

Exercise 35 COLOURING MY SUBTLE-ENERGY SYSTEM

You will need: a set of coloured pencils or pens (all colours, including magenta); keep the book open, ready to colour in the body outline opposite, which represents you (sign and date it before you begin).

- **To begin**, take five minutes sitting in a quiet place, breathing slowly, relaxing and closing your eyes. Now start to sense your body and your aura. Release any emotions that arise. Forget anything you have ever heard or read about chakras and auras. You are simply 'sensing' how your own unique energies are flowing at present. Check from your feet up to your head to pick up any little clues that your body is giving you. Sense your auric energy field around you as well. What is it 'telling' you? Does your auric field feel fluid and open — or have you shut off all feelings and thoughts of it? Check through your chakras one by one. How are they feeling?

- **When you feel ready**, open your eyes and — immediately and without thinking — quickly colour in your complete chakra system of the seven main chakras, plus any of the higher head chakras and minor chakras or parts of the body (and the surrounding page) as you wish. There is no right or wrong place to apply the colour: it is entirely up to you.

- **There is no need** to interpret this drawing of your chakras and auric field. It represents a snapshot of where your energies are flowing at the present time. Just write any comments below the picture on the next page, date and sign it.

My colouring in my subtle-energy system experience

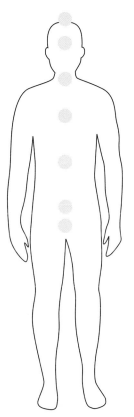

Date _____ Signature _____

BODY OUTLINE
CHARTS

Use the following body outline charts to record your
impressions when you sense the condition and balance
of your chakras.

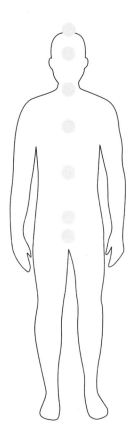

Date _____ Signature _____

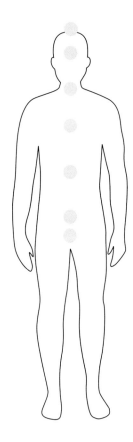

Date _____   Signature _____

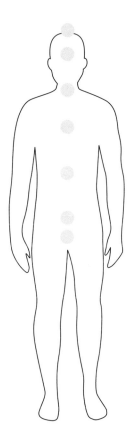

Date _____   Signature _____

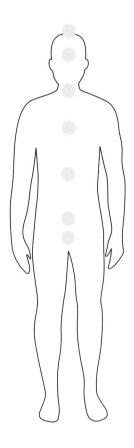

Date _____   Signature _____

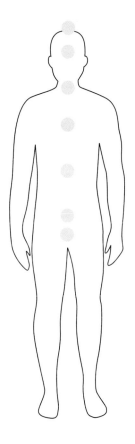

Date _____   Signature _____

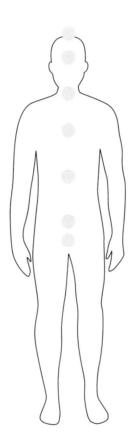

Date _____   Signature _____

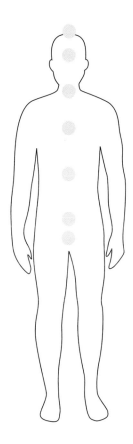

Date _____   Signature _____

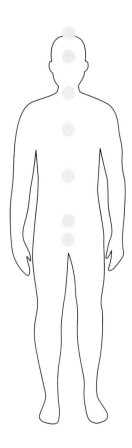

Date _____ Signature _____

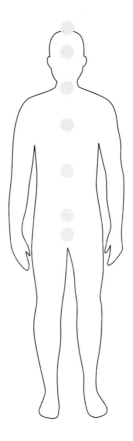

Date _____ Signature _____

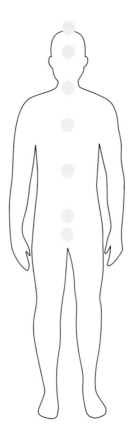

Date _____   Signature _____

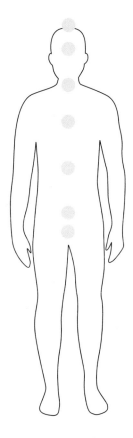

Date _____   Signature _____

Glossary of terms

Ancestral light body An aspect of our multidimensional self connected to our auric field.

Aura/auric field A subtle bio-energetic field of light surrounding a physical body, which, although not easily seen, may be sensed.

Being of Light An incarnate or disincarnate being or person, vibrating at high frequencies of light.

Body language Movements or expressions indicating our state of wellness and ease or disharmony and dis-ease.

Chi/ki A generalized type of subtle energy, identical to *prana*; a Chinese and Japanese term.

Clairvoyance Clearly seeing non-physical realms; closely associated with intuition.

Dis-ease Not being at ease in our body, and our body demonstrating that we need to rebalance it.

Ego A psychological term meaning one of the three main divisions of the mind; written here with a small 'e' to reduce its power.

Emotional imprint A subtle-energy pattern in the auric field and chakras.

Energy Medicine A wide-ranging and diverse holistic type of healthcare and healing, which provides treatment by balancing the human energy system; sometimes called Vibrational Healing.

Field of Life Part of the Quantum Field relevant to Earth life.

Force of Grace Force is an active energy, Grace is a special spiritual endowment or influence; in Hinduism, Grace is 'kripa', the ultimate key required for spiritual self-realization; in Buddhism, a state of Grace is attained through advancement on the Eightfold Path.

Healing crisis A rapid release of underlying causes of dis-ease that temporarily worsens a condition.

Inner child The vulnerable or playful part of our inner life/mind.

Karma Traditional: 'The wheel of cause and effect'; modern: an outdated attachment to Time, embedded deep in the fabric of our ancestral light body, causing compliance with archaic control mechanisms.

Kundalini Primal life energy, normally dormant at the base of the spine and having its roots at the Base Chakra.

Light Divine Spiritual Light, as compared to light (with a small 'l').

Luminous body/light body An 'awakened' and active human auric field.

Nadi A subtle-energy channel through which *prana* flows – similar, but not identical, to acupuncture meridians.

Prana A yogic term for a number of different types of subtle energy; sometimes called 'life-force'.

Quantum Field Interconnecting and interpenetrating energy fields of cosmic complexity and proportions.

Reiki A living path of spiritual healing rediscovered by Dr Mikao Usui.

Resonance When a particular body or system oscillates in its natural frequency as a result of impulses received from some other system that is vibrating with the same frequency.

Sanskrit A classical Indo-European language in which scientific, philosophical and religious ideas were expressed.

Subtle body An alternative expression for a person's auric and chakra energies; also the auric field, or a part or layer of it, such as the Lower Mental Body.

Superconsciousness Elevated human consciousness, both individually and collectively.

Yogi/yogic A dedicated practitioner of yoga/ pertaining to the practice of yoga.

Index

Acknowledgements

I would like to thank all the participants in my courses and workshops who, over the years, have helped me to develop and test the exercises in this book. Thanks, as always, to my husband and sound therapist Mikhail, who advised, researched and supported my writing.

Picture Acknowledgements

Alamy/Michael DeFreitas Asia 152; /Tetra Images 150. **Corbis**/Ocean 85, 125, 187. **Fotolia**/Coqrouge 29; /diez-artwork 1; /dngood 189; /Liv Friis-larsen 122; /Gorilla 55; /Barbara House 21; /Kathrin39 27; /kohashi 6, 215; /Mahesh Patil 91; /Richard Robinson 185; /Valua Vitaly 213; /WavebreakMediaMicro 88; /Zilotis 180. **Getty Images**/Martin Barraud 119; /B. Blue 127; /bravobravo 53; /Pascal Broze 116; /George Doyle 149; /Marcy Maloy 7; /Tom Merton 32; /moodboard 183; /Dejan Patic 157; /Trinette Reed 61. **Octopus Publishing Group** 63; /Colin Bowling 95 left; /Frazer Cunningham 13, 192, 221; /Janeanne Gilchrist 186; /Russell Sadur 17, 19, 57, 62, 93, 123, 191, 216; /Ruth Jenkinson 11, 21, 59, 159.

Commissioning Editor: Liz Dean
Managing Editor: Clare Churly
Deputy Art Director: Yasia Williams
Designer: Cobalt ID
Picture Library Manager: Jennifer Veall
Production Manager: Peter Hunt

DIARY OF A VAMPIRE

DIARY OF A VAMPIRE

GARY BOWEN

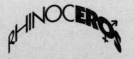

First Rhino*ceros* Edition 1995

First Printing August 1995

ISBN 1-56333-331-7

Cover Photograph © 1995 by Robert Chouraqui

Cover Design by Dayna Navarro

Manufactured in the United States of America
Published by Masquerade Books, Inc.
801 Second Avenue
New York, N.Y. 10017

DIARY OF A VAMPIRE

TO PETER FOR PATIENCE;
TO GREG FOR PASSION

"LOVE, FATAL CREATURE..."
—SAPPHO

Chapter One
RUDE AWAKENING

The Lord of stealthy murder,
facing his doom with a heart both craven and cruel.
　　　　　　　　　　　　　—Theodore Roosevelt

Budapest, October 1957; Baltimore, 6 October 1991

Kneeling in the damp earth I picked an armload of white frostflowers from where they grew among the ruins of the cemetery wall, then carried them to Valentin's grave. It had been a year since I had buried him. In those desperate days when all our friends were imprisoned, dead, or in hiding I carried out that gloomy task alone. His abandoned body had lain putrefying on the floor of our flat until I recovered enough to carry him to the old cemetery and inter him. He became one of the anonymous poor, buried a half-dozen to the plot in homemade shrouds with no coffins. In time water pressure forced their naked bones to the surface to nestle forlornly among the weeds and tall grasses. To spare my beloved Valentin the same fate I had heaped his grave with stones from the fallen wall, and now I covered the bleak stones with flowers, their soft petals blurring the sharp gray lines.

9

In ancient days men kept the dead in the earth by weighing them down with stones; only recently had gravestones become monuments.

Rap, rap, rap. By the sound of the mallet I knew that someone had found sterner measures to be necessary to keep a restless corpse in its grave. The sound mesmerized me and I followed it, the ground giving forth a charnel vapor that swirled around my ankles as I threaded my way through the tilted tombstones. The phosphorescent fog shifted constantly to reveal and then conceal the sunken graves of the poor. I skirted them carefully to avoid stepping on the protruding bones of those less fortunate than myself. Still I hurried. I was certain I would be too late, but I had to try.

The glow of an electric lantern illuminated an eerie scene: A grim old man stood in an open grave, lethal mallet firmly in his grip, while a young man in a woolen shirt held a shovel in a menacing way in case the immortal one offered any resistance. An innocent-eyed boy sat on the heap of earth from the violated grave, the shrouded lantern steady in his lap while exhumed skulls and femurs lay scattered around him. Without looking, the old man tossed the mallet aside to rattle among the ivory bones. Then he took some earth in his hands and bent into the grave to fill the corpse's mouth with dirt.

He stood up and stretched his back, then he removed his handkerchief from his pocket and bent down again. He was tying the corpse's jaw closed so that it could not chew its way to the surface. He reached for the shovel and the young man passed it to him. The shovel rose and fell, then rose and fell again. Small bones crunched and shattered at each blow. The corpse would not dig its way out either. The old man picked up the severed fingers and tossed them to the foot of the grave. They landed with a splash.

A gasp of horror escaped me. I started to retreat, but the

boy caught me in the beam of his lantern, the electric glare blinding me.

"Who are you?" the old man demanded. After eight years in the country my Hungarian was good, but I could barely understand his uncouth dialect.

"What are you doing? Dismembering the dead to make black magic, or just looting them for their rings?" I knew perfectly well what they were doing, but I pretended ignorance lest suspicion fall on me.

"Neither," snapped the old man. "We're not graverobbers, and we're not witches. We're her family. We've come to put her wandering soul to rest."

The smell coming from the grave was fresher than the usual miasma of the necropolis. Quelling my uneasy stomach I looked into the pit. The grave was awash with blood: The cerecloth was crimson with it. A white hawthorn stake pierced the corpse's stomach and anchored her in the muddy hole. Slashes allowed her arms to escape the sodden winding sheet and float freely on the red tide. Her fingerless hands bobbed in the ripples of blood as the old man climbed out. I was relieved that I did not know her.

"I've never seen such a thing! What is it?"

"Vampyr," he answered. "An undead monster that walks by night. Three weeks ago she scorned God's law by killing herself. Now she is killing us. Twelve people are dead or dying from her poisonous bite."

"Superstitious nonsense! This is 1957, for God's sake!"

"It's true!" the youth protested. "I've seen her!"

"It's your own guilt that haunts you, not some specter. This girl's suicide is a tragedy, not a horror."

"Maybe you will believe this!" The old man pulled his collar aside to reveal four puncture wounds next to his collarbone.

I had often seen such marks, but for my life I must admit

no knowledge. These three knew too well what they were about.

"Ridiculous! If this girl walks by night, why is she in her grave now?"

The grim one picked a wooden cross from among the debris of death. "We laid this on her grave!"

I recoiled.

The young man hefted the shovel in a way I did not like, his shoulders bulging with lethal strength. "Why are you here?" he demanded.

"I couldn't sleep so I brought flowers for the grave of a friend."

"You're too pale, stranger."

The three peasants formed a line. I retreated but the cold wall of a tomb blocked my escape.

"Mercy," I beseeched them.

Distantly I heard the wailing of a siren drawing nearer. I was a fugitive from the law; I did not want to meet the police any more than I wanted to stay with these barbarians. I tried to slide along the cracked wall of the tomb, but the boy with the light moved to cut me off. On my left the old man held up the cross while he quoted the Twenty-third Psalm at me.

Suddenly I knew how to disarm their hellish suspicions of me. I prayed in unison with him. "…Yea, though I walk through the valley of the shadow of death, I will fear no evil: for thou art with me; thy rod and thy staff they comfort me…." Each of us was sincere in our desire for deliverance.

The old man wavered.

"I'm a Spaniard, for God's sake! Not a monster. Just a foreigner."

"Someone's coming!" warned the burly youth.

The old man growled, "Run!"—but not to me. He and his sons fled into the fog.

The siren continued wailing. Groggily I realized it was the burglar alarm and switched it off. Nightmare. Only a nightmare. I was safe in my sanctuary, I need not fear.

The alarm! Shock sent me to my feet. The distant rapping had been the sound of someone forcing his way into my house—the dream had tried to warn me. My chest constricted, my breath stopped, the sense of disaster was suffocating. Pain numbed my brain and made me frantic. I held my head in my hands and ground my teeth to quiet the rising hysteria. Somewhere in the back of mind was a little piece of sanity that said I must remain calm and think. I tried.

I was in my vault under the house, steel separated me from the intruders. They could not take me by force—even if they could find the hidden door. I was safe against any disaster that might befall. Except suffocation. The vault was cunningly ventilated, but what if the ventilation failed, or was deliberately stopped? I would suffocate to death in a tomb of my own making.

I paced madly about the confines of my cell. In the grip of paranoia all dangers seemed possible, and disaster seemed imminent.

Hunger.

The desire for blood screamed through my withered veins: Liquid, red, hot blood that would rebuild my shrunken flesh. The hunger knotted my entrails and laced my veins with cold agony. My legs buckled, toppling me to the floor where I lay while a great weight pressed me against the concrete so hard I could barely breathe. My pulse raced in irregular fits while my heart palpitated and my head ached. Sudden anxiety filled me: I was going to die. The edge of doom was near, and I was about to tumble into the abyss. I knew it for a certainty.

After a few minutes on the cold floor it occurred to me

that things were getting no worse. I raised my head cautiously, but the movement plagued me with vertigo and nausea. I rested, then concentrated. The spinning of the darkness steadied and I could discern the shadowy shapes of the furniture. Carefully I commanded my limbs to lift me, but they felt distant and uncoordinated as if I were a marionette pulling my own strings. Grabbing the corner of the bedstead for support I staggered to my feet. My breathing was better, my heart tapping out a more stable rhythm, but I was still aware of the horror lurking just out of my vision, something lethal and inescapable should it choose to claim me. I shook my head against the madness, but the delusion of impending disaster remained.

I had become a revenant: An insane, ravenous monster doomed to shamble through a miserable unlife until the sun caught me or a whitethorn stake impaled me. What a fool I had been! I had trusted the Long Sleep to make me better than I was, but instead I was wracked with the worst hunger I had ever known, my higher faculties dull and unreliable. I had tried so hard and lost so much! Immortality was pointless if it was nothing more than crude survival for all the days of eternity. Now I understood why Valentin had not tried to escape his fate. He had given up on everything, even me.

I could not give up.

I would not quit, I would not remain in my fastness under the house. I would hunt those that dared to hunt me. Their hot blood would warm my cold flesh, strengthen my limbs, and settle my mind. I would sate myself at the blood feast and all would be well.

I drew back the bolts that sealed me in my vault, the door swinging silently open. Like a puma on the trail I crept silently up the stairs one turn behind the intruder so that even if he glanced over his shoulder he would not see me. He snapped on the lights as he climbed but most of the lamps remained dark and that made the stairway a dim place full of odd shadows.

I would flick off the lights, then seize him while he was disoriented in the darkness. I would strangle him into submission and drag his unconscious body to the basement. When I had glutted myself I would be able to think better. I would dispose of his body then.

He quickly checked the bathroom and library. He rattled the knob of my bedroom door then his shoulder thumped heavily against the wood veneered steel door. It held against his assaults, which was why I had installed it.

"Rafael!" he shouted. "Can you hear me?"

The sound of my name shocked me. Why did he call to me? Did he know me? Was it James? No, not James. James was a tenor, this man a baritone. It was not my brother Roberto, he would have called to me in Spanish. No one else knew where I lived.

Who was he?

"I'm calling an ambulance!" the stranger shouted, which bewildered me even more. He rushed down the stairs and I barely managed to dodge without being seen. As I ducked into the music room I slapped the light switch and plunged the hallways into sudden darkness. He halted in mid-flight.

"Uncle Rafael? Is that you?"

Uncle? If he spoke English, he must be one of Violeta's boys, either Michael or Alexander, but he was too old to be either of them.

"Who are you? What are you doing in my house?" I had lost both my composure and my silence.

"Michael, Michael Duran, your nephew. Violeta's son. Are you all right?"

His answer made no sense. Michael was in the Boy Scouts, not a grown man.

"You have no right to enter my house!"

"I'm sorry, but I thought I heard you scream. I thought you needed help."

His answer confused me further. The vault was nearly soundproof, and I had not screamed. Or was I deluding myself?

"I didn't scream." I clung stubbornly to what I hoped was the truth.

"I did hear something. I was worried for you, an old man all alone in a bad neighborhood."

Old man? Me?

"How old are you?"

"Twenty-five," he replied in a puzzled voice.

Impossible! I could not have slept fifteen years!

"If you really are Michael Duran, what did I send you for your First Communion?"

"A silver pen." He patted his pocket. "I still have it. It's sort of a good luck token for me."

"Throw it down."

A silver dart glimmered and bounced, then rolled across the hallway into the deeper darkness of the music room. I recognized the pen. Michael was kin.

I spoke harshly. "Why are you here?"

"I need your help," he said. "Mother doesn't approve of me being an artist. You're a musician, you know what it's like. Please." He descended several steps as he spoke.

"Stand where you are," I commanded.

He stopped on the lower landing.

"What do you want from me?" I demanded.

"Just a place to stay while I go to the galleries. I need to sell some paintings."

"Use a hotel."

"I'm broke, I can't afford a hotel. Please, I won't get in your way."

He was already in the way.

"Sleep in your car."

"In this neighborhood? Are you crazy? No offense, I'm sure it was a lot nicer when you moved in, but not anymore. I'll be surprised if I still have a car in the morning."

For your own safety, go away. I did not have the mental stamina to win an argument with him, nor protect him if he stayed.

"Please go," I said, but my voice was tired and lacked conviction.

He sighed and sat down on the edge of the landing.

"Nobody's heard from you for ages. At least tell me how you've been." With the toe of his boot he doodled in the dust.

The disturbances in the thick dust appalled and fascinated me. By that evidence he knew all was not well in this house. I had to stall him while I thought up a good explanation. My affairs would bear neither investigation nor gossip.

"You may sleep on the sofa in the library, provided you mind your own business. Discuss my affairs with no one, most especially not your mother."

If Violeta knew what was happening here she would appoint herself the manager of my affairs and I would end up in a lunatic asylum. I had already done one stint in the hospital, courtesy of my family, I did not care for a second visit.

"Thank you." He advanced towards my voice. "Tomorrow I'll help you fix up the place. I'd like to help."

"Go to bed and stay there!" I roared.

"Yes, sir," he replied meekly. He stepped upstairs immediately, much to my relief. The guise had never worked on his mother.

I let myself into the chilly night with no need for keys. My house was a part of me even as my flesh was part of me; the locks obeyed my will. There was a small covered patio beside the stoop, a blind area between the kitchen addition and the windowless brick wall of my neighbor's house. I had built it deliberately so I could do what I had to do in privacy.

Underneath the invisibly hinged steps was a black metal box fastened with a corroded padlock. With my mind I could feel the stiffness of the tumblers and solid immobility of the barrel. No cheap piece of metal was going to thwart me: I willed it open.

The lock burst. Pieces flew through the air, bounced off my skin without hurting me, then tinkled and rang on the pavement. I gaped at it in astonishment, for such a thing had never happened before. I must have misjudged the amount of power necessary. The error unsettled me; I needed to be able to depend upon my senses and power when I hunted. Bad miscalculations could have fatal effects. But if I hunted animals instead of men mistakes would be merely inconvenient. I would be all right.

Pawing through the spare clothes I found that they were all spotted with mildew. When I turned to dump them in the garbage I discovered that one of the trash cans was missing. A quick search revealed that Michael had moved it under the kitchen window, which he had broken open and climbed through, thereby setting off the burglar alarm and waking me. He had to have been both agile and strong to gain entry that way. I had underestimated mortal ingenuity.

The small lawn was rife with weeds while the rose garden had become a bramble patch. The two vegetative forces were doing battle for possession of the driveway. A poison ivy vine crept up the brick, and the mortar needed repointing. The green shutters were peeling, and one set flapped open—the pair that Michael had violated. With a flick of my mind I closed them. They slammed shut, making me jump. Again I had used too much power without even realizing it.

None of the row houses of my block was in pristine condition, but mine was the worst by far. James was supposed to have maintained the house while I was asleep, but he had not. He had my keys, he had control of my money; there was no excuse for not maintaining things properly. But I was hungry; finances would have to wait until more pressing needs were answered.

I stripped off my clothes and placed them in the box and closed the steps. My physical form melted and shaped itself to my will and I dropped to my hands and knees to better accommodate my emerging shape. My shrunken body was easy to change; I could rearrange it without adding or subtracting any mass. My face lengthened into a blunt snout and my ears grew triangular and erect while my legs and arms shortened until I stood on four strong paws. A long tail grew while thick tan hair covered my body. I felt strong and breathed easily. The cougar shape was more comfortable to wear than my own meager flesh. Unfortunately, the hunger remained. Some things never change.

The trees held scarlet and gold banners of autumn leaves, their black branches webbed across the face of the gibbous moon. Brown weeds crunched and rustled underfoot as I went to stalk deer in the park. The cold dew wetted my paws while a chilly mist hung among the tree boles. Frostflowers held up blooms of white, yellow or purple in defiance of the cold death that claimed all around. The white ones reminded me of Valentin. I threw back my head and howled in a strange, unfeline voice, notes beginning as a bass rumble swelling in volume to an ear piercing shriek, then slowly dying away. The neighborhood dogs knew something awful was afoot; they howled back at me.

Eternity is a long time to be alone.

Some time later I heard laughter. A blond man and a brunette woman were strolling down the path with their arms around each other. Their breath steamed around them as they laughed together, paying no attention to the sere autumn world that surrounded them. Envy ate at my heart, envy for the simple human contact that they shared without thinking how precious it was. My lovers and I had had to hoard our intimacy in secret, careful not to show affection for fear of those who denied us what they themselves enjoyed.

It was so unfair! I had keener senses than they; when I made love I could feel the pounding pulse of life throughout every nerve of my body. Kissing was an exquisite pleasure that aroused me so that my fangs extended, then when my teeth sank into softly resisting flesh and blood thrilled across my tongue I orgasmed, power spreading through my limbs as the life of another warmed and strengthened me. Like a fish on a line I followed a lure I could not resist; I wanted the mortal heat they gave each other without any appreciation for the value of what they squandered.

The two of them stepped off the path and threaded through some shrubbery until they came to a hollow surrounded by trees. It was a private place softly carpeted with grass. There he took her in his arms and kissed her slowly while his hands went under the back of her jacket. She put her arms around his neck and pressed her body against him. After a long kiss, he slipped his hand between them, cupping her breast. She pulled her blouse out of the way, revealing a small braless breast. When he bent and kissed it, she moaned and knotted her fingers in his hair.

The hunger was a conflagration that burned my mind and animated my limbs. In the back of my mind I felt regret, but there was no other choice. The hunger drove me.

I bowled him over, jaws snapping at his face. The

woman screamed his name, but I silenced her by tearing out her throat. Crimson splattered everywhere, the aroma of hot blood distracting me while her lover scrambled to his feet. I knocked him down again, pinning him with my weight, feeling my cold groin against his hot flesh.

I want you!

Sex and blood, blood and sex. They were one and the same to me. I felt my sex lengthen and harden as he writhed frantically under me, his hand pushing at my jaw, trying vainly to turn aside the teeth that grinned at him. My upper fangs extended to a truly terrifying length while he watched in spellbound horror. The lower ones extended also, but not so impressively.

With a whimper of sudden terror he renewed the struggle.

I was pleased that in spite of my decrepit condition I was much stronger than he, and more agile as well. He lay trapped beneath me, wiggling pleasantly while I lapped up the blood welling from his wounds, rasping away the bloody tatters of his shirt and jacket with my rough cat tongue. His skin was salty with sweat, acrid with fear, and best of all, musky with sex. I liked his masculine scent and taste, liked the hot blood flowing over my tongue, liked the way my body pressed full length against his, my erection grinding into his belly. I began to rock slightly, massaging that hard flesh between us.

His gasp of horror and sudden slippery movement startled me. I realized that my claws had lost purchase on his bloody skin because I no longer had claws, I had hands. I had become so entranced in fantasies of fucking him that I had reverted to human form, and he was taking advantage of the momentary confusion to slip away from me. My hand snaked out and grabbed his arm, and jerked him back to me, his eyes rolling in fear.

"No!" he cried.

For answer I sank my teeth into his throat. In manform my fangs were much smaller than in feline, but still they were large enough to pierce him deeply. Blood spurted in my mouth with each pulse of his heart. He could not escape me now, not unless he were willing to tear out his own throat. I sucked up the libation with fierce pleasure.

The power of his pulse intoxicated me; the rhythm of its pounding dictated the beat of my own heart. I wanted to couple with that strong flesh, to be one in the body even as we were one in the blood. I slid my naked knee between his. He resisted but I forced his legs apart. I traced the swell of his pectoral muscles, found the knob of his nipple and played with it. His hand pushed feebly against mine, but I had taken his strength from him. He could not resist me. My hand crossed his flat belly and found the soft hot flesh of his manhood but I had hurt him too badly, his flesh did not respond to my caresses.

His heart stumbled and resumed its cadence, then stumbled again. It was a strong heart that did not want to die. My heart echoed every beat as a gentle lassitude stole over my limbs. The pain in my breast eased while the coldness in my veins warmed a little. I was as comfortable as if I slept with a lover. It was so tempting! Just lie down and sleep the never-ending sleep.

I jerked my head away. Almost I had surrendered to the false temptations of death. I was dead already, death offered me nothing new.

Hours passed unnoticed. Once I had known how to reckon time by the celestial clock, but no longer. I was not far from home. If the stars melted into a silver sky I could still retreat to my sanctuary in time to escape the burning dawn. I rested drowsily, listening mindlessly to the distant growl of traffic as well as the nearby pounding of my own pulse. I fancied I could hear Michael shifting in his sleep. If my ears were that keen the city noises would deafen me. I could not tell which were the phantasms of my own brain, and which were dimly perceived realities, and I wondered at my sanity.

When the city glowed with predawn light and a few lights showed where early risers were leaving their beds to begin the day I transformed once again to cougar shape and slipped from the shelter of the trees. As I trotted along the sidewalk I checked behind me to see if I was leaving a bloody spoor, but the pavement was clean. No one saw the gory animal that vaulted into my backyard.

On the patio I became human again. I knelt nude beside the faucet and rinsed the incriminating blood down the drain. Dead skin and dirt peeled away with it, running in ugly brown rivulets down my body, and dripping to the pavement. The condition of my body disgusted me. Did Michael think I stank? Or was it only my own overly sensitive nose that was offended?

My hair and beard were long and matted, and my long curved nails snagged repeatedly as I washed them. I slapped them against the wall, breaking them off at jagged angles and scratching the bricks. I bit them with sharp teeth, shortening them to a respectable, if ragged length. The parings I dropped down the drain so that Michael would not accidentally discover them and wonder.

By the time I was done I was chilled, but I did not shiver; that was a human reaction. At least I was clean, if not presentable. I dressed rapidly, the clothes sticking to my damp body.

The back door opened without a touch. Just across the threshold I paused and felt for Michael's presence, found him sleeping upstairs on the library sofa. I stole quietly along the hall to the music room—another difference between myself and the mortals. They had dining rooms to indulge their gustatory pleasures, but I had a music room.

I pulled the white covers off the furniture and stashed them in the credenza. Next I placed the silver candelabra on the harpsichord, my hand tingling at the touch. A longer contact would burn. The tarnish vanished with a thought and the candles flamed with warm light. Always I have preferred the romantic glow of the candle to the harsh and unforgiving glare of electric lamps. Truly I was out of place, residing in a century and a country unsuited to my nature. Why was I not born four hundred years ago when the harpsichord was king?

I seated myself on the bench and lifted the cover to reveal gleaming ivory keys. I ran my fingers across them, but no music sounded, only the twanging complaints of the strings. It was a fine old instrument brought all the way from Vienna, but badly out of tune. Fetching my tools from the credenza I replaced the broken strings, then tuned it. The meticulous work soothed me.

When the work was done I put away my tools and I settled on the bench once again. With my hands arching over the keys, I tried to play a piece of my own composition, a piece I had written for Valentin so long ago. The music was indelibly imprinted on my brain, yet I stumbled. I could force my hands only halting through the patterns of the music. A bitter coil of fear encircled my heart. What if the music would never be mine again?

For decade after decade, no matter what difficulty assailed me, I had come home to the comfort of the keyboard. Music was the solace that made my exile from the human race bearable. I had written reams of it, music heard only by the walls of my house, music that had never been published. Total abstinence from public notice was the only way to keep my secret safe, and my life with it.

Yet though I must be my own audience, the music was still my reason for existing. It was the one thing that distinguished me from the undead monsters that created nothing and destroyed everything. Without music there was no reason to live.

The soft sound of Michael's bare feet on the stairway interrupted my dreary reverie. I blew out the candles—the darkness was my protection. He continued down the caliginous stair, his hand on the railing to guide him.

"I'd like to hear you play," he said gently.

"No."

"Please, I'm an artist. I know how hard it is to be true to yourself when our whole family is against us." He descended another cautious step. I retreated to the curtained archway.

"Our family doesn't understand us, but we can understand each other. We are both creative people."

"We have nothing in common."

"How can you say that when you don't even know me?" he asked with a touch of asperity.

"How can you say that when you don't even know me?" I countered.

"Please let me try."

His plea tempted me. I had been alone for a very long time, and I needed help. But he was a stranger. Yet he was kin, and those of our blood took our obligations seriously. I could ask him for help, ask him for understanding, ask him to be as great a man as his grandfather was. No. I could not, I dared not, the hunger would return again tomorrow, and the morrow after that, through interminable years. As an alcoholic I cannot yield just a little to temptation, so I feared I could no longer control myself and my lusts.

He sighed in frustration. "Uncle Rafael," he said tentatively. I made no answer. "Please, I'd like to talk to you."

"Don't call me 'Uncle,' just 'Rafael.' I haven't been anyone's uncle in a long time."

"All right, Rafael." We stood in silence for a time. "You're a stubborn man."

I chuckled. "It runs in the family."

"It does indeed," he agreed ruefully. "My mother and I are constantly at loggerheads."

"Why?"

He leaned on the railing. "She doesn't approve of art. I suppose you got the same flack about music. What did you do? How did you get them to take you seriously?"

"I never did. I simply moved far enough away that they couldn't interfere in my life."

"New York's not very far away."

"Well, yes, but I was here first. When I settled in Baltimore I had no idea that Violeta would marry an American and drop down practically on my doorstep. It's taken diligent effort to keep her away from me."

"Why aren't the two of you on speaking terms?"

"She kept trying to get me married to one of her girlfriends, and I kept refusing. Speaking of which, are you married?"

"No," he replied, diverted by the question about his own life—as I intended. "I guess I know what you mean. She's always asking me when I'm going to get married, settle down, get a job, have kids, get an ulcer, get divorced...well, you know what I mean. She refuses to believe that I can make a living from art."

"Can you?"

"Yes," he said in some embarrassment. "I mean, I haven't so far, but I could. I have sold stuff, and I have a commission right now. But I have no place to work. That's why I came down here. My contract won't let me put paintings in galleries within two hundred miles, so I had to find someplace else. I need the exposure, that's what gets commissions. And new gallery placements often mean quick sales, at least that's what my friends tell me."

"You must have been pretty desperate to come to me instead of your mother."

"Uh, I owe her a lot already. She didn't take it too well when I told her I was broke again."

"Do you intend to borrow money from me?"

"No," he said stoutly. "I've got twenty bucks. I figure I can get some groceries and go home when they're gone."

I imagined that he had intended to live off my larder—never guessing that I did not have one. Now seemed like a good time to cover that point. "You're lucky I was here. I've been away for a long time. I arrived just before you did. I've had no opportunity to do anything." It sounded reasonable. A little lame, and a little too strong on coincidence, but a rational mind will seize at any plausible explanation rather than entertain thoughts of the supernatural.

"I wondered about that. I confess, I thought maybe you were getting a bit dotty."

"I apologize. You woke me from a sound sleep, and I am always irritable when first awakened. Not to mention I thought you were a burglar."

"I'm sorry. I knocked a couple of times, but you didn't answer. I thought something had happened to you."

My head ached, I was weary. The sun was close to rising. Soon the enchanted sleep would claim me. If I dallied too long I could slip into sleep right where I stood.

"Good night, Michael."

"Good night," he replied. After a few moments he took the hint and withdrew. I slipped quietly up the stairs behind him.

The door to the library was open, and the library window was open as well. Silver light streamed into the hallway. Michael's shadow momentarily blocked it as he passed through the door. I waited for him to settle before passing the open door. I heard the thump as his boots hit the floor one and after another, and the zip of his zipper, followed by the rustle of clothes as he stripped off his jeans. Then a fluffing sound as he shook out the blanket, and creaks as he settled on the leather sofa. He yawned and settled into slow, soft respirations.

I advanced cautiously. A band of silver light lay between me and the sanctuary of my bedroom. I had to cross it to reach my bed. And I wanted my bed, the soft comfort of silk sheets, the rich appointments of antique furniture and modern luxuries.

The autumnal sunlight was weak, a ghost of its summer self. I touched one toe into the pallid light. It did me no harm. I stepped into it, stood with one foot in a pool of light. Vortexes of dust whirled in the breeze from the open window, then gradually wafted out and scattered in the freedom of the morning aurora. I stood a long time, stood until the pink fingers of the dawn appeared at the left edge of the window frame and my eyes began to hurt. I yawned, and let myself into my room.

I pulled back the curtains on my box bed and dust billowed. No wonder Michael had opted to sleep with the window open. The sheets were musty too. I stripped them off and fetched fresh linens from the closet. I would clean the room tomorrow; tonight I wanted only sleep. I locked myself in, closed the curtains of the bed, and burrowed into the bedclothes. Sleep claimed me immediately.

Chapter Two
SHOCK TREATMENT

The many men, so beautiful!
And they all dead did lie:
And a thousand thousand slimy things
Lived on; and so did I.

> —Samuel Taylor Coleridge

Baltimore, 6 October 1991

Every evening when I wake I am always a little surprised to find that once again Death has stayed his hand. Blood stirred in my veins, my lungs inflated. Slowly the coldness passed from my limbs. Bit by bit memory returned and with it came the loneliness of another day. I lay bleakly staring at the wooden canopy of my bed wishing for the uncertainty of natural life. Other men might die peacefully in their beds; not me. Murder was the only thing that would send me down to Hades.

Voices. My lethargy evaporated in an instant as adrenaline surged through my withered veins. I threw off the covers and crouched on the bed desperately extending my senses to locate the intruders. Nothing. I could hear their voices but I could not touch their minds. Like a cat I dropped lightly from my bed and padded to the closet. With a speed no mortal could match I donned jeans and a navy turtleneck to camouflage my pale skin. I would ambush the intruders while they thought I slept. A coil of hunger stirred in anticipation of the hunt.

My clothes chafed and restricted me and I realized I was melting into cat-form without conscious thought. I balked, and the transformation stalled, leaving me caught in the intolerably uncomfortable positions of being half man and half cat. With concentration I regained human shape. As effective a hunter as a cougar might be, I needed my intelligence to reconnoiter the situation and choose the best course of action. A hungry cat will kill whatever prey crosses its path. Rat or man made no difference. Blood was blood.

No board squeaked and no footfall sounded as I prowled quietly through the upstairs hall. Even in man-shape I was faster, stronger, and more ferocious than any human. I grinned in feral delight: I liked hunting. I slunk down the dark stairway with all senses alert and muscles coiled to spring.

Flickering blue light bathed the living room and spilled into the hall. Several voices bantered bad jokes about a foot-ball game, then the lilt of voices gave way to inane music. Television! I was stalking electronic ghosts.

In chagrin I crouched on the lower landing to watch Michael. He was slouching on the sofa, his head drooping and his legs splayed before him as he stared at the television. The television had lulled him into mindless passivity verging on sleep. No wonder I had not been able to sense him, there was no mental activity to detect.

My eye fell on the dirty dishes he had left on the cherry butler's tray. Chagrin turned to indignation. The dishes would scratch the fine cherry finish. I fumed. A butler's tray was normally used for carrying dishes; technically Michael had done nothing wrong. It had remained inviolate throughout the years of my ownership because I did not eat. I used it as a coffee table.

The wooden floors gleamed gently and smelled faintly of oil soap. They were not waxed, but washing away the accretion of years had freshened them considerably. The green, rose and ivory of the draperies and rugs glowed cleanly against the dark wood. Made of good materials and protected from the light they had survived in respectable condition. A faint odor of naphthalene perfumed them and preserved them from attack by silverfish and moths. Light softly reflected from the curvaceous legs and heart-shaped backs of Queen Anne chairs. Already two centuries old when I bought them, fifteen years of neglect had not noticeably aged them.

Michael had cleaned the house as thoroughly as soap and hard work could manage, and I was grateful. I could forgive some scratches on the butler's tray. My nephew had done his best to erase the deterioration of the years.

James had failed me. Before going to sleep I had arranged with him for the upkeep of my property. He was duty bound to see the house cleaned and the lawn mowed on a regular basis. He had not. The absence of vermin (animal, insect, or human) suggested that he had made some effort to carry out his obligation, but the peeling wallpaper bespoke minimal concern. He had control of my money, there was no reason for him to stint in the maintenance of my property. Worse, he had not wakened me when I failed to appear on schedule. We had planned on a short sleep, four years at most. He had let me rot for fifteen years! Michael did not even know me, but he respected the bond of kinship between us. He had worked hard on my behalf. James was bound to me by all the ties of emotion and law that I could manufacture and still he had failed me. Truly blood was thicker than water. Convenient or not, Michael was kin. I had to help him.

Michael yawned and stretched, his clean white tee shirt pulling tight across his chest, biceps bulging then relaxing. From his battered cowboy boots to his tight jeans with the silver belt buckle he was a prime hunk of American youth. His skin was smooth except for the five o'clock shadow of beard, and his muscles were supple and firm. The features of his face were regular, even pretty. But his eyes! They were large, dark and lustrous with long thick lashes. He had everything I liked in a man: Good face, good body, and good personality. Maybe not too bright, but from my viewpoint that was a bonus.

Sleep, I silently commanded him.

Emotions flitted across his face as he tried to follow the news and failed. His eyelids fluttered, the long lashes brushing his cheeks.

Sleep, I urged again.

His eyes closed and his breathing deepened as he succumbed to my slumberous influence. I watched the rise and fall of his chest in fascination as each inhalation stretched the thin fabric and briefly outlined the small bumps of his nipples. I crawled closer to crouch beside his legs, felt the heat of his body radiating from the jeans, and yearned to slide my hands under his shirt, tweaking the nipples hard, making them stand up, then lowering my mouth to each of them in turn, kissing turning into biting.... The ache in my teeth brought me back to reality. I enjoyed looking at Michael's perfect body, but my fantasy was impossible. I had promised Papa that I would not harm the family, and I had kept my word. I lifted Michael's hand to my lips and kissed it good-bye, then let go and rose. At least, that was my intention. Instead my fingers tightened their grip. My other hand slipped between his legs, pulling his thigh against my groin. A thrill of pleasure went through me to feel the hardness of his body against my soft sex. I would lie in his lap and his heat would warm me as I drank his blood.

No. Not now. I was too hungry; I would kill him.

But I want him! Blood and sex and death, I want him! I was acting like an idiot; I had friends I could go to, there was no need to throw myself at the first warm body that came along.

I want him.

I crawled into Michael's lap, my legs straddling his while my hands walked up his chest. He stirred under the strange weight, eyelids twitching with the effort to open.

No! Do not look at me! His body went limp, consciousness gone. I should get up, leave him, not molest him as he slept.

But I liked the feel of his groin between my legs, liked the feel of the blood pulsing through the arteries of his lower body. With my fingertips I traced the blood vessels to the great heart that fed them all. My hand curled as my fingers tried to bite into his chest. I wanted to crack his ribs and devour his voluptuous heart. With horror I realized that my fingers were pressing hard enough to bruise, fingernails biting into the thin fabric of his shirt. Whether I wanted it or not, the hunger would glut itself on anything it could catch, and it had caught Michael.

I dropped my head and sank my long teeth into my own forearm. The sleeve tore, and a widening stain of wetness seeped through the fibers, the blood a blacker darkness than the color of the fabric. Pain shot through my arm, but numbness quickly followed, then a pleasant tingling as the analgesic injected by my fangs took effect.

A rush of energy swept through me. Mortal blood always gave me a glow, but my own blood was like lightning. It tasted salty like mortal blood, but sweeter, and it made the room spin. I lost my balance and toppled over, falling into the narrow space between the coffee table and the sofa, scarcely aware of the impact of my limbs upon the floor. Such pleasure! No wonder it was taboo for immortals to prey on one another. We would destroy each other, or worse, deliberately beget more like ourselves to enslave for their blood.

After some moments the room ceased its spinning and I was able to rise. I had drunk enough blood to distract the hunger for a while, but not so much that I had done myself any real harm. The hunger would not destroy its host. It diminished me to know that I was the pawn of a force I could not control, but what could I do? Death or hunger, and neither was an option. Yet with hunger I could hold Death at bay, and so my course was clear.

I bent and kissed Michael's brow in gentle apology, then betook myself to the stairway, letting loose my hold on his mind.

He stirred, limbs tightening as he regained conscious control of them again. Would he remember any of the nightmare that had visited and nearly consumed him? I doubted it. Yet one hand retraced my touches on his chest, while his eyes slowly opened. He pinched his nipples lightly, catching his breath sharply at the sudden pleasure. His fingers moved slowly over and around the bumps in the fabric, then he licked his dry lips and stripped off his shirt in a sudden movement. His chest was hairless, the pectorals clearly defined. The abdominals were hard and smooth. Two little brown nipples stood erect.

He caressed his nipples, then his hands slid across his washboard belly to leisurely rub the length of flesh lying along his thigh. After a moment he stood up and slung his shirt over his shoulder with casual grace. He turned off the television and the house darkened. In the gloom of the hallway I was almost invisible, but to be sure he did not see me I stepped into the music room.

As his tread sounded lightly on the steps I slipped behind him, my eyes following him every step of the way as he sauntered up the stairs. His back was just as gorgeous as his front with his shoulder blades composed of strong triangles of muscle and bone, and his spine a subtle valley between the long muscles on either side. Helplessly I followed him up the stairs, lured by the temptation of his fresh, young flesh.

The library door closed between me and him. A hollow thump was followed shortly by a second as he doffed his boots. I plastered myself against the door, ear pressed against the wood so that I could hear every creak of the leather sofa, every soft breath.

And became aware of the growing lump of flesh between the door and my usually quiescent groin.

Immortality had its price: loss of sexual potency. I often became hard while necking, but it was only the blood lust, the desire to sink my teeth into firm, hot flesh. And when that consummation came it was far more intense than the orgasm of mere sex.

Yet I envied Michael. It was such a normal male thing to wake up horny and do something about it. Sadly I peeled myself away from his door and retreated to the bathroom. I had to make myself presentable and catch myself some dinner before the hunger recovered from the trick I had played upon it.

Michael's car keys were hanging on the hook in the kitchen. I pocketed them. He had not asked my permission to enter my house so I did not bother asking permission to use his car. Besides, if I spoke to him about the car then he would wonder why I wanted it, and I did not want to explain either my dietary habits or my sex life.

The car was an aging gray Corvette parked next to a fire hydrant. A ticket fluttered forlornly under the wiper while a freezing rain spit down from an ugly sky. I pocketed it to pay later. Anyone who hopes to escape the attention of the law should be scrupulous about upholding it in trivial matters.

I slid into the driver's seat, accidentally knocking off my fedora, but snatching it out of the air before it had fallen more than a few inches towards the runny pavement. I tucked my trench coat around me and slammed the door shut, then discovered that duct tape held the upholstery together and fast food wrappers carpeted the floor. After several complaints, the car grumbled and coughed, then roared to life. The dash lights came on and told me the gas tank was nearly empty, while the oil pressure light flickered on and off. The windshield wipers streaked, and only one headlight worked. The brakes went all the way to the floor. In short, it was a rolling death trap.

I nursed the car over to Billy Town, the white working class neighborhood on the eastern side of the city. When I was within a few blocks of my goal I eased it into the first open service station I found.

"My car needs some work," I said.

The bored mechanic was ready to go home. "Sorry, the pumps are open but the garage is closed." I opened my wallet and took out a hundred dollar bill. "I would be happy to pay overtime for you to stay and fix it." A crisp green hundred dollar bill works a special kind of magic. People will do things for one that they would not do for five grubby twenties.

"If it needs any work it'll cost more than a hundred," he said.

I pulled another Franklin out of my wallet. "Whatever it takes."

"You got it."

I stayed on the sidewalks as I cut across the damp and

windy expanse of Patterson Park. The weather was vile, nobody would be cruising tonight, though perhaps a desperate john might be hanging around the men's room. I had been here often in the past; the anonymous sex and men without names had provided a regular part of my diet. But tonight I had another goal in mind: Clement.

Dodging puddles I wended my way through a twisting dark alley to the back of a shabby apartment building. A stick propped open the back door in blatant violation of the faded sign that said, FOR YOUR OWN PROTECTION, THIS DOOR TO BE KEPT CLOSED AND LOCKED AT ALL TIMES. I stood looking at the building in trepidation. Was it more decrepit than I remembered, or was that the additional effect of fifteen years of neglect? A miasma of decay oozed from the place, making my skin crawl. But I had to go in, had to at least look and see if Clement still lived here. My stomach turned to think that I was seeking out a creature that could abide such filth and dilapidation. But I had no choice; I needed to eat, and I needed Clement's special skills.

I slipped carefully through the sagging door to avoid snagging my trench coat or dirtying it by contact with the building. Unidentifiable brown splatters marred the dingy beige of the walls while the odors of sour laundry and stale marijuana smoke permeated the air with a stench that clogged my lungs. It was hot inside, a temperature I normally relished, but the air was stifling, hardly relieved by the open rear door. I unbuttoned my coat, but did not remove it. It was my armor against the filth of the place.

I picked my way down the corridor, its threadbare carpet stretching over a hump running the length of the hallway. The carpet was the same dirty brown carpet that had been there fifteen years ago, the additional stains blending perfectly with the ancient decrepitude I remembered. Door number fourteen was surrounded by posters announcing the resident's political opinions: Anti-war, anti-government, pro-feminism, pro-ecology. Many of them dated to the time of my last visit more than fifteen years ago. A few posters of more recent vintage but similar sentiment had been added. Clement obviously still lived here. I rapped on his door with a black-gloved hand.

"Come in, the door's open!"

I pushed the door open as wide as it would go. It stuck on some dirty laundry. A skinny, gray-haired form I recognized as Clement turned in his chair, his mouth opening in a silent O of amazement. On my right a woman was sitting smoking Kools on his rumpled, sagging bed.

"Good evening, Clement. I have business with you." I tried to suppress the sound of disgust in my voice.

"Angel," he said in a choked voice. "I thought you were dead."

"That was naive of you."

I turned to the female on the bed. She had limp brown hair and wore a black tee shirt advertising a rude rock band. "If you will excuse us, Clement will make it up to you later."

"Hey, he's supposed to take me out to dinner tonight!"

Knowing the kind of females that associated with Clement I knew it was the loss of a free meal, and not the loss of Clement's company, that concerned her. I took a twenty dollar bill out of my wallet. "Get yourself some dinner." She snatched the bill.

"Hey, thanks mister. Take your time." I closed the door behind her and locked it.

Clement looked at me nervously from under shaggy brown hair streaked with gray.

"So what's with the suit, man?"

"This is a business call." He flinched, but his eyes glittered with the memory of what I had to offer.

"Whatcha want?"

There was no place that I dared to sit. Books and magazines were piled everywhere. On top of the refrigerator, on chairs, on the floor, on the counter beside the sink, over the rack where a few presumably clean clothes hung—no place was devoid of printed materials. The center of the room had a small clear space to enable him to reach his bed, his computer, and his refrigerator. I stood there.

"Do you still work for the university?"

"Yeah."

"I need a college transcript. Tonight."

"It'll cost you."

I opened my wallet and took out a hundred dollar bill. That was his usual fee for altering a grade.

His eyes fixed on the greenery. "More," he said. He was perpetually short of cash because of the way his mercenary girlfriends spent it. I pulled out a second bill. He licked his lips and kept watching. I pulled out a third bill. His lips parted and he started to breathe harder. I pulled out a fourth bill and his mouth worked in soundless protest. I pulled out a fifth bill.

He looked up at me. "How come you always have so much money?"

I fanned out the five hundred-dollar bills and held them in front of him. "Do you really want to know?"

He emphatically shook his head "no." He took the bills with a trembling hand.

"I want you to fix the records tonight. I'll be calling tomorrow for transcripts."

"No problem. What years?"

I thought about it. I had allegedly graduated from high school in '83. That would mean college graduation in '87—too many years to fill between then and now. "Eighty-five to '89." He typed, the ineffable numbers and letters scrolling past, then asked, "Name?"

"Rafael Guitierrez, Junior."

"How do you spell that?"

I spelled it.

"This you?"

I tensed. I had not wanted Clement to know my real name, but there was no help for it. "Yes," I said reluctantly.

"Birthday?"

"December 27, 1965."

"You're older than that. You're at least as old as I am."

"You're aging prematurely." He winced.

We filled in all the personal information, then proceeded to fill in the details of my education. It took hours of looking up classes in the on-line catalog, and then cross referencing them to make sure they had not been dropped or changed. Once we had the classes picked and grades assigned, it would be a number of more hours for Clement to enter them into the record and make sure it agreed with all the other records. I was running out of patience. "Make sure all my bills are paid," I grumbled.

He laughed. "No problem. Want to join a club or anything?"

I reflected a moment. "A big club. Anything musically oriented, or artsy, or literary. But big enough that nobody would remember a shy guy who never said anything."

"Theater?"

"Too cliquish."

"Movie club?" Lots of bodies sitting quietly in the dark, reviewing obscure foreign films, with discussion afterwards.

"Perfect."

"Anything else?"

"I think that finishes the education part." His weasel eyes swept over my suit and tie. He was not used to seeing me like this, and it made him nervous.

"You have something else in mind?"

Food.

It was too late to go elsewhere. The hunger would not allow it.

"Blood."

"You know what you have to do to get it."

I knew. I had done it with hundreds of men, preferably men I did not know, but Clement's hobby of computer hacking had come in handy often enough for us to get to know each other rather well. Or to put it more accurately: We knew one another's vices well.

I dropped to my knees before him as he unzipped his beltless beige polyester pants. I hated him for the way he smelled, hated myself for needing such a repulsive specimen of humanity. I did not remove my gloves as I pulled the pants down his legs. He pulled down his dirty underwear, the sight of which made my stomach turn.

I took his flaccid flesh in my black-gloved hand and fondled it. With the leather of the glove between my hand and his flesh I could almost pretend it was not what it was. It felt like overripe fruit. Then it hardened, and juice dripped from the tip, making a shiny spot on the black leather.

I put my other hand on his thigh, caressing it, while avoiding looking at his face, or his crotch, or his room. I closed my eyes; self imposed blindness was the only way to get through what I had to do. I bent my head into his lap and took his flabby little hard-on into my mouth. The taste of his dripping juice aroused my hunger, and I sucked him hard.

"Oh God that's good!" he said. "Nobody does that as good as you!"

I sucked him eagerly, wanting the hot liquid of his body squirting in my mouth. I clasped his hip in one arm while I cradled his balls in my other hand. I went down hard on him, sucking him down my throat, massaging his cock with my tongue, squeezing his balls with my fingers, wanting the consummation of my need as fast as I could get it.

Clement grabbed my hair and thrust his cock deep into my throat. I gagged, my nose buried in his smelly pubic hair. He liked fellatio; why would he not perform the elementary courtesy of shaving? But that was too much to ask of a man who wore the same underwear for a week.

I pulled his hands off my head and tried to sit up, but hot sour fluid oozed from his cock into my mouth, and my resistance melted. My need latched me tight to his flesh while he raped my face with violent strokes. He was going to come soon, and I was going to get what I wanted and be free of his filthy embrace.

A sudden eruption of sour liquid filled my mouth, and I sucked eagerly, devouring every drop of the liquid of life he let me have—and craving more. My fangs extended, brushing against the sides of his cock, making him whimper in fear. I lifted my mouth and sank my teeth savagely into his thigh.

"Ow!"

I was not gentle with him; no tender embrace to reassure him that I cared for him and would not harm him, no soft sensual sucking like a baby at his mother's nipple, no sensual communion of blood and desire; only the animal feeding upon his prey.

I wanted to kill him, wanted to wipe out his witnessing of how my need overrode my self-respect, the way it dragged me to the lowest levels of humanity, the way I would pay any price to keep myself alive. And most of all, I wanted to destroy him for understanding nothing but that he could exploit my lust to gratify his. Better that he should die than humiliate me this way.

He beat futilely at my head, whimpering and moaning

in fear. He could not hurt me; he was a spineless geek. I could drain the blood from him like a giant leech and he was powerless to stop me. I could bloat myself with blood, fill myself with so much blood that I would not need to eat for a week.

But only for a week. I would have to eat again—the hunger never ended. If not Clement, then somebody like him. A drunk at a nightclub, a bum sleeping in the park, a prostitute; these were the inevitable companions of my hunger.

I sat up abruptly, his blood dripping down my chin. I rubbed it with my gloved hand before it could spot my white shirt or stain my expensive suit. Clement stared at me, the fearful confusion in his face showing that he sensed but did not understand the danger he had barely escaped.

I rose and went to his filthy sink and ran the water. I put my gloved hands under the flow and washed them clean with plenty of melting green soap, then washed my face and mouth. I washed them again, then washed them a third time. I rubbed clean a circle on his grimy mirror and inspected myself carefully. Satisfied that my clothes were unspotted, I put my gloves under the water and washed them again. I would never feel clean.

At last I turned to him. He had righted his clothes and was crouching on the far corner of the bed, as far away from me as he could get in the chaotic confines of the room. He was pale, and had one hand on the wall to keep his balance.

"I'll apply for transcripts and a copy of my diploma tomorrow. The records had better be ready by then." He nodded compliance with my will.

I stalked out of the claustrophobic room, retracing my steps to the cool, fresh air of the park. Loamy smells of decaying leaves and the perfume of ever-present frostflowers cleansed my nose of human pollution. I leaned against a leafless tree for a long time with the rain beating down and dripping from the brim of my fedora.

I did as I always did when I was unhappy: I settled at the harpsichord and played. My playing was brittle and slow, but my old music came back to me. I heaved a sigh of relief, and began to hope that maybe the Long Sleep had not done me any permanent harm. Tomorrow I would seek out James and settle things between us, then everything would be the same as it had been, the gap of fifteen years stitched closed as if it had never been.

Weariness tugged at my soul, and I found myself improvising in a minor key. What was the point of living? I had deceived myself to think that my musical talents made me any different from those other immortals who cared nothing for civilization. We were alike—natural predators that took and never gave, lurking on the edges of human society, destroying its vulnerable members: Bums, winos, prostitutes, runaways, the poor, the lost, the lonely, and the unlucky.

What use were our gifts? We hoarded them to ourselves, neglecting them in favor of the hunt, the perpetual struggle for survival, the selfish urge to defy our natural end.

The soft sound of Michael's tread on the stair interrupted my meandering thoughts. The strings sighed into silence. From his place on the stairs he could not see into the music room. "Please play some more," he asked.

I folded my hands in my lap, embarrassed me that he had heard me give an inferior performance. My career might be dead, but my vanity was not. "I'm out of practice."

"It sounded good to me," he said, descending a step. "I'd like to hear more."

It had been a long time since I had had an audience of

any kind. His request tempted me. "Perhaps later. But not tonight."

He descended a second step. "I liked that music. Is it one of your pieces?"

"Yes. An improvisation."

"It's different. Moody and emotional, very evocative."

"Ah, you flatter me."

"I don't know enough to flatter you. All I can say is it moved me."

"Did it?" My heart trembled. Perhaps he could understand me...no. I was not even human. It was foolish to even think it.

"Yes." His voice was a low throb in the darkness; he was edging toward the doorway.

"Stop!"

"I'm your nephew," he said painfully. "Why won't you let me see you?"

"I don't want you to see what time has done to me."

"Everyone grows old."

"Some more gracefully than others."

"That doesn't matter!"

"It matters to me."

"You've let vanity ruin your career! You should still be in concert!"

"You don't understand," I began.

"I do understand! It's hard to be true to yourself when people are nagging you to conform, to settle down, get married, have kids. We can't live like normal people do. We have to be true to our art."

"Yes, but—"

"No buts. Art is all that matters. It's bigger than humanity, it survives even when civilizations fall. Art is stronger than science because it speaks to the soul. Science falls with the civilization that invented it. Only art is eternal." He turned on his heel, paced two steps, turned and paced back to where he had started.

"Sometimes it's hard. Sometimes I don't have any idea how to paint what I see. Then I want to quit, but I can't. I keep trying. Suddenly the ideas flow and the paint goes on the canvas like magic. I get a glimpse of something greater than myself, something I can only reach through art. I try to paint it so that other people can see it, and sometimes they do. Some of them.

"But however frustrated I get, I can't quit. I'd always be painting in my head and wondering if I could have made it if I'd stuck with it long enough." His hand wrenched at the doorframe. "Don't you understand? Art transcends everything."

"I do understand," I whispered. "When the music possesses me nothing else matters. I can't eat, I can't sleep, I can't stop until the music is done." But it had been a long, long time since I felt that way.

"Then why did you retire?"

"I had no choice."

"I don't understand. Are you sick?"

"No. Just old. I've seen too many people die. There's no one left that really matters anymore."

"What about your friends?"

I hesitated. "I've been alone a long time. I don't know if I have any friends left." I leaned wearily on the harpsichord.

"You have family."

I laughed harshly. "I'm the black sheep of the family. They don't want anything to do with me."

"It's not that bad. They just don't understand that us creative people need a lot of freedom."

"They didn't approve of the company I kept."

Michael laughed. "Mother hates every woman I ever

dated. I haven't even bothered to introduce her to my gay friends."

"You have gay friends?" I asked in astonishment.

"They're nice people, and good artists," he replied defensively.

"I know that."

"Do you?"

The burden of secrecy weighed heavily on me. Papa had imposed it to protect the family from scandal. Michael, on the other hand, did not seem to need protecting. But he might tell his mother, and Violeta was a meddler.

"I don't think I should discuss it with you."

"Discuss what?"

I plinked a key, B flat. Michael was open-minded, but that did not mean he could tolerate living under the same roof as a queer. He might leave. That would solve many problems for me. My chest ached. I did not want to lose his company.

"I can't say," I replied softly.

"We're family, you can tell me anything. That's what families are for."

He tempted me. Maybe he could accept me—even a little bit of acceptance would be enough to let me drop one of the heavy secrets I carried.

"You must promise not to tell anyone, not even your mother."

"I promise."

I plinked middle C. "Michael," I took a deep breath. "I'm a homosexual."

Michael was silent.

"You don't approve," I said painfully. I was an idiot, I should have kept my mouth shut.

"No. I mean, I'm just surprised. From the way you talked I thought it would be something terrible."

"Doesn't it bother you?"

"No. Why would it bother me?"

It dawned on me that Michael did not share the family's attitudes about sex. I sat up straighter. "Aren't you afraid I might make a pass at you?"

"No. You're my uncle." His voice was astonished. "Rafael, I'm not a bigot. I don't believe all that nonsense about gay men being sex perverts and stuff. They're just people."

I took a deep breath. I did not know what to think.

"I figure love is always a good thing, and it doesn't really matter what the bodies involved look like. It's none of my business."

"Thank you," I said humbly.

"Rafael," he said gently. "Is that why you won't let me see you? Because you're a queen or something? Because if you are, it's okay with me."

"No. Not that."

He sighed in frustration.

"Do you have a girlfriend?" I wanted to turn the conversation away from me and my peculiarities. What had just happened changed how I thought about Michael, and even how I thought about myself, and I needed time to figure it out.

After a long pause he accepted the change of subject. "No. Not anymore. At first she thought it was fabulous living with an artist. I even did a painting of her. But she made more money than I did, and she thought I was mooching off her. She threw me out. That was yesterday. I went home to mother, but she drove me crazy in less than two hours. When she said one bohemian in the family was enough, I decided to visit you. I figured you were the only person in our family who would understand."

"I suppose you have a point."

"How did you do it? How did you get them to respect your music?"

"I ignored them."

"I can't. Mother is always dropping by or calling me up. She's always trying to run my life." He shifted restlessly.

"Be rude to her. Say 'not now' and hang up the phone or shut the door in her face."

"I can't do that, she's my mother!"

"That doesn't give her the right to drive you crazy."

"You're right." He paced a few steps down the hall and back again. "Just because she's my mother doesn't mean she owns me."

He was so young! I hoped he would never grow old and parsimonious of his affections like his mother.

"Michael," I said hesitantly. "There's a couple of rooms in the attic. You can use one. It's small, but at least you'll have privacy. You can stay as long as you need." Having him here would drive me crazy. He would always be within reach, and always off limits. But sending him away would be worse.

"Thank you, Rafael," he said gratefully. "I really appreciate the way you're putting up with me."

"If you can put up with my eccentricities, I can put up with yours."

"It's a deal!" he said with enthusiasm. "And please let me know if there's anything I can do for you. I don't want to be a problem, and I'd be glad to help you any way I can."

He was young and his heart was still generous. He had not yet learned to be wary of giving promises other people might require him to keep. Papa had taught me that lesson well. I admired my father, but his shadow was a cold place to grow up.

"I'll hold you to that," I said. "If I ever need it."

"Count on me," he said.

"I will." After a moment of silence I added, "The key is on the hook in the kitchen. Why don't you go move your things? Let me know if you need anything."

"I'll do that." He hesitated. "Good night, Rafael."

"Good night, Michael."

Chapter Three
A DEBT OF DISHONOR

Man is to be held only by the slightest chains; with the idea that he can break them at pleasure, he submits to them in sport.

—Maria Edgeworth

Baltimore, 7 October 1991

The "attic" was divided into two rooms with sloping ceilings and dormer windows. The front room was the piano salon and music library. It had a splendid view of the river park with the State Penitentiary on the far shore. Within walking distance the other way was the venerable neighborhood of Mount Vernon, its tree shaded square bounded by the Peabody Conservatory and the Walter's Art Museum, plus many other ancient buildings worthy of note. I considered it a sign of human progress that the Conservatory occupied the site where two hundred years ago young men had met at dawn to kill each other over imagined slights.

Michael had adapted the smaller back room to his use. He had set up a drafting table with a tubular black lamp. An easel stood in the middle of the floor, but a cloth covered its picture. Various size blank canvases leaned

51

against the wall, waiting for inspiration while paints and brushes occupied the window sill and the floor below. Dirty laundry was heaped at the foot of the cot, and blankets trailed over the side. The room was small, cold, and dusty, but I envied him. He was at the start of his life; love and career both awaited him. He could not help but be fired with the ideals of youth, and the arrogant self confidence that he would be the next Monet or Renoir. I had no causes anymore, no ideals. Personal comfort was my only goal in life.

His suitcase lay open on the floor with clean tee shirts, jeans, underwear, and socks all jumbled together. The socks were not even matched. Compulsively I knelt and started sorting things. I hated disorder. Besides, it would annoy Michael to see that I had gone through his personal belongings. I needed to put distance between us, needed to give him second thoughts about staying with his dotty old uncle. The less comfort he was in the sooner he would depart.

In the course of organizing his clothes I discovered his sketchbook. I lifted it carefully, a large, heavy pad of paper bound with a wire spiral. I hesitated, for his sketchbook provoked in me the same feelings as if I had found his diary. That is to say, it seemed an intensely private and personal thing, something I ought to set aside without looking. Yet if it had been his diary, I would have done the same: I opened it.

The first picture was of the block of row houses, mine the derelict one at the end. All the other houses had open shutters, but the shutters of my house were closed against the world. The other houses had neat little postage stamp yards, but weeds choked the front yard and the foundation shrubs were grown so tall they obscured the lower part of the windows. Worst of all were the sinuous twining vines clambering up the face. He had even done a botanical sketch of the leaf cluster and berries, and labeled it "Poison Ivy."

He was from New York, he did not understand realities of life in the Tidewater Basin. The balmy climate encouraged all vegetation to grow luxuriously, which required constant pruning to keep it in check. Poison ivy was merely a pernicious weed, not the eerie and unnatural thing he had portrayed in his picture. It would not help me if Michael was superstitious. I turned the page in annoyance.

It was me. I stared at the sketch, heart palpitating as if I had suddenly turned a corner and met a twin I did not know I had. In the picture I wore an old fashioned black frock coat with a high, white shirt collar and black cravat. My hair was braided into a queue and tied with a black ribbon. He had given me hollow cheeks and piercing black eyes even though my eyes are gray. My lower lip was full, my lips parted, almost pouting. The expression on my face was both stern and sensual. The likeness was superb, yet inaccurate. Once I had been handsome, but no longer. Whatever old photograph had given him my features was badly out of date. But still, I used to keep my hair short. It was only since waking from the Long Sleep that I wore it long. He must have caught a glimpse of me, and it made me uneasy to think I had not been as nimble as I thought.

I could not take my eyes from the sketch. Michael had an uncanny talent: he had drawn the emotional details of his subject as well as the physical. The portrait was so life-like it seemed as if it were about to move or speak. And if it could speak, what would it say? I could no more fathom the thoughts behind the penciled features than I could read the mind of a stranger. It was most disconcerting to see myself captured so well, and yet so alienly.

In his picture my long hair was elegant, with a certain archaic charm. I looked like a gentleman of the Enlightenment, and I was a great fan of that era. Not just harpsichord, but literature, history, philosophy, technology, discovery—all of it. It was a time of great achievements, when one man could forward the body of human knowledge through his own efforts. In those days one man mattered: One mind could enrich humanity.

Michael had persuaded me. I would keep the hair.

James had prospered. Flanagan Ventures, Inc. occupied the entirety of a three story office building in a good neighborhood. I sipped coffee in a restaurant across the street while I waited for the lights to go out. He worked long hours, partly to avoid his wife, and partly because his business fascinated him. Outwitting the law was a source of never ending challenge and entertainment for him. When one light remained I dropped a dollar on the table for the coffee and tip, and wondered if it was enough. Then I wondered what inflation had done to my finances. The cache in my safe would not last long.

I walked around the block to the back of the office building. A new Cadillac was the only car remaining in the parking lot. I laid my gloved hands upon its hood. James. I could smell his pipe smoke and aftershave lingering in the car.

When I met him he had been trying to live the life he wanted, only to be shunned as a social climber. I was rich, good looking, well traveled, cultured, European, and a member of the social class he desperately wanted to join. Under my tutelage he had shed his gaucherie and learned good taste. But he was heavily in debt and when his son died he had had no money to bury the boy. I had given him the money he needed, and he had been grateful. That gratitude had served me well—until now.

I stood a moment studying the rear door of the building. A lock and burglar alarm secured a plate glass door—I could see the ribbon of silver foil on the glass. If the glass were broken it would disrupt the foil and set off the alarm. Contacts, probably magnetic, sensed whether the door was closed or open. There must be a slight delay before the alarm sounded so that a legitimate entrant could deactivate it. Scanning the wall I noted a small panel that no doubt contained the mechanism to deactivate the door alarm.

Confidently I laid my hand over the door lock and the tumblers tripped in well oiled precision. I allowed myself a small smile: I still had the knack. Then I pushed rapidly through the door and crossed to the panel. It was locked, but I had it open in an instant. Underneath was a small pad of numbers and letters like a calculator pad.

What would James choose as a password? Suddenly, I knew.

"P-e-t-e-r." Seconds slipped past in silence; then I sighed in relief. I had guessed right.

Peter was the son James had buried.

I made sure the building was deserted, then tracked the sole remaining light to an office of dark paneling, brown leather furniture, and large, leafy plants. As usual James was the last to leave. He was working at a massive oaken desk, his blond hair shining in the light. The lines in his face and the thickness of his waist had aged him prematurely, but the unique smell of pipe tobacco and aftershave conjured up old images of a younger, more virile man. I leaned in the doorway, and the soft rustling of my suit caught his attention.

"Rafael!" He blanched. "I've been expecting you." He did not look happy.

"Really? Why?"

"I watch the news. When I saw a weird killing done in High Hill Park, I guessed who had done it and why. I drove by your house, and the lights were on. Then I knew you had returned at last."

I shrugged. "Coincidence. I know nothing about it."

His blue eyes raked me. "You're in the worst shape I've ever seen you. You must have been pretty desperate to lower yourself like that."

"You're a clever man." I advanced into the room, my gloved hands curling into fists. "That's why you're my lawyer. But I'm not happy with the way you've maintained my property. I hope my finances are in better condition."

"No."

"No?" His candor startled me. Circumspection had been one of his more endearing qualities.

"I took it. I had to have it after the divorce. Lauren took me to the cleaners."

"Just how much did you take and when did you take it?"

"All of it, about ten years ago."

I put my hands on the desk and looked him in the eye. "How much is it worth now?"

His cold eyes locked on mine. "About three million."

"I want it back."

"You're legally dead and I made myself your heir. You can't touch it. I doubt you could find a judge in the land who would believe you're sixty-five-year-old Rafael Guitierrez."

"He doesn't have to believe that. All he has to believe is that I'm Rafael Junior."

He smirked. "I helped you corrupt the doctor, remember? Your birth certificate wouldn't hold up in court, and neither would the rest of your evidence."

I gnashed my teeth. "How could you do this to me!"

He squirmed. "All that money, going to waste. You were gone for fifteen years!"

"What about my house? Did you take that too?"

His gaze broke. "It's still yours. I paid the taxes."

"How very kind of you. As long as you were stealing my property, why didn't you make a clean sweep of it?"

He fidgeted. "I knew that if you ever came back, you'd go there."

I blinked. "I didn't go anywhere and you know it."

"Liar! I went through the whole damn house looking for you, and you weren't there! That's when I realized what a fool you'd played me for." His glare was venomous. "And I decided that turn about was fair play."

I had not told him about the vault in the basement. And a good thing too, my wiser if nastier self replied. "All you had to do was ring the doorbell, you idiot! We tested it! That thing would wake the dead!"

His hand cracked across my face, the knuckles leaving stinging bruises. I gaped at him in shock. "Bullshit!"

Gingerly I felt my face. "You hit me!"

"You deserve it."

"I don't!"

"You lied to me."

"I didn't!"

He reached across the desk and caught my lapels, dragging me halfway over his desk. His mouth closed over mine, and the old fire was there, the old need: Blood and sex and power all wrapped together in an irresistible bundle. I closed my eyes and gave myself to his kiss, knowing that sex would put us back in our proper relationship, sealing the breach of fifteen years.

His lips parted and his eyes widened. He swayed slightly on the balls of his feet. "You're so damn seductive!" It sounded like a complaint, but he didn't let go.

"James, neither of us is perfect," I said placatingly. "I'm sorry things didn't work out right. Let's put it behind us and start over again." I saw the desire in his eyes. He knew what I was and he wanted me in spite of it. Or perhaps because of it.

"Yes!" he whispered, then bent his head, hot mouth questing for mine. I lifted my chin and our lips met in hungry impact.

Michael's image hovered faintly in my mind, but I ignored it. James could give me everything I wanted, everything I dared not take from Michael. My hands slid around his neck and pulled him closer into my cold embrace. I would give my body to him, then he would give his blood to me. Everything would fall into the old pattern; the same old lonely pattern.

His tongue darted into my mouth and I sucked it eagerly, devouring his ferocity as he mauled me with his mouth. My fingers dug into his back as I pressed myself more ardently against him.

"I can't resist you," he whispered. "I thought I could, but I can't."

"You want it," I purred confidently. I caressed his ear with my lips.

His head came up. "You want it worse. You're like a junkie that has gone too long without a fix. You need the blood."

I did not like the comparison.

"I can control my desire."

"Can you? Did you control it in High Hill Park?"

"I already told you it wasn't me. I know nothing about it."

"Liar. I know you. I know what you're capable of doing."

"I don't have to listen to your insults. I can leave right now." He put his hand between my legs and grabbed. The fire of life blazed through my veins, and suddenly I was alive like I had not been for many years. It was a false life, for when the moment of truth came I would not be able to perform as a man, but I tried not to mind. The illusion was pleasure enough.

"Don't you want to bite me?" My pulse pounded in my temple like a jackhammer.

"Yes," I whispered.

His mouth was close to my ear and his warm breath blew across my cheek. "Don't you want me to fuck you?"

"Yesss—"

"Who wants it worse?"

"I do." Our eyes met, hunter to hunter, and I saw in James the reflection of myself. Whatever had gone wrong between us had happened because I refused to acknowledge him as my equal, had denied the hunter within the mortal frame. We were two of a kind, and all it would take was a few drops of my blood to eliminate the weaknesses of his mortal flesh.

Our arms locked around each other and electricity crackled. I devoured his kiss, lips parting, tongues probing. My fangs extended, and he caressed them with his tongue, not flinching from the sharpness of the monstrous teeth.

He pulled his mouth from mine and kissed my neck. I let my head fall back, baring my throat to his ministrations. He loosened my tie and unbuttoned my collar, pulling it wide, exposing the notch of my collarbone. Then he nipped me. A bolt of white hot passion shot through me, making me gasp in pleasure. He continued nuzzling and nipping my neck while pulling my coat down to my elbows. Then his lips teased across my shirt front until he found my nipple. He bit hard, my back arching and a wild cry escaping my throat. Only a virgin would have thought I cried in pain. He sucked my other nipple and my back arched again, wet shirt clinging to the hard bumps of my nipples. He unbuttoned my shirt, trailing a line of kisses down the front of my body as he knelt before me.

With well practiced movements he stripped off my shoes and pants, leaving me naked from the waist down. I waited placidly, willing to let him take the lead as he always liked. To my surprise he knelt before me, sucking first one half of my scrotum then the other into his mouth, biting gently, which sent violent shocks of pleasure through my body. I spread my legs wide for him, his fine hair brushing the inside of my thighs with unbearable tickles of pleasure.

He licked and lightly nipped the length of my cock, the not-quite pain intensely arousing. Then his tongue laved the head of my shaft, circling the foreskin which slowly retreated as my cock swelled and hardened under his ministrations. He caressed the small slit in the top of the glans until I could not stand it any longer, and fell back upon the desk, small objects denting my back.

His skillful mouth sucked my foreskin, eating my cock bit by bit, the length of it disappearing into the hot hole of his mouth. It was like losing my virginity all over again, only this time I had the knowledge to relish the experience. He sucked me deeply, his lips pressing closer and closer to my short hair. I wanted to drive myself deep into his throat, but he would choke and the spell would be broken, so I kept still, letting him take me at his own pace, no matter how badly I wanted to plunge myself into his body.

James lifted his head. "Will you let me do what I want?" His blue eyes were calculating.

"Oh yes!" I breathed. "Do anything. Do everything. Make me come!" He smiled. We both knew ejaculation was impossible for one of the undead. But at the moment I felt like I was going to erupt through every pore of my body, and I was not in a mood to worry about technical details.

He lifted my legs so that my heels rested on the edge of the desk, then opened the drawer and took out a flimsy synthetic line. He wound the line around my ankles and wrists, securing it to the desk so that my feet and hands were immobilized. My lust took on a greater intensity as the clothesline bit into my flesh. Bondage. I adored bondage. The restraints gave me the freedom to thrash and kick as I liked, secure in the knowledge that I was not going to accidentally hurt my lover. And besides, I was strong enough that if I wanted to get free no cheap piece of clothesline could hold me.

"I know what you want," he taunted me.

I nodded dumbly.

He spit on his fingers then forced them into my ass. I arched and cried out, his rough handling exciting me.

"Harder," I moaned.

He thrust his fingers as deep as they would go. The pleasure was intense, and I badly wanted to come.

"More!" I cried.

He forced three fingers into me. Wordless cries escaped my lips as my ass devoured his hand, sucking it inside of me, all five fingers penetrating my body.

"More, please, more!" He pushed his knuckles inside me, his fist deep in my bowel. It registered faintly in some far off part of my mind that he was not being very careful, but my preternatural flesh withstood his invasion while I convulsed with pleasure.

My need to come was desperate and impossible, yet it tantalized me with the possibility that maybe this time it would happen.

"Harder!" His fist pounded the inside of my body, and I teetered on the brink of unbearable stimulation. Just a little more and I would make it…

"You like it," he taunted me again. I could not even nod.

He withdrew his hand.

"NOOOO!" I cried.

He walked around to the other side of the desk and I looked upside down at him. He unzipped his pants and put his hardness in my mouth, my fangs passing on either side of his shaft. My ass writhed in unfulfilled lust, then the hot, salty taste of his precum dripped upon my tongue and I sucked him madly. I wanted to have his hot elixir of life filling my mouth and flooding down my throat. I loved the salty, manly taste of it, the euphoria it gave me. I would lick him all over, lick the sweat from his skin, the tears from his cheeks, the blood from his wounds. I neither sweated, nor cried, nor bled; I could only share his humanity by taking it from him.

James retreated.

"Come back," I moaned. Once again he had left me on the edge of orgasm, my fangs aching in my mouth as the blood lust swept unabated through my body. "Damn you," I whispered.

He ignored me. He was busy with something else, something below my head that I could not see. Anticipation was an unbearable goad to desire. Whatever it was, I knew I would enjoy it.

He wrapped a rope around my neck.

"No," I said.

He kissed me. His tongue probed my mouth, seeking out the hungry fangs and toying with them. I bit him convulsively, and a drop of his blood oozed into my mouth and I sucked it. I was helpless to control myself. The rope lay loose across my neck.

He broke our kiss. "Too bad," he said.

I tried to sit up, but before I had moved more than a couple of inches the rope tightened around my neck. He had tied it to the legs and left enough slack in it to put a loop around my neck. If I struggled, I would choke myself.

"Enough," I said in annoyance. I flexed my arms, but the bindings held. I flexed mightily, all my sinews cracking and bulging, whipcord muscles standing up on my body, veins prominent upon my pale skin. Not a strand yielded.

James smiled contentedly down at me. "I know this rope won't break—it's tow rope. Each strand will hold up to four thousand pounds, and you're encased in a web of the stuff. You can't escape."

"You planned to do this to me!"

"Yes."

"Why?"

"For once you're going to know what it's like to be completely controlled, to have your desires used against you no matter what your wishes are."

I stared at him wordlessly.

He inserted the tip of his penis in my anus. Once he had the proper position he slammed it home. I groaned. He planted his hands on either side of me and leaned into the strokes. My body leaped to the peak of pleasure again, responding instantly to the rhythm of his thrusting. I twitched and moaned, the ropes chafing me cruelly as I thrashed in their web. Through it all burned a thread of fear that goaded me toward climax. This time he had taken me farther than I had ever gone, and it might be far enough... James jerked out of me as he felt the clenching of my muscles as my body gathered itself for orgasm. Once more I teetered on the brink, and sobbing in frustration fell back.

He opened the drawer and held up a thick black marker. "You'll do anything for the blood, won't you?"

My face burned scarlet. "Yes."

He wrote "slut" on the inside of my left thigh.

He laughed. "I'm going to give you blood. Would you like that?"

"Yes!" I said too eagerly.

He wrote "whore" on my right leg, and laughed again. "Your price is cheap." He shoved the marker into me. I arched with this new penetration and my muscles went into spasm. Each clench against the unyielding mass of the marker caused a shudder to go through my body. Leisurely he moved the marker in and out as I panted with humiliation and helpless desire. He watched me carefully, pushing me toward orgasm again, playing with my need, manipulating my body for his own amusement. When my ass muscles clenched wildly, he removed it, leaving me lying limp and sore and panting.

"I've threatened you and humiliated you but you like it." He rummaged through his drawer again and pulled out a sword-shaped letter opener. "Now I have to hurt you."

My eyes widened. "James, we're lovers. Don't hurt me!"

"You never loved me," he said coldly. "You used me. You're using me right now."

"I did love you," I protested. I fought my bonds but it was no use. The ropes were as strong as he said, and the desk that anchored them was mercilessly solid oak.

"You're not capable of love. You encircled me with your vampire powers and kept control of me, but you never loved me! That's a human emotion, and you have no heart."

"No James, I didn't! I swear I didn't!"

"When you left me I took man after man trying to find what I thought we had. That's what ruined my marriage. But it also made me realize I didn't want men, I wanted you." He put the point of the letter opener against my anus. "And most importantly, it made me realize that the only way to be free of you was to kill you." I whimpered as he slid the blade millimeter by cold millimeter into me. I held very still, afraid any movement would cut me, feeling the slim length sliding deeper and deeper, wondering when it would pierce a vital organ. It was short, too short to reach my heart, but would a puncture to liver or spleen be equally fatal?

"Vlad Tepes, the real Dracula, impaled one hundred thousand Turks. They were bound with a stake in their ass and the stake was planted in the ground. Over the course of hours or days the weight of their bodies dragged them down until they died. It was worse for the strong ones, their strength only prolonged their anguish as they tried to resist the pull of gravity. It would take you a long time to die that way."

"Mercy," I whispered.

"You have never given mercy to anyone." He plunged the blade up to the hilt in my body, and I screamed.

He watched me writhing uncontrollably, all sense of reason and dignity eaten away by the agony of my body; supersensitive nerves delivering an equal measure of pain where formerly they had given pleasure.

"I can't endure it," I moaned.

He put his hand on the hilt and twisted it. I shrieked again, my blood oozing from the wound and dripping from my body. I grew faint, but the pain did not recede. "Kill me. Don't torture me. If you want me dead, do it," I begged.

"I've hardly hurt you." He worked the blade back and forth slicing me internally, blood gushing from my body to puddle upon the floor. Death was very near at hand and there was nothing, absolutely nothing I could do to stop it. Valentin's image appeared before me then, and I sighed in understanding at long last. There comes a point when further struggle yields only suffering, and it is better to give up and die.

Valentin.

"What did you say?" James demanded.

His voice came faintly to me. A veil of darkness covered my vision.

Beloved.

The blade clattered to the floor.

"Damn it, you bastard! You still love him, don't you?" He was weeping with rage. "Why don't you love me? I gave up everything for you!" My body began to repair itself as soon as the knife was gone. The bleeding stopped, the pain eased a little, and the darkness in my brain receded slightly. My head lolled and I felt sick, my ears registering only noise when James babbled at me.

"What?" I said dully.

He untied me. "I'll give the money back. I always intended to. It's just that other things got in the way, and as long as I thought you were dead, it didn't really matter." He gathered me in his arms and sank to the floor. He kissed me hungrily, forcing my mouth open with his tongue and I was too weak to resist. His kisses insisted that I forgive his cruelty and embrace my ravager. I lifted one hand weakly to his face. He kissed my hand.

"I trusted you, James," I whispered. "I put my life and fortune in your hands. I never thought you would do this to me. I never thought it even when I saw how the house was neglected."

He bowed his head in shame. "You left me! You left me in the worst way! I had to wait and wait and wait and never know if I was waiting for nothing! You were gone too long!"

"I'm sorry."

He pulled my shirt onto my shoulders and buttoned it. "Why did you let me hurt you? Why didn't you try to save yourself?"

"Couldn't. Can't make you do what you don't want to do."

"Dammit! I told myself you were a monster, that I had to destroy you before you destroyed me." His voice cracked.

"I forgive you."

He gave an anguished cry. "That's worse. If you hated me I could kill you." He picked me up and sat me in his chair. He straightened my coat, put my pants on my legs.

He dressed me as if I were a big rag a doll. As he tied my shoes it occurred me that maybe I could have freed myself. Whatever I had done to disassemble the rusted lock might have burst the ropes. He had kept my attention so firmly fixed on him that only belatedly had I been able to think about my predicament.

James folded up my crumpled tie and put it in my pocket. "Will you be all right?"

"You promised me blood," I whispered.

Something far back in his eyes closed against me. He extended his arm anyway. "Drink." I needed the blood desperately, too desperately to worry about what he might or night not do next. He shuddered as I bit into his forearm. Blood flowed in my mouth and I sighed in relief. My cramped muscles relaxed as the hunger eased, and the pain settled to a dull internal throb. James wobbled, and I continued sucking him. I wanted him so weak he would not be capable of causing trouble while I recuperated. He tried to pull his arm away, but I held on. He could not free himself except by shredding his arm. His knees folded.

"Rafael," he pleaded. "Let me go." I let him drop to the floor.

"I want my money back," I said savagely.

"You'll get it," he mumbled.

"I'll be back in a week."

My home was my refuge and I was glad I still had it. I crawled out of the taxi and staggered to my door. The cab had been a danger, but collapsing on the streets of Baltimore would have been worse. Normally I considered muggers fair prey, but in my current condition I had doubts about my ability to deal with them.

I was hurt, I was stiff, I wanted a drink. I stumbled through the dark to the kitchen. I had several bottles of wine in a rack in a cabinet. I opened one. Past its prime. I opened a second one. Also past its prime. I despaired; they had sat too long. I opened the third. Crimson red and pungent it poured into the crystal goblet. I swirled it around, sniffed it, then sipped it gratefully. My unusual physical attributes were supported by a highly efficient metabolism. The alcohol took effect rapidly and I was tipsy after one glass. I refilled it and took it upstairs with me where I fell down fully clothed on my bed, too numb to mind the crimson splatter.

I had been a fool to trust James with my money, but James had been a worse fool not to kill me while he had the chance. In a few days I would recover while he would still be prostrate from blood loss. I would force him to return my money, then I would drink from him until his heart faltered and collapsed. His death would be blamed on a heart attack and not investigated. It was necessary and just that he die.

Sleep claimed me.

Chapter Four
"NEW YORK BY NIGHT"

Whether at Naishapur or Babylon,
Whether the Cup with sweet or bitter run,
The Wine of Life keeps oozing drop by drop,
The Leaves of Life keep falling one by one.
                                    —Edward Fitzgerald

Baltimore, 9 October 1991

I woke with a dry mouth and an itch between my legs.
Bleary eyed I dragged myself upright, winced at the pain in
my posterior, then stuck out my tongue in disgust because
of the vile coating upon it. My clothes were rumpled, and a
wine stain marked the side of the coverlet. Stale wine lay in
a dark pool on the wooden floor. I stripped off my clothes
and tossed them into the hamper, then fetched a hand
mirror from the dresser and lay down on the bed to examine my awkwardly placed wound.

It itched like mad and I scratched it, inadvertently knocking off the scab to reveal clean red skin beneath. The wound
was healing without any puss or inflammation. My bowel
and bladder were useless vestiges of my human existence,
there was no danger of infection from that source. And since I
had resisted every external infection I had ever encountered,
it seemed unlikely that I would experience any complications.

I glanced at my watch, which was still strapped to my wrist, and noticed that a day had slipped past without me waking. That was not unusual; activity would slow down the healing process. Better to simply sleep through it. I laid aside the mirror and burrowed into the bedclothes.

Hunger slithered inside me and I groaned into my pillow. I was going to have to get up whether I liked it or not. What was I going to do? Shapechanging was much too strenuous an activity to undertake while seriously injured. That meant I could not don feline form to go hunting. Picking up a kinky date in a bar or buying a prostitute both had the drawback of requiring a certain amount of activity on my part—getting up and getting dressed at the minimum. I pulled the pillow over my head.

Food.

It hammered at me, the hungry beast wanted out. I did not want it out. And so, deliberately, I lifted my arm to my mouth and sank my teeth into my own flesh. The blood was warm and sweet, intoxicating in its power. Simple, easy, addictive...I could ruin myself this way. But it served a purpose: It let me gathered myself together to plan a sensible dinner, rather than taking whatever crossed my path.

I cleaned up the spilled wine, then showered, shaved, and dressed decently in black slacks and sweater I descended the stairs, ready to face Michael, the day, and the prospect of dinner, albeit not very enthusiastically. And got a shock.

Michael had hung his paintings along the length of the downstairs hall, driving nails into the plaster (Had he bothered to find the studs, or were they in danger of crashing down, ripping the plaster away from the walls? I should have packed him off to a hotel that first night.) All but one of the paintings portrayed city scenes at night, or in rain, or fog. They were dark blue and black and gray highlighted with luminous colored lights. Details such as streetlights and neon signs told me that they were real places; large brush strokes and blurring colors made them seem fantastical and foreign.

The best of the scenes was the largest, almost as wide as my outstretched arms and about three feet tall. Wraith-like figures drifted through the fog toward the colored lights of a distant nightclub. However much I stared at them I could not make up my mind as to what they were. Men? Women? Ghosts? I lifted the painting away from the wall and found a label taped to the back that said, NEW YORK BY NIGHT: $1500.00.

One other painting impressed me. A voluptuous nude female reclined upon a blue cloth. With his paints Michael had made the fabric shine in contrast to her warm and touchable skin. She stared back at me with strong eyes as if she were a little contemptuous of me. Artists do not usually paint pictures of people who look contemptuously upon potential buyers. It tickled me. But I thought I would soon grow tired of it. I went back to the big cityscape. With his paints he had made the ordinary extraordinary.

Art was the key to Michael's seduction. He had come all the way from New York to talk to me about it. If his parents understood and supported his work he would have had no need to come to me. I wondered if he had ever shown them his work. Probably not. It was too ambiguous for the average person to enjoy. Besides, if I had painted a nude, I would not have shown it to Violeta either. The woman should have been a nun.

I went up to the library and counted bills out of my safe. Fifteen hundred dollars made a considerable dent in my emergency funds. I put them in an envelope and added a short note. I knew a gallery owner—at least, I hoped I did. I dialed information and was relieved to hear that the gallery still existed. It even had the same number.

A strange male voice answered my call. "Ponchartrain Gallery. May I help you?"

"I'd like to know if George Ponchartrain is still the owner of the gallery," I said.

"This is Damon Greyson. George Ponchartrain and I are partners in the gallery. May I help you?" I wondered how extensive their "partnership" was, and whether it could tolerate an old flame of George's asking for a favor.

"I'd like to speak to George, please."

"Whom shall I say is calling?"

I took a deep breath.

"Angel," I said. That was the nickname George had given me in college.

There was a pause and then George's breathless voice came on line. "Angel?" he asked dubiously.

"Hello, Achilles," I replied, using my own pet name for him. George had had red hair and muscles, just like the hero of the *Iliad*. "Who was that?" I asked.

"Damon Greyson, my partner. And my lover."

"Really? For how many weeks now?"

He sighed. "Years and years."

Tempus fugit. Even the wild and wanton George had settled down. "How's the art business?"

"Good enough. Why do you ask?" I wondered if Damon was listening to our conversation. If George had told him anything about the mischief we used to make, my call must be worrying him.

"I have a favor to ask."

"What kind of favor?"

"My nephew is in town. He's an artist. I'd like you to take a look at his work."

"Sure," he said cheerfully. He seemed relieved that I had not asked anything nefarious of him. "Send him down. I'm always looking for new talent."

"George, don't just look. Take something. Anything. Encourage him."

"I could do that," he said dubiously. "But you know I try to be honest with my artists."

"Yes, I know. He's good, George. Not great, but it won't embarrass you to hang his stuff in your gallery. Give him a chance, please?"

He sighed deeply. "All right."

"Thank you, George. I appreciate it." Then I said, "I'd like to drop by some time, catch up with you."

"Maybe."

"That's not very encouraging." A possible explanation for his reserve occurred to me. "Have you been talking to James?"

"No, why?"

"We're having a fight. If he calls, would you let me know?"

"Of course. What's up?"

"He's having one of his jealous fits again."

"Oh." He sounded relieved.

"Well, I doubt I'll hear from him then. He knows Day and I are monogamous."

"You? Monogamous? Since when?"

"Since AIDS."

"Oh," I said. I was not enlightened. "What's 'aids'?"

A long silence. Then, "What have you been doing for the last fifteen years?"

Oops. "Sleeping," I admitted reluctantly.

"Sleeping?"

"Remember back during the Bicentennial when I decided to take the Long Sleep?"

"Yes."

"I just woke up."

"That's incredible!"

"It astonishes me too. James has not taken it well."

"I bet he's tied in knots!"

"No, I was the one tied up." George whooped with laughter. Before he could recover I spoke again "What did I miss?"

George adapted rapidly. He always had. "AIDS. The Teflon president, Ronnie Raygun. The meltdown of the Chernobyl nuclear power plant. The disintegration of the Soviet Union. The massacre of democracy in China. The War in the Persian Gulf. Gay Lib. Yuppies. But for you the most important thing is AIDS."

"None of that means anything to me." I felt hopelessly antiquated.

"The only thing you need to worry about is AIDS. It's a disease, Acquired Immune Deficiency Syndrome. Basically, if you get it, you die. But you can have it for ten years before you know it. Once it starts bothering you enough to notice, you're going to be dead shortly. A few years, maybe longer."

"How do you get it?"

"It's carried in the body fluids. Blood and semen are the usual transmitters. Condoms help, but they aren't perfect. And for you, they're useless." As somebody who lived on blood and promiscuous sex, I was not happy. I had enjoyed the madcap freedom of American night life. It had helped me forget the dreariness of Hungary without Valentin.

"Are you all right?" I asked. George had been one of the more reckless lovers I knew.

"Yes, both Day and I tested negative. County health does anonymous testing if you want to get tested."

"I suppose that would be a good idea." But I felt no sense of urgency on my own behalf; I had proved invulnerable to hepatitis and cholera, I doubted that AIDS could be any worse.

"I wish you well. You certainly made my life interesting. It would be a pity if anything were to happen to you."

"Thank you. I could continue making your life interesting if you like."

He sighed. "Rafael, I'm sixty-seven. I quit dying my hair after you disappeared. Nowadays my idea of an evening's entertainment is watching the news on PBS."

"You dyed your hair?" I asked in astonishment.

"Rafael, Rafael, what good are your eyes if you don't use them?"

"But, I thought you'd be my red-haired Achilles forever! It never dawned on me that you were going gray."

"Gray and fat, sweetheart," he said softly. "I wish I had died before you returned. Then I would have been your red-haired warrior forever."

I swallowed hard. "I want to see you."

"I don't want to see you. I said good-bye to you a long time ago. It's better we hang up now, before the dreams are irrevocably ruined. Good night, Rafael. Good luck. And good-bye."

"Good-bye," I said just before the phone clicked and buzzed.

After hanging up the phone I went and stared at "New York by Night." Its tenebrous colors suited my unhappy mood. George had been my best and last friend. Now I had no one. No one but Michael, as tenuous as that connection was. Grimly I decided to move the painting to the music room. I wanted it to be perfectly clear to Michael that I was not giving him the money; I had bought the painting. I was his patron now. Very soon I was going to have to trust him whether I wanted to or not, and I wanted every hold on him that I could manufacture.

I plucked the nails from the wall, then took them to the music room where by sheer perverse strength I pushed them in like thumb tacks, leveling the painting on the first try. ("What good are your vampire eyes if you don't use them?") Then I sank onto the window seat while I lost myself in contemplation. Surely those phantom forms were envious souls, haunting the world they could no longer enjoy. Like me.

I needed a friend. The people I had trusted had fallen away from me. Silently I ticked them off on my fingers: My family was estranged, no longer even speaking to me. Valentin was long dead, buried under the frostflowers. James wanted me dead, but lacked the nerve to actually do it. George had said good-bye forever. And if George had not exaggerated, AIDS had eliminated the casual acquaintances and freewheeling sex I had exploited for food. An arctic chill went through my soul. Why had I even bothered to wake up? Michael. Michael had awakened me.

He was new, tempting, dangerous, interesting, exciting. What would life be like without him? I removed Michael's meteor bright presence from my mind. All that was left was cold, dark silence. I shivered. A gale wind was blowing through my soul. Before the Long Sleep it had been a cool and taunting breeze, but now it roared through me.

Suicide.

I opened the lid of the harpsichord and hit random keys. Music. Music was the wall between me and oblivion. I did not know what I played, I improvised. Anything to hold back the darkness.

A long time later I lifted my head and hands. The walls vibrated with the echoes of dying music. Nobody heard, not even Michael. My heart was empty and barren. Music was the most important thing in the world, but music had to have an audience. One old recluse slowly driving himself into madness with endless improvisations did not qualify.

Maybe, just maybe, "Junior" could go on stage and play his "father's" music, resuming the career aborted thirty-five years ago.

No, do not think it. It was too dangerous.

I was broke, I had to do something to bring in money. My nocturnal habits allowed few opportunities for employment. Night watchman, night shift hospital orderly, night cashier, movie projectionist. I did not have the skills for anything else. Music was my sole area of expertise, unless I counted my criminal skills. I would make an excellent cat burglar, mugger, gigolo, or assassin. I put my head down. What would I have to do to survive? My money had insulated me from such hard choices.

But I had two drawers full of finished music scores. As Rafael Junior I could posthumously edit and publish my father's work. And with my father's work to bolster me, I could begin a new career as a composer, safe in my study, isolated (insulated) from the world. James had done me a favor by declaring me dead: I did not need to fake my own death.

I had no choice, I had to publish. I went to the credenza and started sorting through the scores.

The recognizable rumble of Michael's Corvette halted in front of the house. I doused the lights. A moment later the front door opened and closed. Michael started up the stairs, then paused. Both feet hit the floor as he jumped off the lower landing. He searched quickly up and down the hallway, looking for the missing painting, then entered the music room. I slipped into the living room. Cautiously I opened a small space between the velvet curtains and spied on him.

Michael glanced at the envelope with his name on it, then turned to face the painting. He stood looking at it for a long minute while I studied his profile, noting the high cheekbones. From this angle his father's Indio ancestry was obvious. Then he turned back to the harpsichord and opened the envelope. He read the letter, but did not pocket the money.

"Rafael?"

I made no answer.

"I know you're there, I can feel you watching me." I withdrew my fingers from the curtains. Even without looking at him I could feel the warmth of his presence.

"You don't have to do this."

I spoke reluctantly. "I confess, when you told me you were an artist I had doubts about your ability, but you are good. I like the painting."

"Do you really?"

"Yes. I've often seen the city like that. It's a different place at night. A place where strange things can happen."

"Yes," he breathed. "I think so. It's like something extraordinary could happen, something that would be impossible by the light of day."

"Do you believe in ghosts?" I asked.

He stepped closer to the curtain. "Yes. I think there's a whole kind of existence we only glimpse. Some people have second sight and they can see it, but the rest of us are blind." He sighed. "I catch glimpses of it sometimes, in dreams or out of the corner of my eye. I wish I could see it, really see it, and paint it so that others could see it."

"George can see it," I replied. "He'll like your work."

The note rustled. "Is this George Ponchartrain a friend of yours?"

"Yes."

"I don't want him to take my stuff just because you two are friends. I want him to take it because it's good."

Ah, vanity. "George is a shrewd judge of art. He knows what will sell. If you ask him for an honest opinion, you'll get it. Some artists consider him brutally honest."

"Honesty I can bear." He sighed. "It's the endless carping criticism that drives me nuts." The print of his fingertips appeared in the curtain as he slowly rubbed the velvet. The movement of the cloth distracted me. I wanted to push myself up against his hand and feel him stroke me the way he was stroking the curtain. He continued speaking.

"Nobody believes I can do it. Not my ex-girlfriend, not my mother. I have artist friends, but I'm not really close to any of them.

"They tell me I'm too romantic. Art today is supposed to have a message. I guess I don't know how to get my message across." Slowly my hand lifted and my fingertips matched his so lightly the plush velvet did not crush. His fingertips through the curtain were warm and my hand tingled. How sweet if I could have the whole of him against me! I would never be cold again.

His hand dropped. After a moment's hesitation mine fell too. He was so close, but impossibly far away. "You have to believe in yourself. That's all that matters." I spoke softly, not wanting him to hear the depths that might be there if I spoke out loud. He was my nephew, after all.

"It would be easier to believe in myself if somebody else believed in me too. People tell me I'm a fool and I think they must be right. But painting is what I am. I just wish I could find somebody who understood that."

"I understand."

"Do you?" he asked doubtfully. His fingers walked up the curtain. I wanted to seize those teasing fingers and devour them.

"Yes," I said lowly. "I had somebody like that once."

"What happened?"

"He died."

He waited for me to tell the story. I did not. Only the nightwalkers of Budapest knew the details of the morbid and futile vengeance I had wrought when Valentin died. My ferocity had frightened even them.

Michael's voice brought me back from my dark reverie.

"Did he understand your music?"

"Oh yes," I breathed. "When I wrote, I wrote for him. When I played, I played for him. And when the crowd gave me a standing ovation, it was his face I sought before I took my bows."

"I envy you," he said in a low voice. " 'It is better to have loved and lost than to never have loved at all.' "

"I've had other lovers since then. But I still miss Valentin."

"Especially in the middle of the night when everything is dark and lonely. That's why you play then, isn't it?"

His perspicacity surprised me. "Yes," I answered. "You're the first person to hear me play in years," I added.

"That's such a waste! You should still be in concert, not sitting around waiting to die!"

"I don't want to die," I whispered. "I want a reason to live."

"Music! Maybe you can't do everything you used to, but you can still do something! Anything is better than wasting away like this."

"I am doing something. I write music. I was deciding which scores to send to Sheridan when you interrupted me."

"Oh. I didn't know."

"You're impulsive. You jump to conclusions. And you're temperamental." I paused. "I like you."

"I'm glad you like me, but I'm not sure I feel complimented."

I touched the curtain with my fingers. "I find you interesting."

"To some people 'interesting' is about as laudable as 'different'," he retorted.

"I like it." He did not know what to say, and I was afraid of what else I might say if I kept talking.

I dropped my hand. "Good night Michael."

"Good night," he replied in bewilderment. After a moment's hesitation he picked up the envelope and shuffled upstairs. Did he pause before mounting the final flight to his garret? Or was my own imagination tantalizing me with vain hopes? I slumped on the sofa feeling the intolerable ache in my soul. It was worse than the pain of my body. The wound would heal and disappear, but the psychic pain went on forever. Perhaps the other immortals were right. Perhaps some day soon I too would see that the gulf between me and humanity was uncrossable. Then I would be free to stop struggling to remain civilized and could live like a ghoul without a conscience, taking what I wanted when I wanted it.

The ring of the telephone interrupted my brooding. I gaped at it in shock, then picked it up. Who would be calling me?

"May I speak to Rafael Guitierrez, please?" a woman's voice asked. I did not recognize it.

"Who's calling please?"

She hesitated. "It's a private call. Do I have the correct number?"

Curiosity compelled me to answer, "I'm Rafael Guitierrez, Junior. Do you want me or my father?"

"Oh. I didn't know there were two of you."

"Who are you?" She hesitated. "Zoæ Flanagan. I'm the daughter of James Flanagan." Little blonde Zoæ was Michael's age. I tried to transform my mental image of a ten-year-old tomboy into a poised young woman. I failed. The two might have the same name, but they were different people to me. "I'm sorry to bother you this late, but I'm trying to set my father's affairs in order. He's had a heart attack."

"Is he dead?"

"No, but he's very ill. He's convinced he's going to die."

James had good reason to fear death. He was going to meet the wrath of an avenging Angel very soon.

"Please, I need to speak to your father about a personal matter."

"My father is dead."

"Oh," she said faintly. "When did it happen?"

"A long time ago." The soft crackle of static on the line was the only sound while she absorbed that news.

"Have you seen my father recently?" I wondered if she was the one who had found the nude and bloody James on his office floor. "Yes," I said neutrally. If Zoæ was handling James's affairs, then perhaps I could get Zoæ to return my money to me.

"I had questions about his handling of Dad's estate. I was a kid when he died so I had no idea what the grown-ups were doing. But now that I've been going through Dad's personal papers myself I see some discrepancies. Perhaps you can help straighten things out for me."

"I'd be glad to do what I can."

Getting back the money I had entrusted to James was probably going to be exceedingly difficult, but there was one matter that ought to be fairly straightforward.

"I've found an insurance policy that Dad took out with me as beneficiary. It's face value is two hundred and fifty thousand dollars. I never received it. I'd like to know if a claim was ever filed and where the money went if it was paid."

"I don't know, but I can find out." If the claim had never been paid, I could collect it. If, as I suspected, James had collected and pocketed the money then Zoæ would be seeing for herself that her father was a liar and a thief. That being the case, she and I could probably reach an accommodation.

"I'd appreciate it if you could. Give me a call when you know something. And please, don't discuss the matter with anybody but me."

"I'm sure we can handle this quickly and quietly."

So Zoæ was worried about something too.

"Thank you." I organized my thoughts. "By going through Dad's papers I've learned a lot about him. Perhaps I could answer that personal question you said you had." I willed her to confide in me. She did not. The telephone was a poor medium for conveying my power; I did much better in face to face conversations. I had to say something.

"I know for example, that our fathers were lovers."

Zoæ breathed a great sigh. "Yes, Dad has mentioned something about that. It bothers him a lot. He seems to feel like he didn't have any choice." I bit my tongue to keep from saying anything rude.

"I had the impression that my father liked James and trusted him too freely. He loaned James money to bury Peter, but James never paid him back."

Zoæ caught her breath. I was the one who had taken her to movies and ice cream every night while her parents were at the hospital watching Peter die. That should mean something to us, but it did not. James had severed that connection by declaring me dead. Rafael Junior was a stranger who had no claim on her. But maybe she would want to honor the memory of Rafael Senior by checking to see that his estate had been executed the way he intended.

"I don't know anything about that."

I had pressed too hard.

"Perhaps I'm wrong. Perhaps I'm reading something into the papers that Dad didn't say or feel. After all, I didn't know him well."

"My father is a good lawyer. I'm sure that we will find everything is in order."

"He may be competent," I said coolly, "But I have yet to see any proof that he is good."

She slammed down the receiver.

James had done me dirt. If she thought he could do no wrong, well then, she needed a rude awakening! I put my head in my hands. I should have agreed blandly to anything she said. My temper could get me in trouble as readily as my other passions. I would have to apologize to her—later.

I considered the situation. By the fact that James had called on Zoæ for help I knew he had not gone to the police. No, James would attack on a different front. He would use his underworld connections to find somebody who would lie for money. A little cash, a little coaching, and suddenly there would be an eyewitness to the murder in High Hill Park. I understood the police game. I could counter whatever moves he made on that front. I had played cat and mouse with the Hungarian secret police for three years—and the Baltimore police were pansies by comparison. They, after all, were bound by the rule of law.

Yet there was another, subtler technique James could use. He could start rumors in my own neighborhood. I envisioned a mob with torches and crosses storming my house. Mobs have no rules of evidence, no careful considerations of testimony. They act on impulse and emotion. Discretion was my defense against them, but if James bruited my secret, I would truly be in dire straits. I had to act promptly to forestall any rumors about undead monsters.

The sun had already dipped below the line of roof tops across from me, but the day was full of lavender light. It was the wan light of winter, but many times brighter than the ghostly light I had tested that first morning. By the light of day I could see that the row houses of my street had deteriorated more than I had realized. Once it had been a neighborhood of scholarly poverty, inhabited in large part by students who attended the nearby conservatory and university. A smattering of actors and good-natured harlots had added spice to the district. Now the storefront tarot reader had been replaced by a package liquor store.

A knot of sullen men and cheaply dressed women loitered outside the liquor store smoking cigarettes and drinking from brown bags. Their conversation was a buzz of bored hostility. I recognized their mood; they'd start a fight just to have something to do. Under normal circumstances I walked right past such gadflies, but tonight I was walking with a definite mince because of my injuries. That would bring them down on me like hounds on a hare. I stayed on my side of the street until I was half way down the block, but then I had to cross the street to Rosie's Deli. I kept a wary eye on them. Some of them watched me, but I was far enough away they could not easily hassle me.

I let myself into Rosie's and was pleased to notice most of the half-dozen tables were occupied. The atmosphere was pleasantly bright and noisy, a welcome contrast to the hoodlums outside. Rosie was not in tonight, instead a young black woman was standing behind the meat counter. It would take a little longer for the gossip to circulate, but once Rosie got the word, the whole neighborhood would have it in less than twenty-four hours.

I walked up to the counter and surveyed the display of cheeses and roasted meats. The smell of dead animals nauseated me.

"What'll it be?"

"What's on special tonight?"

"Reubens, plenty of sauerkraut, and a pickle on the side."

"I'll take two, one for here, one to go." She built the sandwich to Rosie's specifications: overloaded. My stomach churned in anticipation of the misery to come. I forced a smile. "My Dad told me about this place. He said you make the best sandwiches in town."

"Really? Who's your Dad?"

I steeled myself to carry through. "Rafael Guitierrez. He owned the house at the end of the block when he was alive. I inherited it and have decided to move in."

"Oh," she said. "I thought it was abandoned."

I shook my head. "In storage. I'll be fixing it up."

"That's good, it needs it." She passed over the sandwiches, one on a plate, one in a bag. "Do you want some chips?"

"Yes, please." Salt would help me keep the disgusting mess down long enough to cross the street and throw up in the privacy of my own bathroom.

She heaped up the chips. "Drink?"

Something that would not be too revolting when it came back up. "Mineral water." The only table open was the one closest to the front door. I set down my food, took a seat, and steeled myself to give a good performance. I started with the mineral water. To my surprise it tasted good. I had not realized that I was thirsty. I drank the bottle comfortably, then bought another. Maybe my body would be happy to get food of any nature, even if it was solid and greasy and cold.

My stomach slowly flip-flopped as I confronted the reuben. Not bloody likely.

I nibbled some chips. The salt tasted good. My body had lost minerals as well as water. The chips themselves were almost null in terms of nutrition. The heavy burden of salt counteracted any disturbance they made in my digestion. I ate them without trouble. I tried the pickle next. It was sour and crisp and juicy. I became a little queasy and put it down. Finally I resigned myself to poisoning myself with dead meat and fermented cabbage. I chewed grimly and forced myself to swallow, while my stomach tried frantically to send it back up again.

"Hi." A young woman slid into the seat opposite me. She was wearing a navy blue sweatshirt with "Hopkins" emblazoned on it, and brown hair fluffed around her face.

"I'm Marjorie. I live next door to you." She offered her hand.

I put down my sandwich and tried not to let my internal distress show. "Rafael Guitierrez, Junior," I said. Americans judge people by their handshake so I gave her cool hand a firm squeeze.

She smiled warmly. "Did I just hear you say you were fixing up the place?"

"Yes."

"While you're at it, could you do something about the poison ivy? It keeps coming over the wall into my yard, then my dog rolls in it and brings it in the house."

I sighed. "There's a lot of work to do to the place. Right now my cousin is here and we're cleaning the inside. But I'll make sure we do something about the poison ivy."

"Thanks. I'd appreciate it. If there's anything I can do to help, I'd be happy to come over for an afternoon."

"Thank you for the offer. I'll keep it in mind." I had no intention of letting her snoop through my house.

"Well, I won't keep you. Nice meeting you. Welcome to the neighborhood." She smiled brightly as she rose.

"Thank you." I watched her exit with a feeling of disquiet. I had the feeling she had just made a pass at me, but I could not put my finger on any particular detail that would prove or disprove my theory. I should have responded more warmly, chatted in a friendly way, told her I'd hurt my leg so there would be something to counteract the nasty talk that was going to go around about the way I minced down the street. I sighed, afterthoughts were useless thoughts.

I tackled the reuben again. With no further interruptions I forced most of it down. I threw away the pickle and walked carefully out the front door. Each step I took made my injury hurt and my stomach gurgle. I avoided the crowd in front of the liquor store again as I glided down the hill trying to make as few motions as possible. Nausea surged. I gritted my teeth and resisted the urge to make a run for it. I had to look like a normal citizen going home from the deli.

Once the door closed behind me I bolted up the stairs and into the bathroom. I knelt over the toilet and vomited. There are times when acute senses are a definite drawback. My guts heaved repeatedly to bring up every bit of masticated meat and strings of sauerkraut. When there was nothing left to bring up my guts heaved up green bile, which tasted like sauerkraut gone rancid. I never liked sauerkraut.

Michael knocked on the door. I groaned. "Are you all right?" he asked.

I washed my mouth out before answering. "Yes. Dinner didn't agree with me. I'm afraid my digestion can't handle reubens anymore." I washed my mouth thoroughly.

"I can fix something else for you."

"No, don't bother. I bought dinner for you, the reubens were on special. But maybe you don't want one now."

"I'll try it. Maybe you got food poisoning and we can both be sick. Misery loves company." His insouciance was despicable. I cracked the door and passed the bag out to him.

"Looks okay," he said.

The paper rustled and I heard him chomp into the sandwich.

"Go away!" I absolutely could not stomach listening to him eat that stuff.

"Tastes okay too. Sorry you didn't like it." My stomach rolled again. He moved away.

I retired to the library and settled gingerly in my desk chair. Before the Long Sleep I had been able to tolerate drinking only if I were thirsty, which was a rare occasion. Tonight I had been thirsty, and hungry too, and had both eaten and drunk. It was the sandwich that had made me ill. Perhaps since waking I was not so much hungry, as thirsty. The years had leached liquids from my body, leaving me a dry and shrunken husk. The fluids had to be replenished.

I unscrewed the top of my mineral water and sipped cautiously. Then I nodded, and drank more deeply.

Chapter Five

REVELATION

A night of endless dreams inconsequent and wild is
this my life; none more worth telling than the rest.
                                        —Murasaki Shikibu

Baltimore, 10 October 1991

My limbs lay limply at my side, cold flesh unresponsive to
my will. My eyes would not open, neither could I draw
breath nor feel any movement of my heart. I lay helpless,
waiting and wondering how long it would be before my
body caught up to my restless mind.

I counted the minutes until one soft beat stirred my
heart. Another beat followed minutes later. Soon beat
followed beat in an ever-increasing tempo. Blood crept
slowly through my veins gradually warming my flesh. My
eyes fluttered open.

I inhaled a shallow, aching breath. My lungs strained to
fill with fresh air, then collapsed as breath rushed out.
Another weak breath inflated my chest, then another. Pain
eased and stiffness melted. Respiration steadied into a natural rhythm and I inhaled each breath with gratitude.

My fingertips twitched in response to my desire to raise

my hand. I dragged them to my chest where I let them rest. There was nothing for them to do until the rest of my body was able to cooperate. Bit by bit my muscles took on tone and strength until I was able to lever myself to a sitting position.

I took a deep breath and stretched my arms, then swung my legs over the side of the bed. Gently I lowered my hands to touch my toes. Muscles pulled and ached, but flexing them felt good. With a little more effort my palms settled flat against the floor. I was sore but mobile.

I listened cautiously before limping into the dim upstairs hallway. On my left the stairs wended their way to the attic, on my right the library and bathroom doors stood open, the rooms empty. Silence hung heavy everywhere. No television, no running water, no soft footsteps. The house creaked uneasily as the wind blew. I swallowed a sudden lump in my throat. Had Michael left me? I hurried upstairs to his room.

The harsh glare of the late afternoon sun poured through the dormer window. Michael's suitcase lay open on the floor. Dirty clothes were heaped in a corner. The cot was unmade. A cloth covered a painting on his easel. Paints were haphazardly stacked under the window while brushes dried on the sill. He would return.

My eyes hurt and my head ached from the brightness of the light. Normally I slept through the sunlit hours safe in my darkened sanctuary. My only acquaintance with daylight was during the cool hours of dawn and evening when the sun was absent, and only its aurora reddened the sky.

I descended to the back door and let myself into the deep shadows of the sheltered patio. Standing there I surveyed the yard. The house shadowed all but a narrow strip along the side wall where the roses had gone wild and become a thorny thicket. Weeds carpeted the ruined lawn, a few of them still holding up ragged heads of blue blossoms. Other weeds grew through cracks in the pavement in defiant proof of the unquenchable spirit of life.

The short driveway emptied into an alley lined with parked cars, garbage cans, and miscellaneous junk mercifully hidden from view by the high brick wall that surrounded my backyard. A stout wooden gate barred the driveway, the four numbered dials of its padlock corroded into immobility. I remembered the combination; it was impossible to forget. 1956, the year of Valentin's death.

I drifted across the dirty concrete and paused in the sheltering shadow of the house. A few feet away the harsh light of autumn gleamed on scarlet rose hips. Long strands of thorns gone wild were beaded with vermilion fruit like necklaces for a giantess. I had planted the bushes in defiance of the old superstition that said roses were anathema for my kind. Each night, just before dawn, I had worked in my garden, pruning and weeding, picking off the voracious Japanese beetles and washing away the aphids, knees damp from the soft, moist earth while sleeves brushed against the large velvet blooms. The heavenly perfume had clung to my clothes and skin so that when I retired to my bed the bewitching scent came with me and perfumed my sheets.

When I die, let them fill my coffin with red roses. Do not let them cover me with the cold white bloom of frostflowers.

Weeds wrapped around my ankles as I waded across the lawn, hands itching to restore order to the briar patch my garden had become. Sunlight tingled on my exposed skin and I dared to look directly at the golden tyrant, the sun. Sundogs blinded me. I bowed my head and covered my eyes, but the sundogs continued to dance through the darkness behind my hands. I used the heat of the sun on my

skin to navigate back to the cool shade. There in the soothing dimness my vision gradually returned. I contemplated
my hands, the faint blush of color rapidly fading in the
comfort of the shade.

The sun was no longer the jailer of my days. No more
skulking behind shuttered windows, no more special
appointments for business after dark, no more racing against
the dawn for the safety of my home; I was free at last.

In the privacy of my patio I stripped off my clothes and
stashed them in the box under the stairs. Vapor swirled
around me as the bonds of my flesh loosened and I shed
excess mass. That was the hard part: To keep my mind
focused on the task at hand when entropy urged dissipation.

I chose a form I knew well: alley cat. If I had tried to
change to something strange to me, say an armadillo or a
penguin, I could have ended up as a dysfunctional approximation of my intended shape. It would not be a fatal
accident, but it could be a painful one.

Chaos coalesced into a small furry shape. I stretched my
brown striped legs before me, flexed my claws, then
reversed positions and stretched my hind legs. My tail
arched over my back in a saucy question mark. I smoothed
my whiskers with first one paw and then the other. Certain
that all was settled the way it should be, I stepped jauntily
down the driveway and squeezed under the gate.

The feline form was well suited to my needs. Originally
a desert animal, the common house cat had dense fur to
protect its skin, and nictating membranes to protect its eyes.
Night hunters, their irises opened wide giving them excellent night vision, but in bright light they narrowed to
immeasurably thin slits. That coupled with strength, speed,
and agility made them one of nature's most successful
predators.

The alley debouched into a four lane blacktop road that

separated my house from the park. When I had bought the house it had been a quiet brick lane. Deer had sometimes wandered into my yard. Shortly thereafter the city had paved over the bricks and widened the road. I had retaliated by building the brick wall to keep out the noise and smell of the new thoroughfare. I darted across, dodging car wheels easily in spite of the nagging ache in my hind end. A horn honked, then the golden eaves of the wooded park closed over me, and I was in the natural world, where the smell of loam and decaying leaves dominated in spite of the taint of car exhaust. I slunk through the underbrush, damp ground chilling my silent paws.

Rhythmic, repetitive music sounded to my right. Three black youths came in sight, one with a radio on his shoulder. Their bodies were lean and muscular, not yet broadened and softened by the weight of maturity. They bantered with one another in the soft, sensuous voices of the native Baltimorean. I liked the dialect, it was part of the moonlight and magnolia mystique of the South.

The three young men turned onto the riverwalk, and I fell in behind them. They walked with a bouncing, energetic step that made their bright colored vinyl jackets swing about their hips. I admired the tight round firmness of their buttocks and the rippling muscles of their legs. My attention centered on the shortest one, who was also the most muscular. I could clearly imagine lying along his naked back, kissing the nape of his neck, then sliding slowly down his spine sprinkling kisses as I went.

My imagination was too vivid. I felt a peculiar looseness of flesh, as if all the bonds of my body were gently dissolving. My steps lost their coordination and I stumbled. It would be embarrassing at best, disastrous at worst to materialize nude on the path. There were plenty of ways to travel through the park. I would take the first cross trail.

My course did not veer.

No, not again. I will not do this.

My paws dragged through several shuffling steps. The youths quickly outdistanced me, but their spoor remained on the pavement as a faint and enticing scent. My nose went down. I put one paw in front of the other. I could overtake them easily if I hurried.

No! Hunger twisted inside me. My head ached. Bile rose in my throat. I turned my head this way and that looking for anything else to take.

A raccoon paused in the shadow of a large tree. He was bigger than I was, but that did not matter. I pounced. The startled raccoon had no idea of his danger until it was too late. Warm blood gushed in my mouth and I sucked it up greedily. I clung to its back with my claws as it writhed and tried to crawl out from underneath me. Then it collapsed, twitched, and lay still.

I threw back my head and yowled. The scant blood had whetted but not satisfied my appetite. I dug my claws deeply into the inert flesh under me. If I let go I would hurl myself down the path in desperate pursuit of those young men. They did not deserve to die simply because I could not control myself. I yowled again.

Suddenly I caught the scent of dog moving my direction, no doubt attracted by the noise I had made. In a moment I was face to face with a Great Dane. The dog lowered his head and bared his teeth in a low growl. No master called him back. He stepped closer, eyes fixed on me. I did not know if he merely wanted the sport of chasing me up a tree or if he had more hostile intentions in mind. I retreated step by step until I was clear of the tangled remains of the raccoon.

The Great Dane sniffed the offal lying beside the path. While his attention was diverted I rapidly changed shape.

Increasing size was easier than decreasing, and the puma shape was one of my favorites. In about three seconds I had become a hundred and twenty pounds of mountain lion. The Dane turned tail and ran.

With one mighty pounce I crossed the intervening distance and landed on his back. My weight drove him sprawling to the ground. Powerful jaws snapped his neck, paralyzing him. With feline instinct I twisted to bring my hind paws into play and clawed his belly. Fur flew. Intestines slopped around me and splashed my legs as I dragged my prey deep into the underbrush.

My rough tongue lapped up blood and hair. I spit out the hair and lapped again, paused, and spit out more hair. I had never liked dogs. The noxious odor of dog filled my nostrils while I ate. I pawed at the dog, turned it over, found a spot of pooled blood, licked it up, and turned the carcass again to no avail. I was still hungry, and the dog was drained. I nosed through the corpse, willing even to eat tainted intestines to satisfy my hunger.

Marrow. Marrow would be good to eat. My long claws peeled the flesh away in thick strips to reveal a pale femur with gobbets of muscle and ligament dangling from it. The thick bone cracked and splintered between my jaws. Luscious, savory marrow spilled into my mouth. The flavor was richer than blood, and more satisfying. I excarnated another bone and broke it.

Suddenly I realized my pale blood-stained hand was holding the bone while my lips closed around the jagged end. I was a man again, and I was lying belly down in the warm, wet, slippery viscera. I got to my hands and knees. Blood and the stinking contents of the dog's intestines clung to my legs, groin, and belly.

There were still bones to be broken and emptied of their marrow. Food was too difficult to obtain, I could not afford to abandon my dinner for some squeamish reason. Men routinely ate the meat of butchered animals, there was no reason for me to flinch at the chore. One by one I took the bones in hand and snapped them into pieces, sucked out the marrow, and tossed the remnants aside.

My chin lolled on my chest as I sat slumped amid the ruins of my dinner. Marrow was satisfying out of proportion to its volume, and I was satiated. Certainly too well fed to spend any energy wishing I had known about marrow in the past. The past was gone, buried behind an avalanche of years. However harsh were the lessons of the Long Sleep, I was learning.

I crawled on my hands and knees through the underbrush until I came to the river. Black water swirled past rocks and rippled over fallen tree limbs. Streaks of almost invisible color and whorls of bubbles added their own variations to the flow of water, the river changing endlessly like a kaleidoscope.

Abruptly I shook my head and shifted my stiff joints, realizing that minutes (hours?) had slipped away in fascinated contemplation of the river. Others of my kind found themselves compulsively counting grains of rice or thorns (an aberration I occasionally indulged in myself), or else found themselves standing hopelessly undecided at the crossroads, capable of imagining a myriad of possibilities, and unable to choose among them. My particular compulsion seemed to be water, and once it had nearly been my undoing when the rising sun had caught me. I had avoided water since then.

Oh no, I was doing it again! I shook my head to clear the river-generated mental fog, then thrust my hands into the icy flow. The shock of cold water splashed upon my body helped fix my attention on the here and now. I scrubbed away the gore, then took tomcat form and loped home.

Michael's Corvette pulled up in front, coughed and rattled a few times, then died. The door slammed as Michael got out. I waited for the sound of the key in the lock, but it did not come. After a few minutes of waiting I concluded that he had walked up to Rosie's Deli for dinner, which vexed me because I wanted to borrow his car again. Searching through his suitcase I came up with a spare pair of keys. I kissed them and blessed Michael for being the sort of fellow who carried extra keys in his luggage, then I drove to the mall.

Double-breasted suits were back in style. The new suits sharply emphasized the trimness of the body under them, in contrast to the old suits designed to give dignity to men with middle-aged paunches. I bought two, plus a three piece suit. Black, naturally. The clerk's eyes popped as I laid cash on the counter to pay for them. After fifteen years of disuse I doubted American Express would honor my card.

"I usually order custom suits," I said, "But I don't have time." While the store tailor altered them to fit I bought six white shirts (a man never has enough white shirts), three silk ties, socks, shoes, boxer shorts (when did they start making them in anything besides white or blue?), belt, gloves, fedora, an overcoat, and a trench coat, updating my wardrobe in the all the important ways.

The ties were hardest to buy. They were the only item of men's apparel not ruled by the laws of good taste. Paisleys seemed the tamest thing offered. I browsed through a bewildering plethora of splatter prints, florals, and picture ties. I looked vainly for regimental stripes. When in doubt, stripes are always proper.

"Do you have any striped ties?" I asked the clerk.

"No, mostly we cater to younger men," he replied.

That told me what I needed to know. I studied the ties. "Who wears paisley ties?" I asked.

"Some of our customers feel they need a more conservative tie for certain occasions."

I quietly gulped. Fifteen years ago a man wearing a paisley tie would have been beaten on the streets for being queer.

I picked up a pale yellow paisley and held it under my chin. It looked good with the suit, terrible with my complexion. I exchanged it for a pale pink paisley. The pink went well with the suit, and added an illusion of color to my face. I put it down.

I could wear a paisley tie if that was the fashion, but pink was too much to ask of me. I might as well write "faggot" across my forehead.

I let my hand wander across some of the floral ties. The clerk's interest revived. "Now that's a nice one." He named a designer I did not recognize. "We sell a lot of her ties."

I smiled. "Women have terrible taste in ties. I'll pass." I looked slowly through dozens of different designs. I used to be able to pick out ties in an instant. At last I chose a pair of abstract prints. One was an elegant gray and black, the other was a saucy bright blue. Then I bought the pink paisley and wondered if I would ever have the nerve to wear it.

I retired to the restroom and removed all the tags from my new clothes. The old clothes went into one of the shopping bags. I dressed, then combed my hair and rebraided it neatly. The gray tie and double-breasted suit made an elegant combination. The new clothes were necessary. An out of date suit would tell a sharp eye that I was short on money, and the want of money has inspired many crimes. When I dealt with the insurance company, police, and lawyers I wanted to look like a perfectly respectable citizen with no need to stoop to crime.

I stopped in a sundry shop and picked up miscellaneous necessities. First, a black velvet ribbon for my hair so that I would fulfill as much as possible Michael's portrait of me. Then shaving cream, toothbrushes, shampoo, soap, dish soap, and toilet paper.

Not that I needed toilet paper, but Michael did. I passed the baby food aisle, stopped, and returned.

Babies eat pap because they cannot digest regular food. I turned down the aisle and paused in front of the section of baby formula. There were half a dozen different kinds, and each of them came as powder, liquid, or ready to eat. I read labels trying to determine if any of them would be tolerable. At last I came across one that proclaimed itself especially for infants with sensitive digestion. It was the most expensive, of course.

"Do you have a baby?" a familiar female voice asked.

I forced a smile and met Marjorie's gaze. "No," I said. "But a friend does. I'm just running an errand for her."

"Boy or girl?"

"Boy." At least I knew something about the male anatomy. I hoped I could improvise on the subject of baby boys.

"How old?"

"Six months." Marjorie eyed me speculatively. Her curly auburn hair tumbled about her shoulders and a bright red sweater slopped off her shoulder.

"It's not mine," I said guessing the direction of her thoughts. "We're just friends." Marjorie's smile warmed. I realized then it had been a tactical mistake to admit being an unattached male. In her sights I was now a fair target.

"Really? In that case I guess it's safe to invite you to my Halloween party later this month."

"You don't have to do that," I demurred. "I wouldn't know anyone."

"You know me! But I know what you mean. I'm sure my girlfriends wouldn't mind if you brought one of your male friends along. Most of them are single. Perhaps something special will happen."

"If I bring a man with me, he won't be available." I put the baby formula in my basket and started to walk away.

"Well, that's okay too."

I paused. "Beg your pardon?"

She smiled lopsidedly and shrugged. "Neighbors should get along. It's a mixed enough neighborhood that nobody would speak to anybody if we let our differences get in the way." Her enlightened attitude startled me. My former next door neighbor had pursed her lips and pointedly ignored me whenever we met.

"In that case, I'd be delighted to attend your party. When is it?"

"The nineteenth, at seven. That's the Saturday after this one."

A party! I had not attended a party in years. The pall of melancholy that had hung over me ever since waking lifted slightly. I smiled, feeling almost shy. "I'll be there. Thank you for the invitation."

She nodded. "I'll see you then."

"I'm looking forward to it."

The mechanics at Sear's said mechanic-type things to me and I nodded agreeably. I paid the bill without a quibble. Michael's car started with a macho rumble. The tune up, oil change, transmission work, and brake work had done wonders for the car. It was clean inside and out. The Corvette handled well enough on the drive home, but I wanted my Ferrari.

Michael's window at the top of the house glowed with welcome light. I had lived alone since Valentin's death because I liked my privacy and my independence. But now I was glad of Michael's presence, glad to enter a warm and living house instead of the desolation of my voluntary exile.

Marjorie's invitation had touched a nerve in me that I thought had been long dead. I wanted company.

I quietly hung my new clothes in the closet, the smell of cedar wafting past me. I switched shirts, then fetched the diamond cufflinks from my jewelry box and installed them in my sleeves. I checked my image in the mirror. I was looking well. Not as robust as I used to look, but quite handsome and distinguished. I adjusted the new gray tie slightly, then turned to make sure my suit coat was lying smooth. I wanted to look my best when I finally showed myself to Michael.

The smell of paints and turpentine drifted down from the attic room. The smells were noxious but they did not bother me.

Instead they were like an enchanting perfume— Michael's perfume. I would not like him nearly so well if he were a insurance salesman, accountant, or dentist. I stepped into the music room, lighting the candles with an easy gesture.

The mirror over the fireplace doubled the candles, filling the room with radiance. Their ruddy light gave my skin an alabaster glow it lacked under artificial illumination, flattering me with a warm and ethereal beauty. I settled at the harpsichord and surveyed the room. Michael's painting and the hall door were to my right, the shuttered bay window to my left. The draped archway was across from me, opposite the brown marble fireplace. It was my favorite room, and the perfect setting for Michael's first view of me.

The music of the Eastern Dances flowed effortlessly out my hands and through the strings. Pleasure flooded through me. This evening was the first time since waking that the endless hunger was laid to rest, and my mind was clear of all distraction. Old skill merged with new emotion, and I played with all the dreamy romance that had won the adoration of Budapest's *beau monde*.

The first movement ended. Michael did not come slipping down the stairs as he had done all the other times I had played. I expanded my senses from music to the whole house and found him engrossed in his painting. I tapped my fingers in annoyance. The mantel clock ticked away the minutes while I waited. Still no Michael. I closed the key cover with a bang and sulked. There was something he found more interesting than me.

Art.

I could compete with another man—a woman even—but not art. Yet I must. Michael was the most important person in the world to me. I had to make myself equally important to him. If he was going to hate me, let me find out now. And if he was going to help me, let me know that too. I could tolerate anything from him except indifference.

Abruptly I jumped up from my seat and swiftly climbed the stairs. His door was closed. I heard the hum of a space heater and felt a warm draft across my ankles. With my ear against the door I could hear his paintbrush slithering across canvas and the soft susurration of his breath. The door squeaked a little on its hinges as I pushed it ajar. The room was warm and brightly lit by several lamps. Michael was stripped to the waist, perspiration gleaming between his tan shoulder blades. Muscles rippled as he deftly applied paint to canvas.

"If you're coming in, come in. If not, don't. But close the door. There's a cold draft across my back." He did not look around.

"Another city scene?" I asked hovering on the threshold. His beautiful back blocked my view of the canvas.

"No." I waited for him to elucidate, but he ignored me.

"So what is it?"

"Rafael, I appreciate your interest, but right now I'm trying to get this finished. I'd prefer to work alone." He remained intent upon his work, not even bothering to glance at me.

"What is it?" I persisted.

"The Gorman commission. I've been trying to get this thing done for weeks. A few more hours and it will be finished and I can take it back to New York."

"You're leaving so soon?"

"I have an appointment to see Ponchartrain in a few days. If he takes any of my paintings then I will have done what I set out to do. I'll be able to go home and get out of your way."

"You're not in my way." Michael tried to peek over his shoulder at me. I stepped into the hallway and out of his sight.

He sighed in frustration. "I know I can't stay. You've been helpful, and I appreciate it. I don't mean the money. What's really helped me is the whole atmosphere here." He continued in a soft, dreamy voice, "It seems like the real world has dropped away, that this house is its own reality. I feel free for the first time in my life, like I belong here. I can do anything, try anything. I don't have to worry about ordinary conventions anymore. I have so many ideas! I've filled a whole sketchbook. As soon as the Gorman's out of the way, I can start painting them. I'll be painting for months."

"Paint them here."

Michael stepped closer to the door. "Do you want me to stay?"

"Yes."

I licked my lips. If he left, my house would be dark and empty. I would have no one left but enemies and lost friends. I would get down on my knees and beg him to stay if necessary.

"If I stay, will you let me see you?"

My heart thumped heavily against my breastbone. "Yes."

"Now?"

"If you like," I whispered. I didn't think he could hear me.

"Yes," he replied.

I hesitated, then stepped into the room.

My eyes went past him to his painting. It was me as he had seen me the other night amid the zebra stripes of moonlight and darkness, but he had taken liberties with the scene. In his painting I sat in the window embrasure, one knee up, one hand resting on it, and my back leaning against the wall. I wore an old fashioned ruffled white shirt open to one button above the waist. My braid tied up with a black velvet ribbon hung over my shoulder. My eyes held secrets my lips promised to deliver.

"That's quite a painting," I said at last.

Michael blushed. "I had no idea it was your face. I thought I was making it up."

"What do you mean? Of course it's my face."

"But I had no idea what you looked like. I've never seen you before."

"Surely you've seen a photograph."

"Not that I remember." He shook his head as he spoke. His eyes stared at me in disbelief. "You can't be my uncle. You're too young."

"I'm sixty-five."

He sat down on the cot. "I believe you. It doesn't make any sense, but I believe it anyhow."

I knelt on the floor before him. "Do you really?"

He wet his lips. "Yes. I've dreamed about you every night since I've been here. And during the day I see afterimages of your presence. Usually when I'm at a new place I lose things all the time. But here when I want something, I just ask myself where you would put it, and that's where it is." His eyes went back to the painting. "I guess I'll have to scrape it off and paint something else."

"No!" I said in shock. "Why would you do that?"

"Well, it's your face. It's supposed to be fiction." He shifted uncomfortably.

I looked him in the eye. "It's the best painting of yours I've seen. It's alive, like the image will step out of the picture at any moment."

He steadied. "Do you really think so?" I nodded.

He lifted one long finger. He hesitated, then poked me in the arm.

I smiled. "Flesh and blood. Not a ghost or a fantasy or a dream."

"How can that be? You seem to vanish and materialize into thin air!"

"Not magic. Just light on my feet."

"I'm light on my feet. You're something else."

"Yes."

"What?"

I chose my words with care. "I am very much a man, but more so. I'm a little stronger, a little quicker, a little sharper of hearing. That's all."

"But you're still young!"

"And healthy."

"You're talking about immortality!"

"Yes."

His pupils widened. "This is fabulous! This means the end of sickness and old age!"

I shook my head violently.

He looked shocked. "You can't keep it to yourself! You have to share it with the rest of the world!"

"I refuse. I've made my contribution to the welfare of humanity. I was on the barricades when the tanks rolled into Budapest in '56. I was shot and left for dead, my lover was murdered, my money and possessions confiscated. I became a fugitive.

"I've done all the good that one man can reasonably be expected to do. It's cost me dearly. Freedom is the only thing I have left. I fully intend to keep it."

It took him a moment to absorb what I said. "I didn't know. No one ever talks about you."

"Nobody knows," I said wearily. "Papa was the only one. When I finally escaped West he met me in Austria and took care of me. He sent me to the States, bought this house for me, gave me money—on the condition that I keep quiet. He did not want the family disgraced by a gay revolutionary."

After a moment's silence Michael asked, "Is that how Valentin died? When the Red Army put down the rebellion?"

"Yes."

"That must have been awful! To be in love and not be able to tell anyone, and then when he died you still couldn't tell anyone!" Michael's empathy surprised me. He seemed to understand my grief at Valentin's death. But Michael was much too nice a person to be able to understand my rage at the savage way they had killed him. Rage had brought me back from the bourne of death to take a bloody vengeance. A vengeance that had accomplished nothing.

"Michael," I said softly. His eyes met mine. They were gorgeous, so clear and so sensitive. I wanted to weep over Valentin at long last while Michael held me in his arms and promised me that everything would be all right. Vain dreams.

"Inside these walls is civilization. Here is art, music, philosophy and personal freedom. Inside this house the laws of the world do not apply; we choose to live as we wish to live. But outside is a savage world. I have to live by certain subterfuges to protect myself. I need you to understand that, and respect it."

"I don't understand," he replied. "You would be a hero if you came forward and revealed yourself!"

"If people knew what I was, they'd burn me at the stake."

"That's medieval! People don't think like that anymore!"

"No, nowadays people would never hate a man just because he's different. They would never beat an Asian man to death just because Japan was selling cars in America. They would never castrate a black man because he was dating a white girl. And they would never arrest a man just because he loved another man."

He started to open his mouth in protest, and I held up my hand.

"Think, Michael. That's simple prejudice of no benefit to anyone. What would happen to me if they knew about me? How could they resist the triple lure of long life, perfect health, and perpetual youth? They'd take me into custody 'for my own protection' while they experimented on me and tried to figure out what made me tick. They would torture me for the benefit of mankind!"

Michael lowered his eyes. "I guess I'm naive. I know such things happen, but I don't expect them to happen to people I know."

"You're a sweet young man. But we live in an imperfect world and we have to deal with it. So if anybody asks, you and I are cousins. My name is now Rafael Guitierrez, Junior, and I'm officially twenty-six." I smiled wryly at him. "I have a lot of things to sort out, so I'd appreciate it if you didn't discuss my affairs with anybody."

"What about our family?"

"Not even them. Especially not them."

"You should tell them! They're your family!"

Michael was the warmest, most human person I had met in a long time. He was strong and sensitive, honest and appealing. I was grateful to have him as a kinsman. I leaned forward and kissed him on the cheek, Spanish style. "I'll think about it, cousin. But not tonight." My injuries ached. I had pushed myself too far tonight. "I'm tired, I'll see you tomorrow."

"*Mañana,*" Michael replied automatically.

"*Hasta la vista,*" I replied.

I limped downstairs and went to bed. I lay awake until dawn wondering what he would think after he had time to consider the matter without the charisma of my presence to influence him. I could only hope for the best.

Chapter Six
MAD ANTHONY

He is gone who knew the music of my soul.

—Hsueh T'so

Baltimore, 11 October 1991; Budapest, 1949–1959

The clock told me it was two-thirty when I woke. I could not conceive of it being that early and concluded the clock was wrong. After fifteen years without adjustments it could not be expected to keep good time. I went to the window and drew the drapes, opened the interior shutters, threw up the sash, and opened the exterior shutters. A leaden sky lowered over the city. Fog dampened everything. Cars drove past with headlights lit. People hurried down the street, eager to reach their destinations and escape the wet chill.

Further up the street a wailing cry sounded. "Aaaaaa-pulls, Syyyyy-der. Aaaaaa-pulls. Syyyyy-der." The clatter of hooves echoed sharply off the walls of the narrow street. The wagon rolled slowly past, horse's head hanging, black driver walking beside him. I had thought surely the days of the street Arabs were over.

Marjorie came out of her house and scampered down

the steps, wet auburn curls plastered to her neck. The driver handed her a gallon of cider and accepted the dollars she gave him. She saw me in the window as she started back to her door. "Do you want one?" she called.

I shook my head. "What time is it?"

"After two, maybe two-thirty. I had the day off today." I nodded and closed the shutters.

Offices would be open, such as the bank and government agencies with whom I had business. I donned a black suit with a white shirt, regimental tie and black fedora. I shaved, but skipped showering. Time in the real world was too precious a commodity to waste.

As I stepped from the bathroom into the hallway the nauseating smell of tomato, oregano, and garlic hit me. I rapidly traced the appalling stench to the kitchen where Michael was stirring a pot on the stove.

"May I borrow your car?" I asked while trying not to breathe. "I have some errands to run."

"Sure. Supper will be ready around six."

"Aren't you starting a little early?"

He grinned. "I make my sauce from scratch. It'll simmer all afternoon. You'll like it."

"Thank you, but no. I don't care for Italian food. I'll get something while I'm out."

"You don't like spaghetti?" he asked in astonishment.

The cloying smell of garlic was making me queasy. I smiled and shrugged. "We all have our quirks." I resolved to stay away long enough for the odors to dissipate. "I'll see you later." I collected his keys from the hook by the door and made a hasty exit.

By virtue of my forged college transcripts I was able to enroll in one class at the Peabody Conservatory. Since I was joining late they would only let me audit the class. That was fine with me, all I wanted was the photo ID.

Long ago James had obtained a fraudulent birth certificate for Rafael Junior. With it and my school ID I was able to apply for a driver's license. The heavy fog proved a boon because it kept people away from the Motor Vehicle Administration. I skimmed the driver's handbook while I waited for my turn to take the driving test. Traffic law had not changed much. At last they snapped my picture and gave me a piece of plastic still hot from the lamination machine. I had the universally accepted identification proving I was who I said I was.

Now that I had a legal driver's license it was time to see whether or not I had transportation, and if so, what condition it was in. I drove to the rented garage just a few blocks from my home. The building had formerly been a small service station cramped between the row houses on one street and the storefronts on the other. The pumps had been ripped out long ago, and the cracked white tile of the facade was missing some more pieces, but otherwise it looked about the same.

Half a dozen cars were parked on the lot, blocking access to the single overhead door. I parked in the only available space, thereby blocking everyone else's access. With a queasy feeling in the pit of my stomach I put my key in the lock then lifted the door.

Emptiness.

Where there should be a black 1972 Ferrari Daytona Spider convertible there was only the aging plywood covering the grease pit. Fresh tire tracks and footprints in the dust showed that the car had been towed away recently. The dusty blue tarp that had covered it was lying in a heap at the back of the garage. James had waited until the last minute to rob me of my favorite automobile.

I had loved to drive that car, loved to cruise the busy streets at midnight with the top down. Hookers had shouted invitations which I ignored, but often when I stopped at a light or parked the car I would find myself surrounded by appreciative young men—few of whom ever refused when I invited them to go for a ride.

An expensive sports car is the most effective aphrodisiac ever invented. The power and luxury of the car made my chosen victim horny while his admiration of me for possessing such a car made him willing to cooperate with whatever I wanted. I had known all the blind alleys, wooded lots, and unpatrolled parking lots in town. It had been in my mind that Michael, who drove a decrepit Corvette, would be particularly vulnerable to the magic of the Ferrari.

I pulled down the garage door and let it slam against the concrete.

The Enoch Pratt Free Library soothed me as always. I walked a circuit among the brown marble pillars while refreshing my memory of its murals and friezes. One mural showed Gutenberg proofing a sheet of print from his press. The other showed William Caxton, the first English printer, presenting a book to his patroness, the Duchess of Burgundy. Below and between the two murals was a double row of printer's marks ranging from the Italian Renaissance's Manutius to America's Doubleday and Company. Below them hung the portraits of the six Lords Baltimore.

Even on this dark and dreary day the library's glass ceiling and two story tall windows lit the interior with softly luminous natural light. Open mezzanines housed different departments, their white iron and mahogany handrails giving the feel of a Renaissance courtyard. All six thousand years of the wisdom of mankind were enshrined in dusty tomes stacked high on its dark wooden shelves. Ladders were stationed here and there to reach the lofty heights of philosophy, history, or science. People stood or knelt or sat with bowed heads, communing with the wisdom of the pages.

Any library is worthy of respect, but I preferred the Free Library to all others. It was built by a man who understood that a library is the temple of civilization. Enoch Pratt was a miser in his own affairs, but in the days when borrowing books was an expensive privilege, he built the library on the condition that the use of the books be free to whomever wished to borrow them, regardless of their race or sex.

A bank of computers stood where once there had been a gargantuan card file. The terrazzo floor was marked with rectangles of fresh tile recently uncovered when the card catalogs were removed. They made a strange map from the past into the future, and I contemplated them for hidden meaning. They told me nothing; they were as disjoint in time as I was. I turned to the task of mastering the new technology with some dread.

I read the instructions, then pecked the sequences of keys as directed. I had never used a computer before. In my day they had been the province of scientists who, like alchemists before them, spoke a strange language understood only by initiates of the mysteries. Operating the machine proved to be disappointingly simple. It was no improvement over the card catalog. It did not find my references any faster than I could have, and its faded ribbon did not print them anymore legibly than I could have penned them.

"So this is the future," I thought. "Different, but the same." Armed with my sheaf of references I wandered around looking up call numbers and sizing up the patrons. Old ladies checked out mysteries by dead authors, and teenagers pawed through the latest science fiction. A black businessman was sorting through magazines. He was about forty-five, and the frayed lapels on his blue suit gave him the look of a struggling salesman. I thought his need for money would make him vulnerable to my apparent wealth.

"Can I help you find something?" I asked pleasantly. Under pretense of helping him find his book I could lead him down a dead end bookrow. Once I had him trapped I could seduce him with kisses, then drink his blood. I was only a little hungry at the moment, but I believed in taking my dinner when opportunity provided it.

He looked dubiously at me. I was too well dressed to be a librarian. "No thanks, I can find it myself." I thought about pressing him into compliance, but people walked to and fro, their heels clattering on the marble. Bright lights shone down and noises echoed painfully in my sensitive ears. Fragments of conversations jumbled together in a meaningless noise. The racket drowned out the supernatural charm of my voice and eyes. It was too hard a place to work.

"As you like." I shrugged and walked away. Later I would go to a nightclub or bar where willing victims abounded.

I sought out the quietude of the rare book room. It was deserted as usual. I laid my books on a table and began sorting through them. I made three stacks: those to return to the shelves, those to skim now, and those to check out.

A young blond man entered the room and set his books on the next table. He was dressed casually in a black duster and torn blue jeans. His blond hair was cropped short except for his bangs and the hair at the back of his head, which curled in a wispy tail. He sat down at the other table and opened a book. I continued reading.

"You must be speed reader."

I looked up from my book. "Just skimming," I said. "Trying to see if they're worth checking out or not."

He grimaced. "I know what you mean. It's amazing the amount of dreck that has gotten into print."

I nodded. "What are you reading?"

"Oh, old magic books."

I focused my second sight. He remained a young man of nineteen or twenty years and no particular distinction. "Really? Why?"

He smiled ruefully. "I wonder if it works. I read fantasy stories a lot. Sometimes magic seems so silly, but other times it seems like it must be an undiscovered law of nature. So I'm trying to figure out if there's anything to it."

I smiled pleasantly at him. "I can't imagine any subject less likely to yield sensible information."

"Are you interested in the occult?"

"Some," I said. "I lived in Hungary for a while, and belief in certain superstitions was very prominent. One night I saw three men dig up and dismember the corpse of a woman because she had committed suicide, and they were convinced she was rising as a vampire."

"Cool! Was she?"

I shrugged. "Who can say? I never saw her walk." My tale of sadism against the dead delighted him.

"Have you seen anything else?" he asked eagerly.

I pulled my chair up next to him.

"Maybe," I said. "When I was in Hungary a rumor went around that Soviet soldiers were being murdered. Supposedly their throats were ripped out. It was a savage thing, so people thought that no living man could have done it. They said that the soldiers had murdered a man, and that he had risen from the grave to take vengeance on them. After a while the killings stopped, but nobody was ever arrested."

His eyes were shining. "It sounds like a vampire or ghoul. Did any part of them get eaten?"

"Who knows? The murder of soldiers was not printed in the paper. It was thought that such reports would encourage sedition and rebellion. Maybe it was just wild rumor. You know how rumors are."

"Too bad. Wouldn't it be cool to talk to a vampire?"

I smiled slowly. "Now why would you want to do a thing like that?"

He pushed his stack of books away. "Because this is a bunch of mumbo jumbo. But if vampires exist, and they have magical powers like stories say they have, then they could tell me how magic works. I'd really like to know." He stared into space.

"Would knowing be enough, or would you want to do something with the knowledge?" I put my arm across the back of his chair.

"Just knowing would be enough. I'm not into power tripping like some guys who screw around with this stuff. I just want to understand it. I like figuring out how things work. I think it would be cool to use magic as another way of doing stuff, stuff they can't figure out the science for. Like AIDS," he said, noticing the rather bold print on one of my books. "Wouldn't that be cool? Vampires are immune to everything. Maybe their blood could be used to cure AIDS!"

"I rather doubt any vampire would let himself be kept in a lab and milked for his blood," I said dryly.

His face fell. "Maybe they could synthesize it."

I put my hand lightly on his shoulder. "But how long would that take?" He did not know quite what to think of my touch.

"Years and years, I guess." Then the light dawned. "Are you coming on to me?" I dropped my hand. He seemed curious, not offended.

"Yes."

"Oh." He thought about it for a while.

"If you want me to go away, I will," I said carefully. "But I'm enjoying our conversation, and I'd like to talk with you some more." I willed him to look at me, and he did.

"Uh, I'm not sure what to say."

I smiled and put my hand on the back of his chair. " 'Yes,' 'no,' and 'maybe' are the basic options. You can say them as elaborately as you like."

He smiled nervously. "Uh, how about later?"

I smiled. "I'd be delighted."

"Uh, I mean, can I answer later?"

"Maybe."

He blinked, then grinned. "Okay, I get it." He took a moment to untangle his thoughts. "Umm, before I answer, can I ask a question?" I nodded and braced myself.

"Do you have a personal reason for those books on AIDS, or are you just on a fact finding mission?"

"A 'fact finding mission' as you call it." He looked relieved.

"Sorry, I shouldn't have asked anything so personal."

"That's all right, provided I get to ask a personal question in return."

He grinned. "Fair's fair. Shoot."

"What's your name?"

He blushed charmingly. Boys are sweet.

"Anthony. My friends call me 'Mad' Anthony cuz I'm interested in weird stuff."

I offered my right hand. "I'm Rafael. My friends occasionally call me Angel, for similar reasons." He took my hand as if he did not know what to do with it. I squeezed it firmly, then released it.

He shook his fingers. "Strong hand," he said ruefully.

"Sorry. I forget sometimes."

"No problem. Wish I had a grip like that."

I slid nearer to him, each of us aware of the closeness of the other's body. He did not move away. I slipped my arm around his shoulders. He watched me out of the corner of his eye, but he did not cooperate by turning his face to me. I had to be careful to push hard enough but not too hard. I brushed a light kiss across the hair beside his ear.

He smiled crookedly. "That wasn't much of a kiss."

"I can do better."

He looked expectantly at me.

I leaned forward and touched my lips to his. I did not close my eyes, I was watching his reaction. He did not close his eyes either; he was watching me. I brushed my lips gently across his. His lower lip slipped between mine and I sucked it lightly.

His eyes changed as curiosity became interest. He pressed his mouth more firmly against mine. I tasted his lips and my mouth became extraordinary sensitive as my lips swelled slightly. My gums tightened so that I had to lift my head before he felt my fangs move.

"That's kind of nice," he said huskily.

I smiled with a closed mouth. I did not speak. My arms went around him and held him gently. The ribs under his dark coat were lean and lightly muscled. I kissed his cheek with soft lips then nuzzled his ear. My teeth slowly nibbled along the lobe while my warm breath blew softly into his ear.

"Oh wow, that's sexy." I returned to his lips and this time I slipped my tongue into his mouth. He tensed a little and I brought it back. We kissed with the lips for a long time, then his arms went hesitantly around me and his mouth opened. I probed gently with my tongue and his fingers clenched spasmodically on my shoulders. Our tongues slow-danced for a long time before we came up for air.

"You're a good kisser," he said breathlessly.

"I like kissing," I said.

My heart was thumping in eager anticipation. A little more seduction and he would let me do anything I wanted.

I kissed him lightly on each cheek, then pressed my lips to his throat. The sound of the blood rushing through his veins was loud in my ears. I pulled aside his collar and pressed my lips against the triangular muscle joining neck and shoulder. I kissed it, my lips pressing warmly against his skin, then sucked it slowly. Next I nibbled him with my small central teeth, great fangs held in reserve until he was ready for the sacrifice.

"Oh, wow. No girl ever kissed me like that."

"Do you want more?" I asked softly.

"Oh yes!" he breathed eagerly into my ear.

I sank my fangs into his flesh. He gasped and stiffened, then melted against my chest. I sucked the blood greedily from his shoulder, ready to stifle him if he screamed or struggled. Predator instinct urged me to take him to his natural end, to drain him dry of blood and leave his empty husk.

Not again, not murder. I do not need his death! It feels so good! Glut myself on the blood I liked best, give myself the tasty treat of marrow from his broken bones, and perhaps savor the sweetness of his bloody brain; that was what the animal within wanted.

Anthony turned his face to mine and kissed my cheek. I lifted my head and met his eyes.

"You're a—"

"Don't say it!" I hissed.

His eyes were not frightened. Startled, yes, but he showed no fear.

"Wow!" he said enthusiastically. "That was great!"

"You liked it?" I asked in astonishment. Foolish of me, of course he liked it. As long as he was under my spell he would like anything and everything I did to him. "Aren't you afraid of me?" That was the more pertinent question.

"It didn't hurt at all," he said rubbing his shoulder. "It's sort of itchy and numb." His eyes glowed at me. "I knew you weren't really hurting me. It was so kinky, it was great. I want more."

He suddenly realized that my eyes were fixed on the pulse in his throat. He covered it with his hand.

"Will I be all right?"

I eyed him judiciously. I had tired him, but I had not done him irreparable harm. Not yet. "Yes. You might be dizzy when you stand up, but no more." I gave him my best bedroom eyes and waited expectantly. He swayed forward.

"Totally awesome," he murmured, his eyes bright with anticipation.

I cupped his face in my hand and kissed it lightly, then pulled him onto my lap. His legs straddled mine and I felt the heat of his sex against me. That part of a man was always the warmest, and the warmth felt good. I put one hand against the back of his pants and pressed him against me. His arms went around my neck and he kissed me fiercely.

He forced his tongue between my lips and I resisted the reflex action of biting. He traced my teeth with his tongue and sucked my left upper fang. The stimulation aroused me so that my gums tightened into a hard ridge of flesh forcing my fangs out to their fullest length.

"It moves!"

"Like a cat's claw," I purred.

"Cool!" I pressed my lips to his throat and felt the seductive pulsing of his veins. One bite, and I could rip them out. One bite, and he would be mine forever. Like a mother cat with her kitten, I would watch over him, waiting for him to open his eyes. I would nurse him with my blood while I taught him how to hunt, then we would go together into the night, taking whatever prey we pleased.

With an inarticulate cry I set my four fangs against the thick muscle of his shoulder and bit him savagely. He flinched, then bit me back.

A lightning bolt of surprised pleasure shot down my spine and into my groin. I ground my sex against his, writhing between his legs. My mouth groped for his bloody wounds, but not even the taste of blood could obliterate the sensations that rocked me as his teeth tore into my flesh.

"Stop," I murmured drunkenly.

He sucked hard at the wounds he had made in my neck, making noises in his throat like a cat gorging itself.

"Stop," I said weakly.

I did not want to make him stop. I did not have the will to protect him from his own folly. Instead I clamped my hands on his hips while feeling his erection growing against my groin. I longed to strip him out of his clothes and consummate the double desire that coursed through my veins.

Anthony tongued my wound, stimulating new pleasure in me. He kissed it, then bit hard again, and sucked with long hard pulls. My head fell back, exposing my throat to his rapacious fellatio. His lips kissed me from chin to collar, teeth nipping my skin while I sighed with pleasure.

"I...feel...fucking...fantastic!" he pronounced. He did not look tired any more. A trifle pale, but crackling with energy.

"You know that, don't you? It's like being high but better! I feel like I'm in the best shape I've ever been! Like I can run the marathon! Like I can do anything I want to do!"

"Enjoy it while it lasts." I felt a little tired myself, but pleasantly so. I did not bleed readily, and his small teeth were ill suited to drawing blood. He had taken very little from me, but gained much.

"Huh?"

"You're still alive. The effects are only temporary. They won't be permanent until you die, and maybe not even then. It's a fifty-fifty proposition whether death will be fatal or not."

"I'm not—"

"No." I said firmly. "You'll feel a little like it, but you won't change until your heart stops." I tried to find the words to explain it. "It's as if immortality is the body's last desperate attempt to preserve life when there is no hope. Sometimes it works, sometimes it doesn't. You can't count on it."

"Oh. You mean, if I leave here and get run over by a truck, I might rise from the dead and I might not?"

"Exactly."

"No guarantees."

"Worse than that."

"What do you mean?"

"Even if you do rise from the dead, you might be insane." His eyes darkened.

"That's not what I wanted to hear!"

"If you had asked for my blood I would have refused you, just as I have refused all others. But you didn't ask, you took. Now you need to know the consequences."

He looked glum. "The odds aren't so good, are they?"

"If it were certain, or safe, the world would be peopled by nothing but immortals." Anthony climbed off my lap and stood irresolute. "I have all this energy, but I don't know what to do with it. And you tell me that I may have to pay for it by going insane. It'll make me loony wondering what will happen!"

"Why? Whether this had happened or not, your future was uncertain. You have no way of knowing whether you will live out this night or not. Ordinary life is fraught with perils. You might have gone insane anyhow, you might have suffered any number of disasters that deprived you of your mind, your health, your happiness, your ability to earn a living, your love. Even your ability to move or to think.

"What we have done will protect you in some measure from all those disasters. You are more likely to live a long and healthy life than before. And you might or might not have to pay for it after your natural death. It has its benefits."

"You've switched sides! Just a moment ago you were telling me how terrible it was!"

"It is. It carries grave risks. I've seen the carnage wrought by a revenant. If you rise as one of the insatiable undead, I will kill you with my own hands." He read his death in my eyes.

"You've done it before, haven't you?"

"Yes."

He let out a great breath. He rounded on me. "You took the risk. You know all this, and you decided it was worth it. You can't tell me not to do what you have done."

"Mine was a desperate decision. Sit down, and I'll tell you how it was for me."

Anthony turned his chair backwards and straddled it. His eyes were intent on mine. I began to speak.

"In 1949 I accepted a position with the symphony in Budapest. During the rebuilding after World War II it seemed like a good idea to get in on the ground floor of what would become a world class symphony. Their dreams of greatness never quite materialized, and I got a second job teaching keyboard at the university. There I met a man named Valentin. He was half Magyar and half German, and it showed in all the wrong ways. He was tall and rangy, with big hands and prominent knuckles. His nose was Asiatically flat, and his eyes were almond shaped, but blue. He had a shock of wiry red hair that stood out from his head. He was quite the ugliest man I had ever met, and I fell in love with him.

"He requited the sentiment, and we moved into a small

flat in an old house. It was small, but decently equipped. I was happy. The chronic shortages of goods did not bother us because I had money from my family and bought the things we needed on the black market. But the rest of Budapest was restive, chafing at the Communist system that failed to deliver the prosperity and equality it had promised.

"Then came the Revolution of '56. It was as if the politics of the city had spontaneously combusted. The entire population—hundreds of thousands of people—took to the streets and seized government offices and communication facilities. Entire barracks of Communist soldiers stripped off their insignia and joined the people in proclaiming a new democracy. The Russian overlords were suffering a paralysis of will. They took no action.

"Valentin was filled with revolutionary fire. He hardly slept. He stayed up all night writing editorials and flyers on his old typewriter. The next day he used the school's mimeograph machine to copy them. Then we walked about the city passing them out. Everywhere we went people surrounded us begging us for news. With the lifting of Communist censorship information came in a flood, and the people drank it up like thirsty men in the desert. Rumors were rife. The West was sending troops to defend us; the United Nations was going to recognize our government. We were not sure who our government was, but we rejoiced anyhow.

"I did not care about politics, I cared about Valentin, so I happily helped him do what he believed in. For a few heady days we walked and talked freely. We even walked arm in arm in public. I laughed at him and said, 'If you like it so much, you should move West.' He refused. 'My country is free now. At last I have no reason to leave and every reason to remain.' Our freedom lasted seven days. No help came from the West. The Red Army rolled in. Tanks smashed the barricades. Nothing and no one could stop the red juggernaut. Step by step, block by block the Communists reclaimed their rebellious city. I begged Valentin to flee, begged him to go West with me to my family in Spain.

"'They cannot arrest us all,' he said. 'We were hundreds of thousands. They cannot arrest us all.'

"'No,' I said angrily. 'Only the writers of editorials and the publishers of newspapers, the ones who threw the censors into the streets. You know they know who we are and what we have done.'

"We were sitting at our little kitchen table debating the issue over dinner when a heavy knock sounded on our door. When I opened it I saw three large men in overcoats. I slammed the door and held it shut as they kicked against it. 'Run, Valentin! It's the secret police!' A gun fired. The bullet burst through the door amid a hail of splinters and struck me in the chest. The door flew open and knocked me sprawling. I lay stunned. I could not move; I was possessed by pain. I could not even close my eyes. Valentin dropped to his knees at my side, but they grabbed him away from me.

"'You'll end up dead like him if you don't tell us what we want to know.'

"'He's not dead! He's looking at me!' The two thugs beat him into silence, but the officer nudged me with his toe.

"'Right through the heart,' said the officer. 'A lucky shot. Unlucky for him though.' They laid him on his belly on the table and handcuffed his wrists to the legs. His head was hanging over the end where I could see it, but I could make no motion to show him I lived. The officer cut his clothes off with a kitchen knife. The officer was deliberately careless—and he smiled as he worked. Valentin refused to cry out as his blood ran down his body, then dripped over the edge of the table to splatter on the floor.

"The officer said, 'You're a pervert. I imagine you'll enjoy what I have planned for you.' Then Valentin cried hoarsely and fought his bonds. I could not see what the officer was doing, but I was afraid I knew.

"'Now, who were your accomplices?' Valentin was silent, his breath coming raggedly. Suddenly he jerked, straining against his bonds to get as far away from the officer as possible, but unable to escape. 'Who were your accomplices?' the officer asked in cold glee.

"Valentin wept. 'Arman Nagy.'

"'Who else?' He made no answer. The sound of dripping blood was loud in the silence.

"'Mikhail Frent!' Valentin suddenly shrieked, tears coursing down his face as his body jerked. The cords of his muscles stood up and his veins showed purple.

"'Who else?' He answered all their questions, condemning everyone we knew to the same fate we were suffering.

"I hated them for hurting him, hated them for making me helpless and letting me live to see what they were doing to him. Worst of all, I hated the way they diminished him in my eyes. As unconsciousness claimed me I swore that it would not finish me. No matter if I had to come back from the grave itself, I would rise and take vengeance on them. I would destroy them as savagely as they had destroyed me.

"I awoke several days later. The first thing I saw was Valentin's body lying on the floor next to me. They had killed him by inserting the knife in his anus and drawing it up through his genitals and belly, up to the base of his breastbone where they plunged it in. His entrails spilled out. Maggots were hatching in his mouth.

"I rolled away in violent revulsion, then brushed frantically at my body until I realized no insects were crawling on me. I kept my back to Valentin's loathsome corpse while I opened my shirt. My wound was firmly scabbed over, with no sign of infection or infestation. I gingerly felt my breastbone. It was intact; but I was sure it had broken when the bullet struck me.

"I was hungry...very hungry. I smelled the old blood staining the kitchen and turned slowly to look at Valentin's body. Flies crawled in the black blood and I felt desire. Fangs slid into my mouth, startling me. I explored them with my tongue, felt my eyeteeth longer and sharper than they had been.

"I knew then what I had become. It suited me. I would be their angel of death, bringing them vengeance and terror.

"I killed several Russian soldiers that night. I glutted myself on their blood and did not try to conceal the nature of their deaths. I wanted them to know that someone they had wronged had come back from the dead to avenge the horrors they had perpetrated.

"For three years I slept in abandoned buildings, or dank cellars, or attics or old warehouses or anywhere. I lived a bleak existence until my desire for revenge withered and my love for Valentin wore so thin I could no longer tolerate the country he loved. I fled West."

I stopped speaking. Anthony stared at me with mesmerized eyes. At last he stirred.

"Awesome," he said feelingly. "I'm glad I met you. You can bite my neck anytime."

I had corrupted him, but I did not feel guilty about it. I had lifted the veils from his eyes and shown him the beauty and the danger of the world of darkness. It was the beauty of the tiger and the eagle, swift predators who were at their most magnificent while they hunted. Who could not adore the lethal grace of the raptor floating in the sky, or the indomitable leap of the tiger as he landed on the back of his frightened prey? He was young to make such a dire choice, but he had made it of his own free will. All young people had to make the irrevocable decisions that tipped them into adulthood, ready or not.

I stopped at a florist on the way home, and ordered thirteen red roses to be sent to Anthony's dormitory room. On the card I wrote, ROSES WOULD NOT BE ROSES WITHOUT THE THORNS. R.

Chapter Seven
KISS AND MAKE UP

Yet dearly I love You, and would be loved in fain,
But I am betrothed to Your enemy.
Divorce me, untie or break that knot again;
Take me to You, imprison me, for I,
Except You enthrall me, never shall be free,
Nor ever chaste except Thou ravish me.
—John Donne

Baltimore, 12 October 1991

I sat at my desk with my back to the bay window, the louvers cracked enough to let the air flow through but blocking the sun. It was of those glorious days of autumn that lied and said the recent cold spell was just a passing temper; the romance of summer was still alive. A carafe of cut crystal held orange juice, its facets casting diamonds of light across my desk. I was dining lightly tonight as I was not especially hungry. I supposed I should be out finding something to eat anyhow, but the day was too beautiful to taint with such bloody deeds. Later, after dark, I would go hunting.

I rolled up my white sleeves to avoid smearing them with ink, then penned a letter of inquiry to Sheridan and Sons, my former publisher. I advised them of my "death," and offered them the opportunity to publish works from my private collection. I anticipated a positive reply—there was nothing like dying to enhance a composer's career. For a few months after his demise he would be honored with a flurry of performances while everybody belatedly remembered what a genius he was; then he would slip back into obscurity. My body of work was too small to garner much acclaim by itself; I wanted the fifteen minutes of fame Andy Warhol said was due me.

A tune started tapping at the back of my mind. In sudden resolution I gathered up the scattered pages and laid them aside. I fetched clean staff paper and started making notes. Tomorrow I would tend to things as prosaic as dinner. Today let me answer the Muse.

I had written five pages of an Italian style sonata when I heard the front door open. I smiled. Michael was home. "Upstairs!" I called.

I added several more measures of music in the time it took him to mount the stairs. His footsteps were slow, which did not bode well. I wondered what was wrong.

"You're up early," came an unexpected voice.

"James!" I exclaimed. It was a shock to see him standing in the doorway when I had expected Michael. He had a Boston fern in his hand. His trench coat was open showing a light weight gray suit and conservative blue and gray striped tie. The brown leather creaked as I sat back in my chair.

"Hello," I said. "Yes. I like the sunshine."

"That's new."

"Time changes all of us."

"It does indeed." He stepped up to the desk and extended the plant to me. "I know how much you like plants, so I brought you this."

"Thank you. It's lovely," I took the basket in my hands. The scent of fresh greenery filled my nostrils with a pleasant perfume and I inhaled deeply. For a moment I was filled with nostalgia for days gone by. "Do you remember," I asked, "the orchids I used to have?"

He slowly shrugged out of his coat and laid it over the arm of the sofa. "Yes, and the roses, too," he said as if the memory pained him. "I thought about you every moment I laid in that hospital bed." I was wary of his motives for coming, especially when he thought I had been asleep. But if he wanted a reconciliation, I was willing to listen.

"I wasn't trying to kill you," I said.

"I know. I'd be dead if you were. Frankly, I'm surprised I'm not. It gives me hope that maybe we can settle our differences peacefully."

"Maybe," I said.

He hesitated, then said quietly. "I'm sorry about all the rude things I said to you. And I'm sorry that I hurt you. Are you all right?"

"Yes. I've recovered."

He settled on the sofa. His gray-blond hair contrasted strongly with the dark brown leather. "It was cruel of you to leave me for so long, and crueler still to return when I'd gotten used to living without you."

"It was cruel of you to pillage my property and reduce me to penury!"

"I'm prepared to make restitution."

I raised my eyebrows. I knew well that what he intended one moment could be erased in the fury of another. I needed a moment to think before I answered, so I climbed onto the window seat and hung up the plant. Hooks still remained from the plants I had had before. While I was up I opened the top third of the shutters. Light washed across the ceiling, lightening the room further.

When I climbed down I rested my hand on the back of my chair and asked cautiously, "Just what did you have in mind?"

He rose, came around the end of the desk, and held out a silver key chain. The prancing pony flashed in the sunlight.

"Are those the keys to my Ferrari?" I asked in sudden hope.

"Yes. It's a classic car now. I've insured it for two million."

My jaw dropped. "You're joking."

He picked up my hand, put the keys into it. "I never joke about money." He pulled a packet of papers from his pocket and thrust them at me. "I've had it restored and paid six months insurance on it. It's registered to Rafael Junior. I assumed you'd be using your new identity."

I accepted the papers and dropped into my chair. I went through the forms carefully. An appraisal paper was tucked in with them, and showed an estimated auction value of two million dollars. The insurance was made out for the same amount. "Where is it?" I asked eagerly.

"Look out the window." I tore open the rest of the shutters, then threw up the sash, ignoring the brilliant sunlight bathing my head and shoulders making them tingle. My car was parked along the edge of the park, its top down. Black paint gleamed and the white leather seats glowed.

James stepped beside me and laid a hand on my shoulder. The smell of his pipe tobacco swirled around me, appealing to the most primitive part of my brain. "A 1972 Ferrari GT/S—original, not conversion. Only a hundred and twenty-seven of them were ever made. Lots of hard top Daytonas have been converted since then, but they don't fetch the same price as the original Spiders."

"I can't believe it," I said. "I bought the car because it was fun to drive. I never thought it would be worth a fortune."

"I never drove it," he said enviously.

"Why not?" He dropped his hand from my shoulder, and I pulled my head in and closed the window and shutters. My face burned. I put my palms against it and felt the stiff tenderness of my skin. I had sunburned already.

"It was your car. Whenever I looked at it, I could feel you invisibly hovering over me, watching me. I knew you'd be angry if I drove it without your permission."

I crossed my arms. "You have a remarkably selective conscience. My car and house you leave to me, but everything else you take."

"I told you I didn't intend to keep it. I just borrowed it." He pulled another paper from his pocket. "Sign this and you're an equal partner in the Shannon Laboratory."

I took the papers and sat down at my desk with them. "What is it?"

"A blood bank and research laboratory. You sign this, you don't pay one penny, but you get all the blood you want. Not bovine blood like Lonny sold you, but human blood. All legal, clean, and free. As much as you like. We sell blood to hospitals and private patients to make money. You draw a salary; I put up the money to make it work." I skimmed through it while he spoke. The document was remarkably straightforward considering that James had drafted it. "What's the research?" He got down on his knees before me. "You are. You're immune to everything. Or so you think. We can test that in the laboratory and let you know if there's anything you need to worry about. But more importantly, by studying your blood we learn more about how disease and aging work, and how a body—your body—protects itself from them. Then we figure out how to duplicate it in the laboratory. Think of it. There are a million and a half HIV-positives in the United States alone. And each of them would be willing to pay a thousand dollars so he didn't have to die of AIDS. That's a billion and a half dollars." I boggled at the thought of a billion and a half dollars.

"Your blood holds the secret. Give it to us and you will be rich beyond belief."

I dropped back against the chair. "It's not just immunity.

It's a dozen things all wrapped up together. Some good, some bad, some terrible."

"Salk invented the polio vaccine by killing the polio virus and injecting it into healthy people. We can do the same. There is a whole new science that can manipulate things, separate them into their pieces, and reassemble them without the side effects. We can make it work."

A lab of which I was part owner of would not be able to exploit me like a government agency, or other institution. "Yes, if we look, there must be many ways to make positive use of what I am," I said thoughtfully.

"You'll do it?"

"We would need strict security. My blood is dangerous stuff. We don't want the janitor deciding to make himself immortal."

"It will be secret and secure. You can be sure of that."

"Well, then, assuming we can work it out satisfactorily, yes." I signed.

He took the paper and separated it into two copies. He left one on my desk and folded the other into his pocket. "What about us?" he asked, his sky blue eyes searching mine, his blond hair a pale halo about his head.

"That depends. Are you still angry with me?"

He sighed and his shoulders slumped in defeat. "No. I'm sorry I hurt you. You know I wouldn't have flown into such a passion if I didn't care for you." His hand slid onto my knee. "You know you're the most important thing in the world to me, and I want you back."

"I'm not an ordinary man, and I can't live by ordinary rules. I won't put up with your jealousy when my survival is at stake."

His brow darkened. "I don't care about the ones that are just food," he said sullenly.

I stroked his cheek while I considered how hard I could

push him on this point and where I would be forced to compromise. "You've offered me all the food I can eat, and I'll take it. But from time to time I will go hunting on my own, and you will not question me about what I do."

His jaw set stubbornly.

"Hunting men, you mean."

"I will not tolerate any discussion of the subject."

His eyes smoldered with rebellion. "I already said I don't care about the ones that are just food. If you want to play with your food before you eat it, well, I don't care about that either. But I won't tolerate any rivals for your affection."

Coldly I weighed Michael against James. Michael was a highly ornamental young man whose company I enjoyed, but he was my nephew. If he ever discovered what sort of fantasies I harbored about him, he would run screaming. It was my own lonely, hungry, sex-starved existence that made him such a tempting target. If I accepted James' offer, life would become much easier. I would have all I wanted to eat, and almost as much sex as I wanted. (Nobody ever got all the sex they wanted, they did not have the stamina.) I would have the income necessary to support my musical studies and composition without the exigencies of finances most musicians suffered.

With a feeling of exhilaration I realized that I had done it: James was firmly under my thumb again. He was obsessed with me, and would not willingly part from me. From time to time he might be angry with me, but in the long run he would have to please me for fear of losing me.

"That sounds fair to me," I said graciously.

He kissed me then, his lips moving against mine in a sensuous slow dance. I cooperated with his lip choreography and the kiss intensified. My lips parted and his tongue plunged into my mouth. He supported my head with his hand while his tongue probed the soft warm flesh inside my mouth. He toyed with my fangs, licking them and sucking them until they extended.

We kissed a long time, then James slipped his hand inside my shirt. He found the bump of my nipple and tweaked it. "Umm," I said involuntarily. My nipple was the "on" switch for a line of electricity that ran straight to my groin. The nipple grew hard as he played with it, and the same signal was transmitted to my cock. He moved his hand to my other nipple, and fire burned through me.

He caught my shirt front in both hands, then yanked them apart. Buttons flew and I laughed. I shrugged out of the shirt and it fell heedlessly to the floor. He bent his head and fastened his mouth to my nipple, sucking with slow, hungry motions while I closed my eyes and moaned in delight. My trousers felt intolerably tight.

He kissed my neck with slow wet kisses. I lifted my chin and he kissed the front of my throat, then worked his way along my jaw. His tongue dipped into the shell of my ear and tickled it, then he blew softly on it. "Ung," I said, and tightened my grip on him.

He slid his thigh between mine while his hands on my ass pulled me forward. I ground my hot sex against his thigh and groaned for him. He held my ass tightly as I humped his leg again and again. He moaned and answered my movements with thrusts of his own. We found the rhythm and clung to each other while we did nature's oldest dance. I groaned and my arms around his shoulders tightened further.

"No so hard!" he complained.

"Sorry," I murmured. In the grip of passion I had forgotten how fragile mortals were. I loosened my embrace.

"Put your hands behind your neck," he whispered with dry lips.

I obeyed. The prospect of sexual discipline excited me

unbearably. James had always been good at it. He unbuckled my belt and pulled down my pants. My erect cock sprang free of my trousers.

"Stand up," he said.

I stood, and he stripped off my shoes and pants so that I stood naked before him.

"Kneel," he said. I knelt.

"Follow me." He walked from my office to my room and I followed on my knees, eager as an animal and not the least bit embarrassed. I understood the game. We stopped in the middle of the green and gold and cream rug that covered my bedroom floor.

"Kneel up." I sat up, legs folded under me, and my weight pressing my ass against the hard bones of my feet. I clasped my hands behind my neck in the prisoner's stance.

"Close your eyes." I did. I heard him pull the toy box from underneath my bed. I wondered what he would bring. Handcuffs? Rope? Clothespins? After what he had done to me last time, did I dare let him play this game again? James returned. He placed a padded leather blindfold over my eyes and tied it behind my head. A perfect choice. I could defend myself if I had to; I was not bound in any way. Yet the blindfold was a powerful psychological restraint. My breaths came in long hard inhalations.

James moved my hands from my neck to the small of my back. "Don't touch the blindfold." The leather tip of a riding crop caressed my shoulders, then caressed my collarbone and slid up my neck. With it he lifted my chin, my pigtail falling far down my back as I tilted my face upward in compliance with his nonverbal command. I was not in the mood for a whipping, but said nothing. I waited to see what game he had planned for me.

The crop traced a line down the center of my chest. It

crossed my breastbone without deviating to either nipple, paused to rim my navel in delicious promise of what else it might do, then caressed my balls, making me quiver. It rubbed lightly along my tall cock while I shuddered and gasped. It slid lower and went between my legs, brushing past my perineum.

Suddenly the cold metal handle of the crop pressed against my anus. My hips moved as I tried to climb onto it. "Stand still," he said authoritatively. He drew a cold line down the inside of my thigh. I groaned loudly in frustration and my hands dropped between my legs.

"Don't touch," he warned me. I turned my blind face towards him and groped in his direction. He walked away. I dropped to all fours on the floor, panting and reaching out for him.

"Kneel up," he said firmly.

I knelt up and placed my hands behind my back again. I locked my fingers together to try to keep the discipline. A wide hard cuff went around my left thigh. He buckled it into place then took hold of my left arm and guided it down. He buckled my wrist against the outside of my thigh. He put its mate on my right leg, and guided my right hand into the restraint. My hands were now imprisoned at my sides.

I pulled futilely at the restraints. They were the padded black Kevlar ones I had made myself; I could not break them. They could be removed in a couple of other ways so I was not trapped. I relaxed. Now that I was securely bound I could let loose and enjoy sex without fear of breaking the furniture or hurting James.

I heard him rummaging through the toybox again. What would he bring this time? More restraints? A vibrator? Hot wax? A feather! I jumped and squirmed as the plume brushed the inside of my leg. Its touch was so light I scarcely knew I felt it, yet the effect on my super alert nerves was indescribable. Muscles jumped and twitched and I cried, "Not the feather!" I retreated, backing hastily across the thick rug. James followed, the feathery tips brushing against my balls and cock. I rolled onto my back with my legs folded in front of me to protect me from the excessive stimulation. The feather brushed my ankle and I kicked violently, narrowly missing James.

The feather touched my ribs and I rolled onto that side. Then the feather touched my derriere, and I put my hands over as much of it as I could reach. The feather dipped into my belly button, sending me into thrashing spasms. I jerked away and rolled face down with my knees crouched under me. The feather did not pursue.

I caught my breath while I realized my tail was in the air and my face was pressed against the rug. James knelt behind me, and I thought he was going to coit me. I was ready for it, I wanted it. I spread my legs with a groan of desire.

He buried his face in my ass, his tongue probing for Sodom's gate. I let out a long inarticulate cry as his tongue found its way to the center of my wrinkled flesh and thrust. He sucked my asshole, then bit the flesh on either side of it. I banged my head against the floor and my feet kicked wildly while I wailed in pleasure. James withdrew.

"You're kicking like a maiden mare, and I think we'll have to restrain you the same way we do the mares."

I grew up on a farm. When the mares fought the studs, we hobbled their legs to the sides of the stall so that they could neither kick nor escape. I let out a long moan.

James rolled me onto to my back. "I'll be good," I said.

"I doubt it," he replied. "You're wild tonight. We'll do it my way because I really don't want to get my skull caved in." He grasped me under the arms and dragged me to the bed. "Bend over," he said. "Farther." He pushed my face against the bed, his hand heavy on my neck. The blindfold did not fit tightly next to my nose and I saw a sliver of yellow coverlet. He slapped my rump. "Stay put, or I'll hog-tie you."

"Yes, sir." I remained quiet while he knelt behind me and fastened ankle cuffs to my legs. They were of the same manufacture as the cuffs that bound my hands and thighs.

"Straighten your legs. Spread them. Wider."

Breath came hard and fast as I obeyed. I felt incredibly exposed and vulnerable, and I desperately wanted James to exploit my vulnerability. He clipped a double-ended hook to the left ankle cuff and the eyebolt in the bedpost. Then he restrained my other leg the same way. George had helped me install those bolts a long time ago; they would not pull out no matter how I fought them.

James stroked the insides of my legs, and they quivered.

"I've had a fantasy about you," he said softly. "I've dreamed that I had you tied down and helpless, and then I got you all hot and horny like now, and you begged me to make me yours. So I put rings in your nipples, and one in your balls, and you screamed and cried, 'Oh yes, James.' Then I clipped silver chains to your rings and you followed me wherever I went, and you were happy to do it."

I did not like where this fantasy might lead. "You don't have to do that to get my cooperation."

"No, I don't, do I?" He sounded pleased with himself. "Just this." He pressed his face against my rump again and slowly licked my anal cleft from top to bottom. I wiggled and panted and jerked in my bonds while he licked with slow, devoted motions. His lips, tongue and teeth teased my anus unmercifully while I shouted wordlessly and my legs kicked futilely. His tongue thrust against the tight opening and I longed for him to force his way into my body. I went into a paroxysm of yelling and kicking and writhing, my mind blank to all else.

If only it were Michael instead of James.

If only we were doing this for love, not money.

I began to fantasize.

It was a hot summer day on the plain before the walls of Troy. I was a prisoner of a group of Trojans. They stripped the golden corselet off my body, my white tunic snagging and coming with it, golden brooches torn from the fabric laying glinting in the dust. I was kneeling before them clad only in golden greaves and vambraces.

"This one's too pretty to put to work in the fields," said one of my captors. He addressed the tall captain, whose face was covered by his helmet. "You should chain him to your bed for your pleasure."

"Maybe," said somebody else. "Just because he has a pretty face doesn't mean he'll be any good in bed."

The tall one looked down silently at me, and I looked up at him. I did not want to end up as an ordinary slave, toiling in the fields until my back was broken and my looks were burnt away by the relentless sun.

The tall one gestured for me to turn around, and I did. His mailed hand fell heavily on the back of my neck as he bent me over the tail of his chariot. Armored hands grabbed my legs and pulled them apart, ropes binding my ankles to the wheels. Then they grabbed my hands and pressed my arms to my sides, binding my hands firmly to my thighs.

I looked behind me and saw half a dozen warriors lined up, and wondered how many of them would take me. My cock was painfully hard, and I was frightened—frightened that I would not please. I did not want to go to the fields.

The leader doffed his helmet and I saw who he was.

"Michael!" I cried.

As soon as I said it I knew I erred.

"Who in the hell is Michael?" James demanded furiously.

"Nobody," I panted, trying to catch my breath. "Just a fantasy." James had an Irish temper that was not so easily mollified. He grabbed hold of my testicles.

"Ouch!"

"Tell me."

I did not struggle. "I'm sorry, James," I said as contritely as I could manage. "My mind wandered."

He squeezed hard. I yelped.

"I know you. Where your mind wanders, your ass follows. I will not tolerate any competition! Do you understand? You are damn well going to be faithful to me if I have to nail your balls to the floor!"

"Yes, sir," I replied docilely.

"Who is Michael?"

"My cousin." His yanked on my balls as if he would rip them off. It hurt and I screamed unabashedly.

"Don't lie to me. You haven't got any cousins. Your family disowned you years ago!"

"They didn't! He is!"

"Your mother pronounced you anathema and cut off your allowance when you failed to show up for your father's funeral. None of your family want anything to do with you."

"Papa is dead?" I asked in bewilderment.

"And your mother too. She died within a year of him." He sounded smug.

"When?"

"Eighty-one."

"You were supposed to wake me if anything important happened!"

"What do you care?" he sneered. "You never cared about anybody but yourself!"

"They're my parents! How can you think I don't care about my parents?"

He picked up the riding crop and thrashed me across the rump. "You're a liar and a lecher and a leech!"

I twisted the thigh cuffs so that my hands were between my legs. I could reach the buckles of the left restraint with the fingers of my right hand.

James kneed me in the crotch, smashing my hands and balls together. I yelled in pain, writhing helplessly in my restraints.

"Put them back or I'll kick you again!" he threatened.

I twisted my hands to the outside and lay still. At the moment he had the advantage, but in another thirty seconds I would be free and I would throttle him.

A rap sounded on my door. "Rafael, are you all right?"

We froze. "Who's that?" James demanded.

"Michael," I said miserably.

"What's he doing here?"

"Visiting."

He kneed me hard. I let loose a soprano shriek that rattled the windowpanes.

"You two-timing bitch!" he swore. Crack! He laid another stripe across my ass. "You lying whore!" Crack! "No rivals!" Crack! "Do you understand me?" Crack!

I groaned a wordless answer. Suddenly the door crashed open, then flesh hit flesh. Michael had come to my rescue. The struggle continued with the sound of thumps and scuffles and James' ragged breathing. I rubbed my face frantically against the coverlet until the blindfold slipped down around my neck.

I looked over my shoulder. Michael was between James and me, standing with his back straight, legs flexed, and hands up in classic martial arts pose. James picked himself off the floor and put his hands up to box.

"Don't hit him!" I called, but they ignored me.

"So you're Rafael's new bimbo," James taunted him.

"I'm not a bimbo," Michael said. "I'm his cousin."

"Liar!" James spat. "I know him! You're the kind of pretty boy he eats for dinner!" I twisted the cuffs again and reached for the first buckle.

"I think you'd better leave," Michael said evenly.

Suddenly James lunged forward, trying to push past Michael to get to me. Michael grabbed him and twisted his arm behind his back. James struggled, but Michael had him locked in a hold he could not break.

James glowered at me. "You bitch queen! You can't cheat on me and get away with it!" The sight of his disordered suit and lumpy body hanging from Michael's hand like some great gray fish disgusted me.

"Throw the garbage out, Michael." Michael let him down.

"You'll be sorry, you cocksucking asshole!" James hissed at me as he grabbed his coat. "I'll get even with both of you!"

"Stupid prick," I muttered in reply.

Michael escorted James downstairs. I heard him yell, "And don't come back!" then the front door slammed. A moment later he came back up the steps two at a time.

He stopped dead in the doorway, surveying my position. "That's quite a predicament you've gotten yourself into," he said blandly.

The hooks held my legs apart, clearly displaying my anus, perineum, scrotum, and penis. Heat curled through my groin. I felt my cock move slightly and knew I was getting hard again. Two points of heat burned my cheeks.

"I didn't hear you come home," I said in a low voice.

He threw back his head and peals of laughter rang out like a great golden bell. "I heard you!" he replied merrily.

The blush spread until my whole face was burning. "Either let me loose, or finish what you interrupted," I said tartly.

He stepped closer to me. "Do you mean that?" I was incredibly hot, my cock and anus aching for the consummation that James had promised but not delivered.

"Yes," I answered hoarsely.

He put a hand on my left hip. I writhed under his touch. "I heard you today," he said softly, "and I envied you. I've never had sex so good it made me scream." His hand gently clenched on my sweating ass.

"I haven't either," I groaned. "It was all foreplay."

"Foreplay makes you yell like that?"

"Everything makes me yell."

"Even this?" He bent and kissed my back.

The touch of his lips against my skin stopped my breath and blanked my mind. He lifted his lips and I breathed again. "That's not where I want to be kissed," I said hotly.

His knees thumped on the floor behind me. He pulled me back to make room, then put his head between my legs and began worshiping at the altar of Eros.

He started by licking my short-haired balls. He sucked one into his mouth, then the other one. He licked a line up the center, following the prominent vein up onto my cock all the way to the head. I groaned deeply as he sucked the prepuce between his lips. Little by little the length of my penis disappeared into the hot moist hole of his mouth. I bent my knees to press myself into his face, but he moved with me, and I was not any deeper than I had started. I cried in frustration, and my hands tore uselessly at the coverlet.

Michael lifted his mouth, his hot breath brushing across my skin while his hand stroked my ass. My legs tensed and my ass quivered as he reminded me that other parts of my body were equally sensitive. I groaned with pleasure as his finger caressed my anus.

"Do you like that?" he whispered.

"Oh, yes," I moaned.

I could smell his readiness, his musky male lust. He unzipped his pants then rubbed his rigid flesh up and down between the hemispheres of my ass. My fangs unsheathed themselves in answer.

"Please," I begged. I wanted everything he could give me.

He set the tip of his hard flesh against my anus, and I tensed with anticipation. He braced his feet, then thrust gently, his hands on my hips to steady us.

"Harder!" I cried.

He thrust a little more forcefully.

"Harder!" I cried again.

He braced his boots more firmly against the floor and leaned into me.

"Oh, harder!" I cried as great waves of passion rolled through me.

"I don't want to hurt you."

"Don't hold back! Never hold back!"

Even though I cried for more, Michael did not give it to me. He paced himself so that he would last, instead of giving in to my incoherent urgings for instant gratification. I writhed wildly, shrieking and crying in animal pleasure while he groaned over my back.

I bucked hard against him, orgasm rippling so intensely through my body that I almost shook him loose. He held tight, and I bucked again, muscles tightening and unclenching in unstoppable arousal. Michael bit my back, and the feel of his teeth against my flesh sent me into another screaming paroxysm. My fangs extended to their fullest length and I longed to sink them into his flesh. I bit the coverlet furiously.

Michael nipped me three more times across my shoulder blades, then thrust with quick hard strokes. My back arched as I felt the tide of passion carrying him to the crest of desire, and I rose with him, wailing like a banshee as his body slammed into mine. He gave a wordless cry as he spurted in me, and I felt the heat of it inside me. The intimacy of it sent me into orgasmic frenzy, thrashing and crying incoherently until at last I collapsed gasping for breath. Michael lay heavily along my back, sweat dripping from his body to mine.

"Is it my imagination or did you have multiple orgasms?" he asked.

"I did."

"I thought only women could do that." I laughed.

"That's why anal sex is so much fun. Ejaculation isn't everything." In my case, it was nothing at all.

He took a deep breath, then raised himself off me. I moaned regretfully. He zipped his pants, then bent and caught my left ankle in his hand. I gasped, but he merely unhooked it. He freed my other foot, and I rested while he unbuckled the restraints from my thighs and wrists. I kept my face turned away from him while I massaged my wrists and waited for my fangs to retract. He lay on his side on the bed in front of me.

I smiled at him with a carefully closed mouth. "That was fabulous," I murmured.

He smiled gently. "I've never done anything like that before. It was fun. Kinky, but fun." His hazel eyes were large and serious, as if something was bothering him.

Worry cooled my ardor rapidly. "I'm glad we did it," I told him earnestly. I did not want him to feel guilty or dirty. "I've been wanting to do it ever since I first laid eyes on you."

He nodded in understanding. "I've been dreaming about you every night. Wet dreams," he clarified with a trace of embarrassment. "Today when I came home, I could hear you clearly, and it made me so horny. Then I had this most intense fantasy about tying you up and raping you." He looked ashamed to admit it.

"You can't rape a willing victim."

He laid his hand tenderly against my cheek. "I don't want to ever hurt you. I can't believe I even thought such things."

I crawled forward and leaned my head against his chest with a blissful smile. His arm went around my shoulders. "Don't worry, fantasies aren't reality," I reassured him. "We fantasize about a lot of things we would never do. Do you like action movies?"

"Yes."

"Would you actually take a machine gun and mow down a bunch of mobsters? Or blow up cars, or houses, or any of the other things they do in movies?"

He quirked a smile. "Probably not. I can't imagine anything anybody could do that would make me that angry. It would be another matter if somebody tried to hurt my sister. If somebody tried to rape her, I'd shoot him in the balls."

"Naturally. You and I are sane. We can tell the difference between entertainment and reality. Whether it's on the silver screen or in the privacy of our own minds doesn't matter. We act according to what we know about the real world, not according to our fantasies."

He took a deep breath. "One of my fantasies just came true."

I laughed. "And several of mine." More soberly I said, "But not all of them do. We're not animals that act on whatever urge we feel at the moment." My conscience gave a twinge, signifying that it had not quite atrophied into nonexistence. It hurt me to realize I was a hypocrite.

He relaxed a little. We lay together in companionable

silence for a couple of moments, then he said, "I have a question."

"Yes?"

"Who did I throw out?"

I looked blankly at him.

"Have you forgotten already? I horned in on your party!"

"Oh. Him. James, my lawyer."

He raised an eyebrow. "He has a funny way of conducting business."

"It's a funny relationship."

"I think you should get a new lawyer."

I sighed heavily. "I can't afford it."

He gave me a sharp look. "You're rich, it should be no problem for you."

I bit my lip. "Not any more. James embezzled every cent of mine."

"Jesus, Rafael! He robs you and you go to bed with him?"

"I was trying to sweet talk him into returning the money. It was working, too," I retorted.

He grabbed hold of my pigtail and pulled it. "Earth to Rafael, Earth to Rafael. On this planet getting your ass whipped means you lost. He's not gonna give you your money back." He let go of my hair. "Or if he did, it would be at the rate of a hundred dollars a lay. You don't need that bullshit. Let the police handle him."

"I can't."

"Why not?"

"I'm legally dead. Not a judge in the land would believe I'm sixty-five year old Rafael Guitierrez. The only way I can get my money back is by creating invincible proof that I'm the dead man's son, and inherit the money. The court action will take years and cost a fortune. I was working on

James personally because I could save a lot of time, money, and effort if I could persuade him to do the honorable thing."

Michael reached into his pant's pocket. "I doubt he'll do the honorable thing, so I will." He stuffed a wad of green bills into my hand.

"What's this?"

"Most of the money you gave me. I'm buying my painting back. I can get the rest of the money when I go to New York and turn in the Gorman commission."

His suggestion shocked me. "No! I bought it, and I never welsh on a deal!" I shoved it back at him.

"It's twelve hundred dollars, Rafael. If you need it, you can have it. Maybe George will take the painting."

I gave him a black look. "You will not sell my painting to George!" When Michael did not accept the money I stuffed it in the waistband of his jeans. He changed tactics.

"You have to let me pay my share of the rent and utilities as long as I'm here."

"How long are you planning on staying?"

"As long as I can persuade you not to throw me out."

"That's a long time."

He grinned and pulled the crumpled bills out of his pants. "How much for rent and utilities?"

"No rent. I own the house free and clear." Provided James had not monkeyed with the deed. "I haven't received all the bills for the month, so I don't know what utilities will run," I hedged.

He peeled off five hundred dollars. "Here. If it comes to more, let me know." I accepted the money, but I did not promise to ask for more.

He stuck out his hand. "Deal?"

I accepted his hand and gave it a warm squeeze. "Deal."

I was crazy to let him stay with me, but I did it anyhow.

Chapter Eight
RUSSIAN ROULETTE

There is a land of the living and a land of the dead
and the only bridge is love, the only survival, the
only meaning.
—Thornton Wilder

Baltimore, 12 October 1992; Roland Park, 1976

Michael hopped out of bed. "Let's go eat."

"How can you think of food at a time like this?" Though
truth to tell, I was hungry myself. The little I had taken from
Anthony the night before was not adequate. Still, Michael
and I had very different ideas as to what comprised "dinner."

"Let's go!" He swung his legs out of bed.

I rolled indolently in the sheets, casting a calculating
glance at the shutters. If I dawdled, the sun would be safely
below the rooftops before I stepped outside. I lay naked
before him, hand on hip, pelvis cocked suggestively forward.
"Are you sure you want to go out?" I asked saucily. "We
could eat in."

He hesitated, then his eyes crinkled in a smile. "Yes, I
need a little time to absorb what's happened. And I am
hungry; I'll think better after I've eaten."

I pouted. "Thinking is not a virtue. It distracts from more

interesting activities." His stomach rumbled. "Sorry. I skipped lunch, and I haven't had supper yet. If you want to keep my strength up, you have to feed me."

"I'd be delighted to keep you up all night." My lewd smile left no doubt as to my meaning.

He laughed. "I don't doubt it." Still grinning I rose slowly, stretching and flexing for his benefit, whipcord muscles cracking.

"You're so skinny," he said, shaking his head.

"I'm not skinny, I'm lean," I said in annoyance. "There's a difference."

"Yeah, about twenty pounds."

I ran my hands over narrow hips. "I have the body of a cat: all muscle and no fat. I don't need to weigh another twenty pounds."

"Is that why you were throwing up last Wednesday?"

I looked at him blankly, not seeing the connection. "What's that got to do with it?"

He bit his lip, then said, "Some people worry too much about their appearance. They think people won't like them unless they're skinny enough, so they starve themselves and throw up when they overeat."

"Nothing of the sort."

"Look, Rafael. I like you, but your grasp of reality is a little weak on certain subjects. I think it might help if you talked to a therapist."

"I'm not crazy!" I said vehemently. "And I will not talk to a psychiatrist or any other kind of meddler. I don't deny that I'm different from other people; I know I'm different. But I refuse to see that there's anything wrong with being my own man." I turned to the closet and grabbed one of my new black suits. I pulled a white a shirt and red tie to go along with it.

"You are neurotic. No sane man would wear a tie when he didn't have to."

"You said you wanted to go out to dinner! So I'm getting dressed for dinner!" I snapped, not liking the way he was needling me about my appearance.

"I'm not going to wear a tie," he said in exasperation. "And you're not either. No double-breasted suits, no white shirts, no ties, and no wingtip shoes. Casual. C-a-s-u-a-l. Do I make myself clear?"

"Perfectly," I scowled.

I did not want to fight with him anymore, so after a pause to control my temper I decided to accede to his request. "What would you like me to wear?"

"Jeans, if you've got them. If you don't, I'll buy you some."

"I have something better than jeans." Giving him a wicked wink, I started pulling pieces of black leather out of the closet and tossing them over the end of the bed. Making sure he was watching me, I wriggled sinuously into a pair of form-fitting black pants and laced them up. They had fit like a second skin when I bought them, but now they had an extra two inches in the waist. Maybe I was a little too thin. But I was certainly not going to admit it to him, certainly not after the way he had just been nagging me about it.

"No underwear? Doesn't it chafe?"

"Not at all," I replied smoothly. I pulled on a thin black leather shirt and zipped it part way up the front. "It's buttery soft, like silk. I only buy the good stuff." I tucked the tails into my pants.

"I never figured you for a leatherman."

"After tonight I should think it was obvious!"

"You weren't exactly in the dominant position."

I deliberately turned my back to him so he would see the leather stretching tight over my ass as I bent to pull on my motorcycle boots. When I straightened, I looked over my shoulder at him and asked, "You think all leathermen are macho guys who have to be on top all the time?"

"Isn't that the biker code? 'Do unto others before they do unto you.'"

"No, just the opposite. Most leathermen like being bottoms. Speaking from experience, the more macho a guy is, the more he likes to be tied up and abused."

He shook his head bemusedly. "Black leather I understand, that's sexy. But why would anybody want to hurt somebody they like well enough to go to bed with?"

"It's not supposed to hurt," I corrected. "It's supposed to be exciting. I don't like getting hurt, and neither does any other masochist I know. What we enjoy is the illusion of danger." I donned my long black duster, and picked up a pair of motorcycle gloves with a multitude of rivets shining in the wide cuffs.

He eyed me dubiously. "But masochists like pain."

I grinned. "Do you like rollercoasters?"

"Yes."

"They strap you in with metal and vinyl restraints, and you're trapped. You have to go where the ride takes you. You go up that first big hill with your heart in your mouth. You come over the top and you start to fall: Down, down, and down, screaming in excitement because it looks like you're going to crash. But you don't. You get yanked through a series of twists and loops until you don't know which way is up. Then it's over. You arrive safe and sound back at the platform. You get out. Your heart is pounding, your blood is racing, your knees are shaking—and you get right back in line to do it again.

"That's what S/M is all about. But it's a lot more personal, and a lot more fun, because you get taken on exactly the kind of ride you want, for as long as you want. Nobody tells you when to get off. Think of it: two minutes on a coaster—or an hour, a night, or a week of S/M." I spread my gloved hands, the rivets flashing in the fading light. "I know which I prefer."

"You make it sound like fun!"

"It *is* fun! Nobody would do it if it wasn't fun!"

He shook his head. "Not my kind of fun. I'd rather go to dinner and a movie."

I put on a leather cap like Marlon Brando wore in *The Wild One*.

"I like dinner and movies too, but not every date. You're an artist; if you tell me dinner and movies is all you ever do, I won't believe you. You're too creative to get stuck in a rut like that."

"I was," he said in surprise. "I never realized it until now, but lately whenever Andrea wanted to go out, I wanted to stay home and paint. I was bored with her."

"Did she ever get into trouble?"

"Her? Never. The most daring thing she ever did was pose for that painting, and then she wouldn't let me show it to anybody."

"I'll tell you something, Michael. People who get into trouble are far more interesting than those who don't. I'd rather date a rogue than a gentleman."

"Like James?"

I winced. "It has its risks."

"What if he had really wanted to hurt you? You would have been helpless!"

I grinned at him, then clamped a shiny silver handcuff on my wrist. "Watch this." I compressed my fingers together, concentrated, then compressed them more. Slowly I pulled the narrow silver bracelet over my knuckles and off my hand. I presented it to him with a flourish.

"You could have gotten loose any time?"

I nodded. "But it was more fun getting rescued by you."

"I don't think I like that," he said slowly.

"Don't like what?"

"Getting set up like that."

I stiffened. "What do you mean?"

"You seem awfully willing to play games with sex, to use it to manipulate people. I don't like that. I don't go to bed with somebody unless I care about them. You seem to think it's some kind of sport."

"It is sport! It's the best sport in the world!"

He crossed his arms and sulked at me.

I pointed at him. "People like you think sex is a sin, that it's wrong unless you're in love with the person you're screwing. So you pretend to fall in love so you can get laid. You even tell your partner that you love her, and she believes you because she wants to believe in romance, not hormones. But you don't love her. You're just horny. After a while the pretending gets too hard, so you break up."

"I pity you. That's an incredibly shallow and self-serving attitude."

"I'm not shallow! You are! People like you are afraid of sex. It intimidates you. So you convince yourself that all you need to know is procreation—everything else is sin and perversion. That way you can feel virtuous for being ignorant and inadequate. But sex is profound. It shatters the psyche then rebuilds it. It condenses all the emotions of our lives into one intense experience that teaches us more about ourselves than a year of therapy ever could."

He was glaring at me. "I'm not ignorant! And I'm not inadequate. I place spiritual values higher than the temporary gratification of the senses."

I put the tip of my finger in his dimple. "With that attitude, why bother with art, or music, or architecture, or philosophy, or anything else that distinguishes the human from the animal? Spiritual values are physical values. You cannot divorce them from the very flesh that created them."

"That's despicable. It's nothing more than pornography. Art must transcend the physical or else it won't have any meaning except to the artist who created it." He jabbed my stomach with his finger. "You're selfish. You don't care about anything except the gratification of your own desires. You change boyfriends even easier than you change your clothes!"

I felt my face grow white and pinched. "You're the one that wanted to move in with me!"

"Jesus, I must have lost my senses! You're my uncle, for Chrissake!"

"I didn't tie you down and make you do it!"

He blanched badly. "You're right. I did wrong and I'm sorry. It won't happen again."

I pulled his money out of my pocket and threw it at him. "Get out of my house! Go home to your mother where you belong, you sanctimonious son-of-a-bitch!"

Slowly he knelt and gathered up the bills. "I'll get a hotel," he said rising. "I'm supposed to meet Ponchartrain tomorrow. Unless you blackball me."

His accusation stunned me. "I told you to get a hotel in the first place!" I howled, but he just turned his back on me and mounted the steps to his own room. I stomped my feet in a fury no words could express. "You don't know what I'll do! You don't know anything!" I was ready to throw lamps, but none were within reach. "Freeloader! Deadbeat! You mooch off me, then you tell me I'm easy! I get you an appointment at a good gallery, and you think I'm playing games with you! You think you're some kind of a king, waltzing in here like you own the place, and passing judgment on me! I won't have it!" His door closed quietly above me. My breath tore through my throat as I gasped for silence, then I ran into my study. The door hit the frame so hard it bounced, latch rattling futilely. I threw myself into my desk chair, glaring furiously at the open door. Then I gripped the edge of the desk as despair replaced anger. Well. Now I knew where we stood. I wanted him, but as soon as he got to know me even a little bit, he decided he did not like me. I had expected it.

I put my head in my hands and cried.

James had just bought a big house in Roland Park, and he and his wife were throwing a party to celebrate. Cars— expensive cars—were parked along the street, and men in suits and women in party dresses were walking along the sidewalks, converging on his address. Lawns in that neighborhood were huge and green, tended by professional landscapers, who allowed no blade of crabgrass to mar the verdant expanses. Old trees graced the properties, partially hiding the houses that were set far back from the winding road. In a city where even the wealthy lived in row houses (large, expensive row houses), Roland Park was a fantasy land, and anyone who received an invitation to its sacrosanct environs was quick to accept.

In the front hall, at the foot of a massive staircase, James was in his element, playing lord of the castle as he greeted his guests. Natalie, dark and slim in her blue taffeta, was on his arm, making kissy face with her old friends. Zoæ was ludicrous, her long blonde hair done up in curls, dressed in a blue dress with ruffles, pinafore, white knee socks, and saddle shoes, like a child half her age. After Peter died, they had not let her grow up.

I took her hand, kissed it solemnly. "I'm delighted to see you again, Zoæ. How old are you now?"

"Fourteen," she said, and the rebellion in her eyes told me she knew she was too old for pinafores and resented it.

"You're growing up fast."

"Too fast," Natalie agreed warmly, the dagger glint in her eyes telling me to move along.

"Natalie," I said taking her cold hand, but not kissing it. "You're in fine form, as always." Her eyes raked up and down the front of my suit, looking for any flaw she could exploit, and finding none. She fumed, and James extended his hand.

"Good to see you again, Rafael." I shook his hand and smiled warmly at him. Natalie watched me like a hawk.

"You have a lovely home," I told him.

"I'll show you around later," he said casually.

"I'd like that," I replied, agreeing to the assignation. Natalie knew something extra had passed between us, and it made her furious. I smiled unpleasantly at her, then drifted into the living room.

I exchanged greetings with a few people I knew, most of them artists or actors or musicians who were sprinkled in among the masses of politicians and businessmen. As might be expected in an election year, politics were a popular topic of debate. The conversation bored me, so I wandered aimlessly, faces blurring, forgotten as soon as I looked at them. The mayor was there, and several other Democratic politicians, stumping for donations. I avoided them, and found myself alone in the dining room with the buffet table.

I hesitated, then reached for a small ball of cheese covered in nuts. It was small and firm in my hand, smelling of cheese and spices. I lifted it slowly to my mouth, touching it with the tip of my tongue, knowing that I would devoutly regret indulging myself.

"Those are good." I jumped, and lowered the cheese ball. Zoë had drifted up next to me, the white bow in her hair partly undone and falling down her back. I picked up a paper plate, put the cheese ball on it, and started heaping it with random pieces of food.

"Can I ask you a question?"

"Certainly," I replied, not anticipating trouble.

"Are you queer?" I flinched.

"What makes you ask that?"

"Mom says you are. She said it was disgusting and we shouldn't invite you, but Dad insisted."

"Your father is my lawyer. Of course he invited me."

"Are you?"

"That's not a word to use lightly."

"I won't tell anybody."

I had lost my appetite, so I dropped the plate full of food into the garbage. "What else does your mother say?"

"She says you're really old, but you dye your hair and had a facelift."

"And what does your father say?"

"He says he doesn't care, you're still better looking than she is!" I gripped the edge of the table. Things were worse than I had thought if they were fighting in front of Zoæ.

"I'll talk to him."

"What about?"

I almost said, "You're too young to understand," but I looked at her again, her young woman's bosom swelling under her pinafore, and long legs with knee socks falling around her ankles.

"It's complicated. People get lonely. Sometimes they get married, but things don't turn out the way they expected. So they feel lonely again. And when you're an adult, you need friends, because you have a lot more things to worry about: Money, business, politics. Personal relationships cement business deals, and help advance careers. Natalie ought to be glad James is so well liked."

She eyed me shrewdly. "Yeah, but he's not boffing everybody."

"That's none of your business!" I snapped, and stalked away.

A waiter in a white jacket passed, and I snagged a glass of white wine. I sipped it, then in a sudden urge, downed it in two swift gulps. The alcohol hit me hard, and I wobbled. I went looking for another glass of wine, found it, and drank it too. I looked around unsteadily, trying to decide whether I should stay and get drunk in the company of society's finest, or whether I should go to a club and get drunk with a bunch of deviants. James had better wine, but the company in the clubs was better.

"I'd like to talk to you." The voice was big and bluff, and heads turned. Mine turned too, and when I realized I was being addressed, I tried to stand up straighter. The speaker was David Focault, grandson of Pierre Focault, founder of the petrochemical fortune, and father of Natalie Focault. In other words, James' father-in-law. I could guess what he wanted to discuss.

"This way." He turned and walked into the kitchen, expecting me to obey. I stared at his broad back, the bullet shaped head covered with iron gray hair, the custom-tailored charcoal gray suit, and knew I was out of my league. He could buy and sell me a dozen times with his pocket change. I thought about running, but decided I'd better face up to what was coming as gracefully as possible, and maybe we could reach a private settlement.

The kitchen was white and chrome, very modern, with white coated caterers going about their tasks, pretending not to notice us as we pretended not to notice them. Maybe they really were invisible to Focault. He was born to the manor, while I was born on a farm. I felt the difference keenly, and wished I had passed on the wine.

He raked me up and down with hawklike eyes. "You've been quite a popular topic of conversation this evening.

People have been speculating a great deal about your love life. Naturally, I've put the quash on such unfounded rumors. They are unfounded, aren't they?" The threat in his voice was unmistakable.

I knew what he wanted me to say, knew he wanted me to knuckle under and tell him it was gossip and lies, that I would never do any such thing, that I would be sure to conduct myself in the such a way that nobody could reproach me in the future. In other words, he would pretend nothing had happened—if I would give up my affair with James.

"My love life is none of your business," I snapped.

His natural frown deepened. "Be careful what you say, young man. Your conduct has already brought a taint of scandal to James. If it gets worse, then Natalie will have no choice but to divorce him. Without my support, he'll be bankrupt. I know you haven't got the resources to bail him out; you'd bankrupt yourself trying. And there are other repercussions to consider: Scandal surrounding a faculty member would hurt Peabody's ability to get grants and raise funds. Consider your position carefully, and don't make rash decisions."

I licked my lips while I considered the possible consequences of defying David Focault. My friends knew I was homosexual, and a few of my musical colleagues, but I kept my private life private. A few words from him would expose me to the glare of public scandal, and Peabody would have no choice but to throw me out on my ear. I would be unemployed, my career in shambles, and my reputation ruined.

And truth to tell, the affair was dying anyhow. What had started as a passionate affair of sex, music and art had degenerated into a series of sporadic flings. It was not worth fighting for; the gratification of defying Focault was too small, the price he threatened too heavy. But I was too proud to concede him the victory.

"You'll be pleased to know I'm going on sabbatical," I said haughtily, the patrician effect undermined by the wine. "I expect to be gone for a year or two, so there's no need to take precipitate action." He turned that over in his mind.

"That might be the most diplomatic solution to the problem." He put his hand in his pocket. "Do you need funding for an extended trip abroad?"

"I'm not a whore you can pay off and be done with!" I hissed through clenched teeth. "Whatever I did, I certainly didn't do it for money!"

"Everyone always needs more money than he has," he said reasonably. "I was simply offering to remove any financial obstacles to an amicable settlement of this affair."

"I don't want your money!"

"Very well. When will you be leaving?"

"By the end of the month. I've been making plans for a while, I can wrap them up quite quickly."

"That'll be fine." He offered his hand to seal the deal.

This was my life he was talking about! But on the Focault scale of existence, it was a minor problem, and easily solved. When I did not take his hand he withdrew it, with no apparent hard feelings. Who would have hard feelings over the squashing of an ant?

"You'd better tell James you're leaving."

I nodded dumbly, and he walked out of the kitchen. As soon as I was alone, I slumped. The wine was no longer intoxicating me, instead it was giving me a pounding headache. What was I to do? I pulled out my car keys, and without saying good-bye to anyone, went home.

As soon as I arrived home, I went downstairs and unlocked the vault. I stood in the room, just staring at it for some minutes, then realized that Focault had not forced a decision on me; he had simply clarified a decision I had already made but was reluctant to put into action. Everything was ready, all that remained were the good-byes, and I did not have the mental stamina to make them in person. I went upstairs and wrote several notes, bidding farewell to casual acquaintances, telling them I was going abroad for a year or two. My last letter was longer, and addressed to James. It was personal; we had already settled the legal matters.

Dear James,

Forgive me for not saying good-bye to you in person, but have talked about it enough already, and you know my reasons for doing what I am doing. I have outgrown my past acquaintances, who are now turning old and gray and marveling at my apparent youth, while whispering behind my back of hair dye and facelifts; such cosmetic explanations will not last much longer. Likewise my stage career is, and has been, dead for some years, and I never enjoyed teaching.

As to my personal life, I am jaded. The life I used to know has faded as my contemporaries have aged, and I am not flexible enough to adapt to the new fashions. I have lived too long, seen too much, and done too much, to be able to adopt the hip ideals of the new generation. I have become a cynic and a curmudgeon and a recluse. It is time to bow out gracefully before I become one of those senile old dodderers who annoy some and excite the pity of others.

Perhaps I shall awake refreshed and revitalized. I hope so; I do not really wish to abandon my life. On the other hand, the *ennui* is intolerable. If I cannot be cured of it, then let me die of it.

Rafael

I had dropped the letter in the mailbox, sealed the house, then arrayed myself in the hidden vault and slept.

Fifteen years later I sat with my feet propped on the plush green cushion of the window seat watching an arc of moon lift slowly above the dark tree line of the park, its golden light making the gothic towers of the old penitentiary seem churchlike and lovely. I wondered which part of the structure housed the gas chamber, and how many men waited for their deaths? Just one.

I shivered. I had been a coward, choosing sleep over death all those years ago. I swiveled my chair back and forth like a leaf in the breeze, my mind turning this way and that until I finally admitted to myself that it was time to make the decision I had avoided for so long.

My feet thumped to the rug, and I reached into the bottom desk drawer to draw out the revolver. It was a Smith and Wesson thirty-eight caliber model favored by police departments throughout the States. Its cylinder contained six chambers, all empty at the moment. I would only need one. I was a good shot, and my target would not be moving. A faint film of oil slicked my fingers as I opened the cylinder and sighted down the barrel. The gun was in good shape—I took care of everything I owned.

I lifted up the dusty box of ammunition and set it on the desk beside the gun. I flipped open the lid and extracted one cartridge. It was slim and dark, its brass casing tarnished with age, the bullet a dull gray bulge at the end of the round. I stared at it for a long time. This little would thing kill me? I doubted even I could survive having my brains splattered across the wall. Yet I had to be certain. On my stationery I wrote explicit instructions for the disposal of my body. If Michael did as he was told, I would be very dead indeed. Then, on another sheet of paper, I wrote my

Last Will and Testament, leaving everything I owned to the nephew who had rejected me.

I put the round into the chamber then closed the cylinder. I placed the tip of the barrel against my hair just above and behind my ear, and made certain it was pointing at the thickest part of my brain. I sat for a long time, sweat breaking out on my brow, but the trigger did not move. My hand cramped and I laid the gun down on the desk.

I was a fool and a coward too. I wanted to die, wanted to take the honorable way out of a losing situation, but I was too craven. I feared the ultimate night, the bourne from which no traveler returned, the nightmare breeding ground of terrors for mankind. I dreaded Valentin's fate, buried alone and unshriven, without the benefit of family or Church, in an unmarked grave, untended, and abandoned to the worms. Surely Valentin, if his soul survived, must hate me. I had left him alone in the earth to save my own life by going West. He'd had the courage to die for his cause, but I had lived on, a monster without honor or purpose. When I met the Grim Reaper, Valentin would be his servant, gleefully awaiting his vengeance.

I lifted the gun again, hesitated, the barrel wavering next to my head. Something hard and cold inside me rebelled against the destruction of my life. I recognized the feel: It was the slimy, ugly compulsion of the hunger. It would not tolerate anything that threatened its survival. It was an evil demon possessing my soul, a huge, hideous monstrosity clinging to my flesh like a gargoyle riding upon my shoulders, a monster that could be exorcised only by the destruction of my flesh. In sudden resolution, I pulled the trigger again.

Nothing happened. My fingers were frozen into immobility. In despair I threw the gun down on the desk. I dropped my head into my hands and tried to weep, but no tears came. I was a slave to the thing inside me; even the most basic human option—choosing to live or die—was denied to me.

Then I had a thought.

When Czarist soldiers stationed in the Crimea had grown bored with their post, they had invented a new game. They put one bullet in the cylinder of a revolver, spun it, then passed it from hand to hand, joking and betting about who would dare to pull the trigger, and who would pass the weapon to his comrade, offering up his neighbor's life to the god of Death that his own might be spared.

I picked up the gun, feeling the weight of it in my hand, and considered the odds. One in six. Not bad. Not bad at all. If I were playing roulette, I would put my money on the table.

I spun the cylinder.

It whirred and flashed with dim reflections of light, then came to rest. Only one bullet, five empty chambers. I would live. I might die, but that was good, because I wanted to die. I could do this. Yes. Live or die, let the Fates decide. I put the gun to my head, slowly squeezing the trigger, feeling the bitter delight as the hammer began to move.

"Stop!" Startled, my hand jerked. The gun roared, the muzzle flash scorching my scalp as the bullet tore through my hair. The smell of brimstone and burned hair lay heavy in the air. I sat shaking, staring with unseeing eyes, feeling only the burn across my scalp and knowing that I had come very close to death. My hand fell slowly away from my head, seeming to take an eternity to fall to my side, the gun clattering dully on the rug.

"Rafael?" Michael asked in fear.

I collapsed face forward onto the desk.

"Ohmygod!" He raced around the desk and dropped to his knees, hands probing gently through my hair. I flinched and lifted my head as his fingers touched the burned trail of the bullet. He cradled my face tenderly. "Are you all right?" he asked in a frightened whisper.

I nodded dumbly, incapable of speech at that moment.

"Oh Jesus! You scared me!"

"I scared myself too," I rasped out. I caught my breath, then sat up straight and shouted, "Damn it! Can't a man even commit suicide without you butting in?"

"No, you can't," Michael replied levelly. "What in the hell were you thinking?"

I shook violently, teeth chattering, a keening wail rising from the depths of my body. His composure broke then, and he wrapped his arms around me.

"I'm sorry, Rafael. I didn't want to quarrel, and I don't want to leave!"

"You want to stay?" I whispered doubtfully.

"Yes, if you'll have me." The lie of my existence twisted inside me, hope and fear knotted together in one tangled, miserable mass. "I want you to stay." He kissed me then, hard mouth covering mine, as if he would breathe life into me. I clung to him, the guilt goading me, but not breaking my grip on him.

"Everyone has left me," I said. "If you left too, I couldn't stand it. There would be no reason to live."

"Your music," he said. "Isn't that reason enough?" I was hollow inside, the sound of my past career a no longer heard echo.

"My career died when Valentin died. I've accomplished nothing worthwhile since then." I sighed. "I finally understand why he didn't try to run from the Secret Police. A life of fear isn't worth living." My head throbbed under the burning streak, and I felt infinitely tired and irrevocably old. "I went to sleep for fifteen years, Michael, sleeping endlessly until you woke me up. I thought I could sleep away the loneliness, the emptiness, and the pointlessness. But I couldn't. It's come back all over again, but even worse. I have even less now than when I went to sleep."

"You have more," he said forcefully. "You have me. And I'm not going to sit here and let you ruin your life."

I smiled wanly, then rubbed the sore spot under my hair. "Meddler."

His hazel eyes flashed. "Whatever it takes, I'll do."

Hope, not entirely dead, reared its ugly head. Maybe he could straighten out the mess I had made of my life...but how many lies would I have to tell? What awful things would I have to do to protect my guilty secret? I should confess my depravity, should tell him what he did not know, should tell him about the bodies, the blood, and my unwholesome need. Once he knew, he would help me die. Death was the only peace.

Cold, hard silence gripped my tongue. My fingernails bit into the wooden arms of the chair, scarring them with little half moons. Dumbly I nodded. The illusion of happiness was better than nothing.

Chapter Nine
ACID TEST

Mal y pense qui mal y soit.
                        —motto of the Order of the Garter

Baltimore, 13 October 1991

When I returned from the shower the evening sun was shining directly on the front of my house. Thick hazy sunbeams forced their way through the shutters of my room, and dust motes danced like a cloud of tiny pixies. The pale birch furniture glowed in the light, and the thick gold and cream rug looked like a magic carpet ready to fly. It was like crossing the threshold into another, better world.

I piled up the pillows and lay down against them, sinking down almost supine, damp ringlets of black hair sticking to my white bathrobe and clinging to my neck. The soft pillows and clean sheets felt good. I was all those things a man is when he has just awakened: a little sleepy, a little hungry, and little horny. I burrowed into the pillows, reluctant to get up and face the day.

Michael's car rumbled to a stop in front of the house, and I bestirred myself. I rolled to the edge of the bed, opened the top drawer of the nightstand, and deactivated the burglar alarm. His key scraped in the lock as he let himself in, and I turned the alarm back on once he closed the door behind him. A few moments later he called, "Rafael?"

"Upstairs!" I shouted back. I settled back against the pillows while he ran lightly up the stairs.

He stepped jauntily into the room, and I smiled to see him home again. He was clad in a red sleeveless muscle shirt whose large armholes emphasized the bulging round-ness of his shoulder muscles, while his jeans were worn to white threads at knees and crotch. Enough skin showed through the holes that I wondered if he were wearing underwear or not. The possible lack of lingerie made my blood simmer, and I grinned up at him with keen apprecia-tion. He was my denim Adonis, and I adored everything about him, right down to the battered brown cowboy boots.

"I saw Ponch today," he said cheerfully.

"Ponch?"

"Ponchartrain. But he's so fat, I call him 'Paunch.' Don't tell him I said that." His twinkling eyes said he meant no harm.

"George Ponchartrain?" I asked in bewilderment. "Fat?"

He leaned against the bedpost. "Well, I guess it depends on how you define 'fat.' Not so bad for an old guy." I cringed. The George I remembered was young and burly, with muscles like a Greek hero.

"How did it go?" I tried to sound enthusiastic, but it was hard. I was distressed about George.

The sparkle in his eyes grew even brighter. "He bought one. And he took three on commission."

"Great! Which one did he buy?" He grinned easily.

"Your picture, of course. The one I just finished. His eyes bugged out of his head and he pulled out his checkbook and wrote. No argument."

George had photographed me a lot of times; I could well imagine his appreciation of Michael's painting.

"I wonder what Damon thinks of it."

"He asked George if he was keeping a tart on the side. I told him not to worry, you were already taken."

"I've been called a lot of things, but that's the first time anybody ever called me a 'tart'!"

He leaned forward and kissed me. "Good to eat," he murmured.

"Glad to oblige you," I replied.

He straightened. "I cashed George's check on the way home so I have two thousand dollars burning a hole in my pocket. We're going out to eat."

At that moment I would have agreed to anything, but the thought of dining (and throwing up) in public gave me pause. I sat on the edge of the bed, looking up at him. "Wouldn't you rather have dinner at home? We could have a lovely candlelight dinner, a little wine, a little music, just the two of us…"

"You're very tempting, but I know if I stay home alone with you, I'll never get my dinner. You have an irresistible way of distracting me. You have to keep my strength up if you want me to satisfy your appetites."

My eyes dropped to his silver belt buckle. "I'd be happy to keep you up."

He shook his finger at me. "That's exactly what I'm talking about! But tonight I'm holding out for steak and champagne before you get yours."

Barbarian, to mix white wine with red meat. But if that was what he wanted, I was willing to go along. "All right. Toss me my suit."

"I'm going as is, and I forbid you to wear a coat or tie." He tried to give me a stern look, but his eyes twinkled and he grinned when I laughed.

"Your wish is my command, O Mighty Sultan," I said reclining upon the bed and pretending to smoke a hookah. "Your slave will wear whatever you desire." With emphasis on the "desire."

"Do I get three wishes, like Aladdin?" I grinned.

"Of course. And until the three wishes are granted, you are my lord and master."

Lying on my side hampered me a bit, but I made an flamboyant bow by touching my fingertips to forehead and chest, then flourishing them in a circle. That might not have been exactly how the Arabs did it, but it was good enough for our little game.

"My first wish is that you go a whole week without wearing black."

I laughed. "Done. And your other wishes?" I asked lewdly.

"I'll let you know as soon as I decide on them."

I could imagine all manner of things worth wishing a lover to do, and the erotic images made me fidget. For example, mutual kissing starting at the toes and working in to the middle. Unfortunately, I had neglected to stipulate that he had to rub my lamp to get his wishes.

Michael was rifling through my closet in search of something not-black when he suddenly seized on a sliver of yellow at the end of the rod, mostly obscured by the other clothes.

"Not that," I said in alarm, sitting up straight.

His hand clamped onto the hanger and pulled.

"No," I said, "I won't wear that in public." He held the dress against himself.

"And you told me you weren't a queen."

It was a yellow frock, covered with coral cabbage roses and olive green leaves, with short sleeves, a wide white collar, and full skirt. It buttoned up the front with yellow cloth buttons. I had it so that when hunting was lean in the gay clubs, I could take female form and hunt the straight clubs. The dress was not a fetish; it was a hunter's camouflage. But I could not tell him that.

"I'm not a queen," I protested lamely, not wanting to explain my promiscuous feeding habits. We could burn that bridge when we came to it.

He was grinning as he peeled the dress off the hanger and tossed it at me. "Get dressed. I want you to wear it when we go out. That's my second wish." With my eyes I pleaded for mercy.

"Go on, I want to see you in it." I let my robe fall, exposing my mostly hairless pale body, then blushing furiously, stepped into the dress. It was tight across the chest as I buttoned it up. I tugged it uneasily, trying to find a more comfortable position.

He pulled a second hanger from the closet, unclipped the white lace garter belt and sheer silk stockings, then passed them to me. My face was burning with fiery color as I pulled up the skirt and fastened the garterbelt around my waist. Then I sat on the side of the bed and pulled up one sheer stocking and hooked it to the garter belt, then the other.

When I was in female form, getting "dressed" did not embarrass me, but with him leering down at me, it was definitely kinky. It dawned on me then that he liked this particular form of deviancy. I glanced coyly up at him and said, "O Mighty Sultan, do you wish your slave to go barefoot, or will you provide her with shoes?"

He tore his eyes away from my legs, and knelt to rummage among the shoe boxes in the bottom of the closet. After opening and closing several, he found the black leather pumps with the four inch heels and ankle straps. He knelt before me, and ignoring his own prohibition on black, slipped the shoe on my left foot, buckling the strap with trembling fingers. I offered him the other foot, and he kissed it softly before slipping it into the shoe. He fastened the buckle, then slid his hand around my ankle and up my sleek calf to the hem of the dress.

"It's a muscular leg," he said lowly. "But with all the women who work out, it's perfectly believable." The baritone tremor of his voice sent shivers up my spine.

I crossed my knees, letting the skirt ride up to my stocking tops, but still preserving my modesty. "You like me like this?"

He nodded. "You look like a beautiful lady, but underneath you're all man. It's amazing; it's like you're twins, one male, and one female." He grinned crookedly. "Twins are a fantasy of mine."

I could readily imagine him in the middle of a three way with a man and a woman, and I wondered if my shape-changing ability could manage to produce two of me at once to oblige him. "I'm a shapechanger," I said huskily. "I could be a woman if you want."

His eyes popped. "You could?"

I nodded. "Want to see?"

He nodded mutely.

I closed my eyes and concentrated, my body softening and reforming, the dress still in place, but fitting properly now. I unbuttoned the four cloth buttons and showed him two perfect breasts.

"Those are great tits," he said in honest admiration.

I uncrossed my legs, and spreading my knees wide, lifted my skirt to my waist. His eyes dropped to my black-haired pussy, then bugged out of his head.

"Is it real?" he asked. "I mean, if I touch, will it feel like it looks?"

"Yes."

He put his hand between my legs, laying his palm over the mound of soft flesh and hair, leaning his body between my knees, face thrust close to mine, lips seeking mine. The pressure of his hand against my pussy sent startling waves of heat through my body, and I lifted my mouth to his. He kissed me strongly.

"I've never done it as a woman," I murmured against his lips.

"I'm good with virgins," he replied.

His mouth ravished my neck, soft lips caressing my skin while I lifted my chin to allow him full access to my vulnerable throat. He nipped it gently, and I let out a sharp gasp of air. His tongue trailed down my neck, then paused as he nestled his lips against the cleft in my collarbone, kissing it devotedly, sucking it lightly, and running his tongue along the bone.

He pulled the front of my dress open revealing a narrow triangle of flesh which his lips followed, walking softly down the cleavage between my breasts while my nipples strained against the fabric, eager for his touch. He peeled the fabric back, exposing my right breast, his hand cupping it gently, then firmly as his mouth came down upon it. I arched, forcing more of my flesh into his mouth, a line of fire burning through my body straight to my cunt. Fluids began to ooze and drip between my legs.

"Oh, stop!" I whispered, overcome by the sensations that were at once familiar and alien. I felt as if reality had taken a half twist to the left, so that everything looked the same, but nothing fit.

Michael lifted his head and looked at me, then pulled himself up so that he could embrace my shoulders and kiss me. His hard groin pushed against my crotch, and rockets of desire shot through me, obliterating minor technical differences between who I was, and who I had been. I wrapped my legs tight around his body, thrusting up against him, groaning in passion, wanting the union of our bodies, totally engrossed in the unfamiliar (yet similar) female sensations.

Michael slid down my body again, using his strength to force my legs and arms to loosen. He slid lower and lower until suddenly he was kissing my nether parts. His lips planted soft, firm kisses on the hairy mound of flesh at the bottom of my belly, and I collapsed onto the bed limp with astonishment, feeling like I was drowning in wet velvet. I could smell myself, the ripe, voluptuous female smell like fruit that would rupture on the vine if it were not picked.

I moaned long and low, my hips writhing, when suddenly his tongue flicked a small bump of intense pleasure. He nursed it with his mouth, electricity shooting down my legs, making my feet tingle, limbs twitching helplessly as he alternately sucked and licked it. My hands clawed the bedspread, and I groaned and tried to drag myself away from him, but he held me fast.

At last he took pity on me, and releasing my clitoris he slid his tongue up and down my dripping wet slit. He sucked on one labium, then the other, then held me open with his fingers while he licked me from hole to point. I buried my fingers in his hair, pulling unmercifully at his head. He deposited kisses all over the softly swollen flesh of my sex while I jerked and twisted.

"Fuck me!" I cried.

He caught my clit in his mouth again, pinning me to the mattress, while one hand slid down my slit, fingers gently probing for my opening. My back arched and I trembled, because Michael was taking me where I had never been before, and I was desperately afraid I was going to like it.

Two fingers sank into the soft, wet, warm opening of my body, and I squirmed, pushing myself onto his hand while my brain ran screaming in the opposite direction.

"NO!" I cried.

He lifted his face and watched my reactions while his fingers found something inside me and tweaked it. A bolt of white heat shot through my body.

"Do you really want me to stop?" he asked mischievously. "I will, if that's what you want."

For answer I groaned wildly, hands beating the coverlet, then spread my legs wider. "Take me!" I cried, too far gone with feminine lust to make any other answer.

He squeezed me gently with his thumb on my clit and his fingers inside my cunt, then rubbed them simultaneously. The internal pressure made me feel like I was going to pee, and I clenched my muscles, trying hard not to wet myself with excitement. But in spite of my efforts, pearly white fluids oozed around his hand, and the aroma of bitch in heat wafted through the air. The coverlet under my ass was getting very wet, and I squirmed, desperately fucking his hand, yearning for the intimate congress of his lust and mine.

Michael removed his dripping hand, then sat up and unzipped his pants. The prick that had given my male self such pleasure now seemed huge and impossible when it was pointed at my newly deflowered flesh.

I scrambled to a sitting position. "Oh no you don't! Not with that!" I cried in sudden panic. This fantasy was going much further than I was prepared to handle.

He caught me in his arms and bore me down, his hard flesh poking against my sopping wet hair.

"I want to," he whispered hotly in my ear, "It's my third wish."

I wanted to change shape and run far away. But at the same time, I would curse myself for a coward if I quit now.

"Please?" he asked.

"Do I have a choice?"

"Yes, of course." He tried not to look disappointed as he sat up. Putting his hand on his cock he began to stroke himself. I watched him enviously because it was a gorgeous cock, and I did want it, even if it scared me.

"I didn't say no," I told him.

He leaned forward so that his breath was brushing my lips. "Will you let me make love to you?"

"Yes," I whispered. The panicked rats started to run wild through my brain, but I ignored them because I wanted to please him.

He stripped off his shirt and pushed his pants farther down his legs, then lay down between my legs.

"Be gentle. I've never done this before," I begged.

He nodded, then sheathed himself in my body. I screamed.

It was a perfect fit, my hot, wet flesh taking him easily as he buried himself to the hilt. He held still, waiting for me to calm down, but I did not. The sensations were indescribable, and I kicked violently, then locked my legs around his waist and thrust my hips against him, nails biting into his shoulders, wild animal noises coming from my throat. I wanted to fuck him senseless, wanted to engulf the entirety of his hard body with my soft wetness, wanted to suffocate him with my thighs, to reduce him to nothing but the hot seeds of sex that grew inside me, swelling my belly from the inside, the ultimate invasion of my flesh.

He began to pump me, his hardness sliding easy through my slippery flesh, his eyes closed, his expression blissful. His arms wrapped under my back and neck, supporting my head so that he could kiss my face. He was a well practiced and skillful lover, pacing himself and not letting the primal thrashing of my body overwhelm his consideration for my pleasure and my comfort. I hated him for it. I wanted to come, I wanted him to come, to crash into the mind-stopping double climax—no, I did not want him to come! How stupid of me, I was female, and we were not using a condom, I could get pregnant! I don't want to be a woman! His body heated up, the expression on his face becoming more intense. Perspiration gleamed on his brow, and his strokes became harder, deeper, more demanding. My back arched, my heels drummed on his ass, and my fingers clawed his back as I fought him, trying to tear him away from me with my hands while my legs locked him tight against my belly. A great pressure built in my body, and I shrieked, having no other way to release the intensity.

Suddenly he slammed me with short sudden strokes, driving the sensations of my body to a higher, intolerable level. A floodtide of sensation rushed through me, drowning me in a maelstrom of velvety wet softness. Suddenly my body went rigid and my breath stopped, my pelvis jerked and shuddered, then my back went limp, and I sprawled in sudden relief, stars circling inside my closed eyelids. Slowly I realized that this was orgasm, female style.

Michael lay languidly against me and I wondered if he had come. He was so relaxed he must have; I had been so busy with my own climax I had missed his.

"Don't you ever do that to me again," I hissed at him as soon as I caught my breath.

"Did I hurt you?" he asked in surprise.

"No."

"What did I do wrong?"

"I'm a man, and you fucked me like a woman!"

"Well, you are a woman, at least for the moment," he replied in bewilderment. "What was I supposed to do?"

I pressed my hands to my head as if to crush my skull. "You like me better this way, don't you?"

"I like you every way I can get you. Yes, this was a lot of fun, but you're also a lot of fun when you're male."

"Which do you prefer?"

"Both."

I glared at him.

"Really, Rafael. I do. I like you both ways, and I like doing it both ways, and I would hate to be stuck with only one, whichever one it was."

"Life would be easier if I were female."

He laughed then. "Who cares? I would rather have an interesting life than an easy one."

"You don't understand how I'm feeling!"

He sobered. "I've fucked you before. Is it really so different?"

"Yes!"

He cocked his head curiously at me. "Wanna tell me?"

"All my life I've been a kinky gay man. It affects everything I do, everyone I meet, everything I feel. That's a very intense and very different kind of life. Now suddenly, here I am, flat on my back, female, vanilla, and normal! It isn't fair! For years I've been persecuted because of who I am and who I love; now suddenly I'm socially acceptable, just because my plumbing has been rearranged. It's the rankest kind of sexism!"

"I see your point, but it doesn't matter to me. I think you're wonderful, and anybody who doesn't agree with me is an idiot."

"Thank you very much. Now get off of me; I want my body back and you're in the way."

He obligingly lifted himself off me, and I sat up, yanked the dress off, shed the garterbelt, shoes, and stockings. Then I squeezed my eyes shut, and gratefully reclaimed my natural masculine form.

Michael pulled up his pants. "Still want to go out with me?"

"Do I have to wear a dress?"

He grinned wickedly. "Are you gonna welsh on my second wish?"

"I never welsh on a deal," I said hotly, then squirmed. "Of course, if you've changed your mind—"

"I haven't."

"You're not going to let me off easy, are you?"

"Do you want me to?"

This was discipline of a different kind, more subtle and more psychological than the discipline James had administered with whips and chains. That was pure physical sensation, like skydiving or other daredevil sports. Michael was playing with my head, illuminating the dark places in my mind where I had never cared to look too closely before. Did I have the courage to play his version of the game? And yet, what courage did it require to play a game I could quit any time? Michael would never force me, never threaten me, never hurt me. Michael was safe.

I smiled, and pulled the dress over my head. "All right, but if anyone gets too close, you have to deck him for me."

He grinned easily. "I have a brown belt in judo. I'd be happy to protect your virtue."

"Hmph. If I had any virtue you wouldn't have talked me into this." I was stronger, faster, meaner, and tougher than him; if there was any fighting to be done I was the one to do it. Yet even though logic told me it was silly, his gallantry made me feel safe. It was nice to have someone looking out for me instead of always having to look out for myself.

He rose and offered me his hand. "Shall we go to dinner?"

I accepted his hand and rose gracefully. "With pleasure."

A weirding wind was blowing, carrying heat and humidity from the south, while at the same time the evening dusk was cold and clammy, simultaneously stifling and chilling me. I turned back for a coat, but Michael had locked the new lock with a brass key and was handing it to me. I was at a loss for what to do with it because I had neither purse nor pocket, then with sudden inspiration I pulled up my skirt to reveal the top of my garter, and tucked the key into the elastic.

Michael smiled broadly at me. "Nice."

"And so we have the truth." The voice was harsh and flat, anger leveling its tones.

We turned to face James where he stood at the foot of the walk, his hands in the pockets of his trench coat. "The drag queen and his pretty boyfriend," he continued. "I wonder how much he would admire you if he knew just what you were." I wondered too, and stepped carefully down the steps in my high heels, hoping I could meet him halfway and talk quietly.

With a savage grin James looked past me and said, "You ought to see what holy water does to your vampire lover." I let loose a deep breath of relief; James was sadly mistaken if he thought a little salt water would hurt me. But let him have his superstitions.

I stood squarely in front of him, hands on my hips, and called his bluff. "Go ahead and try it. I think you'll be surprised at the results."

A crafty look slipped across his face. "I think I will. You deserve it, you bitch." He pulled a glass bottle out of his pocket, pointed the spray nozzle at my face, and depressed the trigger. A stream of cold wet stuff hit my face, unpleasant at first, then growing into an awful fire that ate away at my skin. I threw up my hands and shrieked, stumbling backwards, turning my face aside while he sprayed me again, catching hands, arms, neck, the front of my dress, soaking me with the fiery liquid, and I lost my balance, the high heels tripping me up, and went crashing to the pavement. My screams went on and on, each nerve of my face, hands, neck, chest shrieking as the evil stuff consumed my flesh, my heightened senses serving only to worsen the agony of the assault.

A door banged suddenly, a noise that barely penetrated my consciousness, and suddenly a massive, hairy shadow passed above me, and I heard the sound of James' dress shoes running across the pavement. His car door slammed, followed by a mighty "Woof!" and scramble of claws as the St. Bernard tried vainly to get at him.

"Acid, oh my God, acid!" Marjorie wailed. "Get the hose!" she snapped, while I writhed on the ground, my scream having climbed to a keening wail so high pitched it was barely audible, the sound of it setting my nerves on edge, but I was powerless to stop. I hurt too much.

Cold water splashed in my face, the stream powerful and shocking. I shut up suddenly, gulping and gasping, blinking my eyes, and rolling my head while she played the water across my face and arms.

Michael knelt beside me, unmindful that he was getting splashed too. "Rafael?" he asked hesitantly.

I sat up, drenched, the dress sticking to my cold flesh, my hands twisted into claws. I opened my eyes and was relieved to discover that I could see. My hands were burned pink as if I had gotten a terrible sunburn, and a few blisters were coming up in places.

Marjorie laid the hose aside, the water running down the sidewalk into the gutter. I blinked at her, noticing the fuzzy brown sweater and the curlers in her hair, but not knowing what to say and or feel. She knelt too, getting her black knit pants wet.

"Are you okay?" I didn't answer; and I was afraid to look at Michael.

Michael lifted my lapel and put his fingers in the holes the acid had eaten in the fabric. "It was acid," he said softly.

"Not holy water." His fingertips brushed lightly across my chest, and I looked down at his hand as his fingers went from hole to hole tracing the path of James' attack. Only then did I dare to look him in the face.

He lifted his hand, but did not touch my injured face. Instead he traced the line of my jaw and brow with his finger a fraction of an inch away. I could feel the warmth of his hand, then his hand slipped around behind my head and cradled my hair. "I'm sorry, I was so stupid. I didn't do anything. If it hadn't been for Marjorie and her dog, he would have hurt you even worse and I would have just stood there. I'm sorry." His hazel eyes were contrite, his expression sincere.

"He fooled us both," I managed to rasp out. My hands trembled and I realized I would be weeping if I were capable. James had lied, but his lie had very nearly parted us—which was his intent. My face and hands hurt badly, but the uncertainty in my heart hurt even more. Were Michael and I going to be all right?

"Oh, Rafael!" he said, arms going around me and drawing me to his chest. I leaned against him, careful not to bump my face or hands, and saw the loiterers in front of the liquor store gaping at us. Awareness of the world beyond my immediate sensations returned, and I realized that I was sitting there on the sidewalk in torn nylons, wet dress sticking to my flat chest, and a man embracing me.

"Well, I'm out of the closet now," I said, trying feebly to make a joke of it.

Michael looked up, noticed our audience hanging out across the street, and said, "I don't care about them. Only you." Relief flooded through me as I gingerly touched my burned face. I was all right. Michael and I were all right. Marjorie was all right. Even the neighbors were all right, because I no longer had to worry about keeping secrets from them. I threw my arms around Michael and kissed him hard, wincing as the pain lanced through my lips. He cradled me gently in his arms, then gathering me to his chest, stood up. I clung to him, startled by his strength, but grateful to let him be strong when I had been so lonely and so brittle for so long.

He mounted the steps to the porch and began to laugh.

"What?" I asked in puzzlement.

"I was all set to make a dramatic exit, but I can't, because the door's locked, and I don't have enough hands to get the key out." I fished under my skirt for the key in my garter, flinching as the fabric scraped across my raw skin. But I got it out and inserted it in the lock.

Marjorie whistled, "C'mon, Bernie!" and the St. Bernard bounded up to her. She scratched him behind the ears. Michael started to step through the door, but I caught the doorframe.

"Marjorie," I said. She looked up. Was that a suppressed bitterness in her expression? "Thank you," I said.

Her face softened. "Hell, I had fun being a hero. I'm glad you're going to be okay; I thought you were being murdered when I heard you scream." I wondered if the acid was James' way of making me helpless while he did something else, like drive a stake through my heart. But he wouldn't murder me in front of the neighbors, would he? Then again, he had sprayed me with acid with a dozen witnesses watching. Who knows what else he might have done? "You might have been right," I said soberly. "You might have been right."

"Thank you, Marjorie," Michael said. "For more than you know." And he crossed the threshold.

Chapter Ten

DAUGHTER OF THE ENEMY

How sharper than a serpent's tooth it is
To have a thankless child!

       —William Shakespeare

       Baltimore, 14 October 1991

Rain rattled against the windows, great sheets of water splashing against the house and sending crumpled brown leaves flying before the gale. Indian Summer was gone, vanished overnight as the mercury plunged fifty degrees, equinoctial gales blowing wildly about the house all night and into the day, bringing sporadic bursts of rain. As sleet mixed with it the rain rattled more brittlely. The music room was dark, the shutters open to the gloomy day, the weather providing no illumination.

The damp chill pervaded the house, and I was too stiff to practice. I could solve that problem quite simply. A careful check with extended senses told me that the chimney was clear—no small animal had built a nest in it. I fetched an armload of wood from the wood box in the basement, then crumpling old newspapers for a base, built a fire in the fireplace. The wood was very dry and caught quickly, burning in a raging blaze. I adjusted the damper and closed the glass, feeling better when the door was shut.

A heavy knocking pulled me away from the fire, and I opened the front door to discover a delivery boy. He was about nineteen, dressed in a blue nylon windbreaker and no hat, his kinky black hair plastered to his skull, his shoulders soaked and shivering. He had a long white box topped with a big red bow in his hands. "Rafael Guitierrez?" he asked, mangling my name.

"Yes."

"Delivery for you."

I accepted the box. "Thank you." He ran down the steps and jumped into his double-parked florist's van, and I shut the door.

The perfume of roses in summer wafted to my nose, the box not secure enough to keep the heavenly smell from escaping. I smiled in appreciation, then started for the kitchen. Michael met me at the bottom of the stairs. He was wearing a tight-fitting white turtleneck and his usual jeans.

"Who was that?"

"Delivery."

His eye fell on the box, and he asked, "Who from?"

"I was hoping it was from you."

"Oh. Sorry. It never occurred to me to send flowers to a guy."

I smiled wanly. "I like receiving flowers."

"I'll remember that."

"I hope so."

I laid the box on the kitchen table, wondering who had sent it. Anthony? It would be logical for him to reciprocate. George? Unlikely. He did not want to see me. James? After what happened? Impossible.

"So open it already!" Michael urged.

"You are a heathen," I said. "Don't you know that anticipation is half the pleasure?" But all the same I laid the box on the kitchen table, then lifted the lid, revealing a massive bouquet of red blooms. The perfume rose in a cloud of scent, pervading the entire room with the smell of nostalgia. I closed my eyes and inhaled deeply. When I opened them Michael was leaning against the doorframe, his arms folded comfortably across his chest, eyes twinkling, and mouth curved in an indulgent smile.

"Aren't you jealous?" I asked.

He looked surprised. "What for?"

"Somebody sent me flowers!"

He sighed softly, and for a moment his expression became adoring and slightly baffled. Then his face fell back into its usual lines of good humor. "I expect you have hoards of admirers, but you didn't pick one of them, you picked me. It makes me vain, not jealous."

I picked up the small white envelope about three by four inches tied to the stems with a small red ribbon. Nothing was written on the outside, and I opened it slowly, wondering who my secret admirer was.

Dear Rafael,

    I apologize for losing my temper with you last night: You know I would not be so angry unless I cared for you. I am jealous, I admit it. I can't bear the thought of losing you to a younger man, not when I thought I had found you again after all these years. Please forgive me, and join me at the symphony. I will take you to dinner afterwards.

James

Enclosed was a ticket for the Joseph Meyerhoff Symphony Hall, dated tonight, showtime, eight-fifteen.

"What does it say?" Michael asked.

I handed it wordlessly to him. He scanned it quickly.

"You're not going!"

"I think I must."

"Why?"

"At the very least to tell him it's over."

"You don't believe this malarkey, do you?"

"I believe that James is obsessed with me, and that I have to make it clear to him that his attentions are unwelcome. As long as he can entertain any hope of winning me back, he will pursue me diligently. Better to finish it now."

"I think you should call the police and have him arrested for what he did to you. That'll get the message across!"

I sighed. "I really don't want to air that kind of dirty laundry with the police. Can you imagine? 'D'ya know why he did it? Because I'm fucking Michael, not him.' We'd all end up in jail on lewd conduct charges."

He sighed in frustration. "You aren't going alone."

The set of his jaw told me he was going to be stubborn about it.

"All right."

"You're not going to argue?"

"I'd love to go to the symphony with you. I think we should get two tickets, so that when I walk out on James I can come sit with you and watch the rest of the performance."

"Okay. Do I have to wear a suit?"

"Do you have a suit?"

"No."

"I guess that answers that question. My suits wouldn't fit you; you're too big a man."

"There's one other problem."

"Yes?"

"If you're going to the symphony, you'll probably run into people you used to know, and they'll probably recognize you."

"I'll tell them I'm Rafael Junior, and it's a family resemblance."

"Might work," he said as if he did not believe it.

"You have something better in mind?"

"Yes. Change your looks. You're a shapechanger; that shouldn't be too hard."

I thought it over. "Shapechanging takes a lot of energy, and it takes concentration to keep the new shape firmly under control."

"I wasn't thinking of anything major, just reshaping your face a little, maybe growing a little taller and a little heavier."

"I used to be heavier. Being thin makes me look different. But I see your point. I suppose if the changes were small enough, I could get in the habit of putting on a new face every day." I made a moue. "But I like my face. It's me, and it's been me for a very long time. I don't really want to change it."

He grasped my arm. "Come with me."

We hiked up to his garret, to the untidy disorder of paints and canvases and dirty laundry. Michael rooted through the mess and found his sketchpad, and we sat side by side on the cot, his only furniture aside from the easel. He quickly sketched my face.

"This is you," he said. I nodded.

"This could be you." He erased the eyebrows with a thick chunk of rubber, then sketched again, leveling the brows, making them thicker and heavier. He paused, considering. I studied the image. It was still my face, but a little different. I made me feel odd. Michael continued sketching, dropping my hairline a quarter inch, and adding a small widow's peak.

I stared at it. Once again Michael had shown an uncanny knack for sketching the emotional features of his subject as well as the physical details. The more prominent hair features gave me a "brooding artist" look that expressed my romantic and volatile personality far more faithfully than absolute accuracy would have.

I took the sketchbook from him and stared at it. "Is this how you see me?" I asked at last.

"Yes and no. I know what you really look like, of course. And I know what you feel like emotionally. And I know what stereotypes our society holds about physical appearance, so I blended them all together to make a new face for you that is still you, but different enough that people will distinguish between Junior and Senior."

I gazed at him with respect. "You're a genius!"

"Thanks. But it's only a drawing. Can you make it real?"

"Yes, I think I can." I closed my eyes and concentrated. The flesh on my forehead crawled, and Michael said, "That's it," so I stopped doing what I was doing. I felt my eyebrows with my hand, but that was not informative enough. I rose and hurried downstairs to my own room to confront myself in the mirror. Michael sauntered up behind me, his image joining mine.

"Yes," he murmured. "Perfect." His arms went around my waist and I clasped my arms over them. Slowly I smiled.

"I like it."

"Now taller, about an inch, maybe an inch and a half."

"My pants will be too short."

"I can sew. I'll lengthen them for you."

"You can sew?" I asked in astonishment.

"Sure, I used to do theater in high school. I did everything—painted sets, acted roles, sewed costumes, the whole works."

"You were an actor?"

He grinned self deprecatingly. "Let's just say I got my

roles because of my looks, not my ability. I had more fun painting sets and making costumes."

"All right. Stand back."

He released me and I doffed my clothes. With an effort I grew another inch, to a grand total of five-eleven. It felt strange, as if I had been stretched on a rack, but there was no pain, only a peculiar loose feeling as if my limbs were slightly too long, which they were. I walked around, shaking my legs and arms trying to get the tingling to stop. Eventually it did, and I started getting used to my new configuration.

True to his word, Michael lengthened several pairs of pants for me. He sat at the kitchen table with one leg tucked under his rump, deftly stitching the hems with tiny invisible stitches. I watched him bemusedly, partly because of the alluring way his muscles rippled as he worked, and partly because he did not look the least bit unmanly while doing it. Sewing was a skill I had adamantly refused to acquire on the grounds that it was women's work. Yet there he was, as macho as could be wished, apparently undisturbed by the affront to his masculine dignity. Young men had changed since I grew up.

I leaned in the doorway, dressed in the upper half of my tuxedo, plus white silk boxers, socks, and garters (masculine style, for holding up recalcitrant socks).

"I appreciate you doing this for me," I said carefully, trying to acknowledge this new breed of masculinity without sounding patronizing.

"You're welcome," he said, then rose and unfolded the ironing board from its wall cabinet. He laid out my tuxedo pants and grinned. "You see, I'm not completely useless."

"I concede the point. In fact, you're the only one of us that's making any money right now. I'm the useless one," I moped.

He spoke while he pressed my trousers with deft movements. "Maybe you could get a job at a piano bar or something. I realize that offends your delicate classical sensibilities, but anything is better than nothing."

"I guess I could apply for a teaching position at Peabody. They have a pretty high turnover in the Prep classes. I've done it before, I can do it again."

Real life. What a strange concept. I had not lived a real life in a long time. I smiled at Michael, desperately glad I was not doing this alone, and equally glad that however much I might love him, he could not support me. We could share our lives with each other, but we could not live them for one another.

Michael tossed my trousers hot off the ironing board at me, interrupting my reverie. I snatched them out of the air before they could hit the floor, then stepped into them, enjoying the warmth against my skin.

"You look good in a tuxedo," he said appreciatively.

I stepped into my dress shoes, then knelt and tied the laces, diamonds winking and twinkling in my cuffs as my hands moved.

"Thank you. Tuxedos were part of why I chose classical music for a career: They were the antithesis of the overalls and farm work I grew up with."

"You promised me a concert once," he said wistfully.

"I remember. I have something special for you, too." Michael followed me into the music room, catching his breath as the candelabra on the mantelpiece flamed into light. He settled on the edge of the window seat, eyes fixed upon me with an expression I could not fathom. I stared wordlessly back at him, my heart full of things I could not readily speak.

"I wrote this music for you."

His face broke into a delighted smile. "I'd like to hear it."

I smiled back. "You will." The sonata was complex and moody, ranging through the treble end of the keys, but underpinned with a bass line that strengthened the lighter passages by virtue of the contrast. I played with my old agility, wrists crossing and uncrossing, fingers stretching to reach combinations of keys impossible for a lesser musician. The demand upon my skill delighted me, for there is no pleasure akin to the mastery of a difficult task.

Michael sat entranced, listening and watching with rapt devotion, the first person since Valentin's death to understand what music meant to me. I did not deserve it, but he loved me, and I was too greedy to let him go. So I played with my heart in my hands, pouring into the keys all the feelings I could not express in words: Love, delight, adoration, and fear; the harpsichord gave voice to the passions that were too overwhelming for words.

When the last note sounded, I sat still, hands poised over the ivory keys, not wanting to break the spell. Michael sat a moment longer, then leaped to his feet and pulled me into his arms. He kissed me passionately, and I cooperated willingly, my mouth meeting his with parted lips. His hands slid under my coattails, pressing me against his body, his groin hot against me. I tightened my grip on his shoulders while he ravished my neck with kisses. I let my head fall back and he nipped my throat lightly, and I groaned wildly, my heart hammering with terror and desire. If only he knew what I was, and wanted me anyhow! He walked me backwards, carefully avoiding the furniture, then hooking his heel behind mine, he knocked me down on the rug before the fire, and fell on top of me. The fire crackled merrily, the heat of it caressing my head, and the rug soft under my back. He pushed his leg between mine, and I wrapped my limbs around him in eager embrace.

He caught my white tie in his teeth and pulled. The bow

tie unraveled, dropping away from my neck. He pressed his mouth against my collar, kissing my throat through the fabric, my neck arching with pleasure, then his teeth closed around the button. The thread gave, and he spit out the button with a predatory grin.

"You're ruining my good shirt!" I was not really protesting.

He laughed. "I'll sew the buttons back before we go out tonight." Then he lowered his mouth, and nuzzling between the lapels of my collar, found the skin over my collarbone, and devoted himself to kissing and sucking it while I panted with pleasure, hands clenching on his shoulders.

When he moved to the next button, I put my hands up and unfastened it myself. He nipped my hands gently, trying to get to the button, but I would not let him.

"Vandal!" I said playfully.

He grinned wolfishly and straddled my stomach, his weight heavy against my groin, his hard-muscled legs trapping me. "Rape and pillage," he said, reaching for my waistcoat. "That's what the Vandals did to the Romans."

"You'll get no resistance to from this Roman," I answered.

"Traitor!" he laughed. I winced, but he did not notice.

He unbuttoned my white brocade waistcoat, pulled my shirttails out of my trousers, and opened my shirt. He ran his fingernails lightly across my bare chest and down my stomach, while I shivered in pleasure. He found my navel and toyed with it, his fingertip tracing a circle around the edge, then gently pressing into it. My libido translated his motions to another part of my body, and I squirmed.

"Roll me over and do it again," I breathed.

"Maybe," he said grinning at me.

He reached over his shoulder and pulled his turtleneck

off with a single graceful motion. His brown nipples stood erect, and I grabbed them. He gasped, and closed his eyes, while I rubbed them between my fingers, twisting them and tugging gently. He began to pant, and his nipples grew larger and harder in my hands, so I tweaked them harder and jerked them firmly. He groaned loudly, leaning against my hands, his swollen crotch pressing against my groin.

I raised my hips, thrusting my hardening cock between his legs, and he pressed down, grinding himself against me, the heat and the pressure making me moan. I clasped his thighs and bucked my hips, getting harder and harder as I banged the crotch of his jeans, while his face contorted with desire. Suddenly his hand went to his silver belt buckle, yanking it open, then he crawled off me long enough to pull off his boots and jeans. While he did that, I unzipped my pants, lowering the waistband of my shorts to the bottom of my scrotum so that my naked cock stood clear of any obstruction. His eyes fixed on it, and he licked his lips. His hungry stare made me even harder.

"Eat it or sit on it," I said. "I like it either way!"

He flashed me a grin. "You wily Roman, you've corrupted your conqueror."

I smiled back at him, lips carefully closed over my fangs. "You're on top. You can leave if you don't like it."

"I like it all right." And he dropped his mouth over my cock.

I groaned and arched my back, enjoying the ministrations of his mouth as he licked me up and down my length, his teeth teasing the frenum, then his tongue stroked the foreskin, inviting it to retract. When it did, he gently sucked the tip of the glans, the sensation incredibly intense. I let out a long low moan, teeth long and hard in my mouth.

He slid along my body, mouth covering me in kisses and sharp little bites until he came to my face. He tried to kiss my mouth then, but I turned my face aside, not wanting him to discover my fangs. His tongue darted into my ear, and his teeth nipped at my throat, making me groan and writhe under him, my teeth aching in their sockets, and my cock rubbing against his belly. He sat up, adjusting his seat, his hand behind him guiding my cock into the crevice of his ass. He rubbed my cock against his flesh until it found the soft spot, then he thrust himself onto my hungry flesh. My teeth extended to full length at the same moment, and I thrashed, impaling him deeply, gnashing my teeth in desperate desire for his blood.

He sat with his back erect, his head tipped back, his Adam's apple bulging in his throat, eyes closed while he lifted himself up and down my shaft, groaning deep in his throat. I clamped my hands to his thighs, fingernails biting into his flesh, drawing blood. I carried the red liquid to my lips, sucked my finger clean, then sank my nails into his thigh again, resisting the desire to rend his flesh from his body. I put my bloody fingers in my mouth again, biting myself so that I cried in pain. I was so hungry! Vampire.

I could no longer live the lie. I wanted Michael to know what he was doing, I wanted him to know what he was fucking, wanted him to know how I had deceived him and used him. Then he would set the stake against my flesh and drive it home with strong strokes, and I would embrace it willingly, eager to make the final peace.

In the moment I accepted my vampire nature and the doom it carried, I came with an intensity that was more pain than pleasure. My head threw back and I howled, my teeth bared to his view, my cock throbbing in his flesh, the vision of death and the sensation of life inextricably bound together in one mind-shattering experience.

He groaned, and hot sticky cum splattered my belly as he came with me.

I had no more pride; hungrily I rubbed my fingers in the sticky white splashes he had left on my belly, then lifted them to my mouth, tasting the sour, masculine flavor of him, and wanting more. I sucked my finger violently, thrusting it in and out of my mouth, trying desperately to gratify my oral need.

Michael shifted his position so that he lay on top of me, throat close to my mouth. "Finish what you started," he demanded.

"What?"

"I can feel the vampire force in me, Raffi. Take me the rest of the way! Drain my blood, take me over the limit so there's no turning back! Make me like you!"

Hunger beat at my brain, urging me to rip out his throat, sate myself on his blood, and bury the remains in a shallow grave where the sun could not reach them. If he was lucky, he would rise again, scattering the loose earth as he sat up in his grave. If not, the dogs that were the enemy of the undead would dig him up and devour him.

No! I used my strength then, tossing him aside to land in a tumble of limbs and a surprised grunt.

Kill.

I dissolved into mist, clothes falling to the floor, while Michael's eyes went wide and his mouth made an O of astonishment. I rematerialized in panther form, the feline body the perfect killing machine if he tried to struggle.

As I loomed over him, his arms went around my neck, and he said, "I love you." He closed his eyes and tipped back his head, waiting with baited breath for me to rip out his throat.

The panther form slipped, and I found myself kneeling on hands and knees, my thoughts in chaos. He loved me? This monster that I was, this thing which would destroy him? How could he? I leaped to my feet, and ran into the kitchen.

I rummaged frantically through the cabinets, knocking

aside small appliances I never used, then pulled out the six pack of baby formula I had hidden the week before. I laid my hand over the top of the can, aluminum squealing in protest as I ripped off the lid. I put the ragged metal against my lips and tipped it up, pouring the cloying chemical concoction down my throat, gulping furiously, formula spilling around the corners of my mouth, running down my chin, and dripping on my bare chest. When the can was empty I threw it away and grabbed another. I belched, then ripped open the second can. I upended it, drinking a trifle slower, but not by much.

Michael looked cautiously around the doorframe. I tossed aside the second can, and it bounced off the cabinets and rolled across the floor. I met his eyes, then looked down in shame.

"Are you going to be all right?" he asked.

I was still hungry, but my stomach was gurgling as it digested what I had given it. I ran my tongue over my fangs, and they were not extended as far as they had been, though the touch of my tongue stimulated them.

"I think so. I wouldn't get too close if I were you." He eased around the corner, and my eyes fell upon the bloody marks on his naked thighs. I licked my lips.

"You should go," I said. "Go back to New York where you're safe."

"I don't want to go to New York."

"You can't stay, I might do something awful to you."

He stepped to my side and slid his arms around me. "No you won't."

"I almost did," I said, standing stiffly in his embrace.

"No you didn't."

"I could have. It was so close!"

He put his hand against my chin and made me look at him. "It's all right. Either way, it's all right."

"I don't want you to die!"

He smiled gently. "I can't die. Not any more. You've seen to that. I can only be born again, better than I was."

"It's not better—"

"If you had a choice, would you become human again?"

His question hit me dead center. "No," I admitted.

"Then why feel guilty about it? I certainly don't regret anything that's happened."

"You don't?"

"You've made my life an extraordinary adventure, and I love you for it."

He had given himself to me utterly, placing his life and death in my hands, trusting me beyond all reason. I was awed by the magnitude of his gift; there was nothing I could do to answer it in kind.

Accept it, Valentin murmured in my mind.

Is it all right? I asked uncertainly.

You have my blessing, he replied.

"I love you, Michael," I said as my arms wrapped tightly around him.

"I love you too," he whispered fiercely in my ear.

There were no other words to be said, so we stood there a long time, listening to the beating of our hearts.

We retrieved our clothes, dressing leisurely in the living room. Michael winced as he stepped into his pants, while I moved with the glacial slowness of somebody in deep shock. I was still a little hungry, but it was a normal kind of hungry.

Just then somebody knocked at the front door.

"I'll get it," Michael said, stuffing his shirt into his pants, and pulling on his boots without socks. A moment later he opened the front door.

"Rafael Guitierrez?" a woman's voice asked.

"No, I'm Michael Duran, his cousin."

"I'm Zoæ Flanagan. I have some business to discuss with him. Is he at home?"

"Just a minute." Michael stuck his head in the living room. "Somebody here to see you."

"I heard. Give me a minute."

I quickly tied my tie over the open collar, the bow concealing the fact that the button was missing. I checked myself quickly to make sure I was presentable, then stepped into the hallway. A tall woman with collar length platinum hair and a black trench coat was waiting on the threshold.

Her eyes raked me up and down. "Rafael Guitierrez, Junior?"

"Yes," I replied.

"I'm Zoæ Flanagan," she said. "We talked on the telephone."

I nodded.

"You look very much like your father," she said.

"Some people think so," I replied. Michael gave me an "I-told-you-so" look. I smiled crookedly in response, admitting that he was right.

Zoæ noticed the exchange of looks. "Did I come at a bad time? If I'm interrupting I can come back later."

"No, not at all," I replied. "Please come in. May I get your hat and coat?"

"Yes, thank you." There was a minor tussle over the coat until she realized I was helping her. Apparently she was one of those feminists who believed in doing everything for herself. I hung up the coat and put the hat on the shelf. She was wearing brown plaid wool pants, a chestnut turtleneck sweater, and a wide brown belt with a fancy buckle over it. Ominously, a silver cross depended from a fine chain around her neck. I wondered what kind of wild stories James had been telling her.

"Would you care for coffee?" I asked as I led the way to the living room.

"If you have it, I'd be grateful. But don't go to any trouble."

"Michael, could you fix some coffee? Café au lait for me, please." I gave him a meaningful look, and he nodded, understanding my need.

"Certainly, be right back." He stepped briskly down the hall, his boot heels thumping softly on the wooden floor.

"Please, have a seat." I seated myself in the white wing chair between the hall door and the sofa. She laid her black leather briefcase on the white velvet sofa beside her, clicking the latches open.

"I must say I had some doubts about your claim, but seeing you in person, I have to admit you're related to Rafael Senior. The family resemblance is unmistakable. And I've checked your birth certificate, not to mention your recently acquired Maryland driver's license. May I ask where you've been these last few years?"

"Traveling."

She waited for me to expand. I smiled agreeably and waited for her to continue.

"I've investigated the insurance matter. The claim was paid to James Flanagan as beneficiary of the policy. I was hoping I could see the original you claim to have."

"Yes, certainly. Anything else?"

"Is it true you have a date with Dad tonight?" Her eyes swept accusingly across my tuxedo.

"It's true your father has asked me out. And it's also true that Michael and I are going to the symphony tonight. I expect to run into him long enough to tell him to leave me alone." My voice was cold and hard.

She studied me. "Can you truthfully say you've done nothing to encourage him?"

"Two days ago I had Michael throw him into the street! Most men would find that adequately discouraging. But yesterday he showed up and sprayed me with acid." I touched my face, which was a little tender, but healed. "Fortunately, the injury was minor. But I think you can appreciate that I don't want, like, or encourage that kind of attention."

Michael drifted in and placed his hand on the back of my chair. "A fresh pot is perking," he said amiably.

Zoæ's eyes narrowed as she looked at him. Then she looked at me thoughtfully. The woman was too smart. I reached up and entwined my fingers with Michael's.

"I tell you truly. Your father's attentions are unwelcome."

At last she heaved a heavy sigh. "I remember your father. A remarkable man. I also remember the profound impact he had on Dad. I suppose it is understandable that the sight of you has roused old feelings. And with your father in the grave, he has transferred his attentions to you, even deluding himself that the old Rafael has returned. The resemblance is uncanny." She rubbed the bridge of her nose, as if she wore glasses and they pained her. "I shall attempt to persuade him to take counseling for this problem."

"He strikes me as the sort of person who would be resistant to counseling."

"He strikes me that way too. Nonetheless, I shall try."

Nodding sympathetically, I said, "I wish you luck."

"Thank you. I'd like to see the insurance papers now."

I rose. "I'll fetch them directly."

When I returned Michael was sitting on the sofa next to her briefcase, pouring coffee from my silver service into blue and white china cups with my monogram on them. I handed the papers to Zoæ and she unfolded them, examining them carefully while I took my seat and accepted a cup and saucer from Michael. I sipped it, and was pleased to discover that baby formula and coffee made a good combination. The sweetness of the formula countered the bitterness of the coffee while the strong flavor of the coffee masked the chemical taste of the formula.

Zoæ took a set of papers out of her briefcase, compared them to my papers, then spoke. "This set of papers was in your father's file at the office. The beneficiary was changed in 1979, which was one year before your father was declared missing and presumed dead." She returned my papers to me, and pulled out another sheaf of documents.

"This is a record of testimony from the court proceedings to determine your father's fate. In it, my father asserts that your father was missing since 1976. And he presents evidence to prove it. The change in insurance beneficiary was never brought up in court."

"How could Dad change the beneficiary if he had been missing since 1976?"

She tossed her papers into the briefcase. "That is the question, isn't it? Answering it will take a lot of digging." She did not sound happy.

I sipped my coffee thoughtfully. "Tell me, is there any testimony from Violeta Duran in that court file?"

"Yes. She signed an affidavit saying she hadn't seen or heard from her brother during the period he was missing."

I looked at Michael. "How does that compare with what you know?"

"We all thought Uncle Rafael was alive and well and living in Baltimore. We had no idea he was missing or dead. We thought he just wasn't talking to us."

"Do you mean to impugn the integrity of the affidavit?" she asked skeptically.

"Yes, I do. If your father was willing to forge a change of

beneficiary, why not forge the testimony from Dad's family? A very neat way to insure that the court proceedings turned out the way he wanted," I answered.

"We don't know that forgery is involved."

"At the very least, my father's family should be contacted and asked to verify the affidavits."

She sighed heavily. After a pregnant pause she asked, "Have you considered obtaining the services of an attorney?"

"Yes. But I'm broke. I can't afford one. That's why I tried talking to your father myself."

She reached into her briefcase and handed me her card. "I'd like to offer my services."

I looked at her card with the elegant silver script, and the words "attorney at law" under her name. "What kind of fee are you suggesting, considering my financial situation?"

"It's a matter of honor. I won't accept a fee."

Zoë Flanagan was proving herself to be a formidable young woman. My respect for her rose several notches.

"I accept." I sat forward and offered my hand to seal the deal.

She clasped my hand strongly. "Tell me everything." So I did.

As I spoke of "Dad's this" and "Dad's that" I felt a great distance between myself and the man I had been. It was easy to think of myself as a separate person; similar as a son is similar to his father, yet different, not doomed to repeat his father's mistakes. I hoped I would prove wiser the second time around.

Chapter Eleven
FUNERAL GAMES

Death is evil; the gods have so judged;
had it been good, they would die.

—Sappho

Meyerhoff Symphony Hall, Baltimore, 14 October 1991

We left early for the Meyerhoff, and I directed Michael
down St. Paul Street, past the elegant four story brick row
houses that lined one of Baltimore's better streets. We were
heading away from the concert hall, but Michael did not
know that. He had not been here long enough to learn his
way around. When we passed the lighted front of Harper
and Klein, I told him to park. He pulled to the left hand
curb (it was a one-way street) and parked.

I smiled at him. "I'll be back in a few minutes."

"Where you going?"

"I'm going to buy a present for you. But it's a surprise,
so you can't come with me."

"What are you going to get?"

I put my black-gloved finger to his lips. "Hush. You'll
find out soon enough." I darted from the car to the shelter
of a doorway, rain splattering on my wool overcoat, the

brim of my fedora protecting my face. I turned and waved at Michael, who watched me through the window. I leapfrogged from doorway to doorway, then let myself into Harper and Klein's.

It was late and it was quiet, with a statuesque blonde girl in a white blouse standing behind the counter staring into space. The bell on the door jangled, and she snapped to attention, smiled warmly at me, and asked, "Can I help you?"

"Yes," I replied. "I'd like to buy a couple of diamond rings."

Her smile became sincere. "Yes, sir. What did you have in mind?"

"I'll let you know," I replied. Harper drifted into the room, looking perpetually middle-aged as always, but having been fooled by George's dyed hair I was inclined to be skeptical about his black locks. I resisted the urge to greet him: Rafael Junior did not know him.

My eye fell at last upon a plain gold band set with two small diamonds on either side of a flat oval. "That one."

She extracted it from the case and set it on the counter before me.

"Can you have it engraved while I wait?"

She glanced at Harper, who replied, "Certainly. I have no other business tonight."

I slid it onto my finger, and it fit well enough. With an effort I remembered to check the price. Six hundred and thirty-five dollars. Two of them would break me, but Michael was worth it.

"Good. I want another one just like it, but in a larger size."

The girl hunted through boxes under the counter, asking, "Do you know how large?"

"Yes," I smiled. "Large enough to fit my index finger."

She studied my hand, then pulled out a box. I slipped

the band on my index finger so that I wore two rings side by side. I held my hand out before me, studying them, liking the way the gold shone against my pale skin, and imagining how it would gleam against Michael's darker complexion. Gold was the perfect metal, for it never lost its luster. The symbolism was apt.

"You have a good eye," I told the clerk.

"Experience."

I removed the two rings. "Have the smaller one engraved with the initial 'M', and the larger with the initial 'R'."

"Certainly," replied Harper, accepting the rings. "You look very familiar. Have you been in here before?"

"My father has. I've been going through his old papers, and came across references that you were his jeweler. So, when I needed a jeweler, I came here. I'm new in town, and had no idea where else to go."

"Ah," he said. "You must be the son of Rafael Guitierrez."

"Yes, I'm Rafael Junior."

"I am delighted to meet you. Your father was a valued customer of ours. We were saddened when he died."

He said it sincerely enough to make me believe it was my father's company, and not his money he missed. I found myself liking him all over again.

"Thank you, that's very kind of you to say."

"I'm glad to be of service." He juggled the rings in his hand. "I'll be right back."

The girl and I settled my bill, and when Harper returned, I put the package into the pocket of my tuxedo. Intermission would be a good time to give it to Michael. Music, a glass of wine, a casual gesture…

"Good night," I said, suddenly nervous. I scarcely heard their good-byes as I let myself out the front door.

I hesitated under the shelter of their marquee, the pale light from the store window washing over me. What if I was being overly romantic? Michael was not the flower-sending sort of man, he was probably not the ring-wearing kind either. It was one thing to surrender privately to me; it was another thing to parade around in public with my initial on his finger, like a tag on a dog.

Valentin and I had never worn rings. Then again, in Hungary, that would have gotten us arrested and sentenced to five years hard labor. Things were different in America. I hoped.

I swallowed hard and stepped into the rain.

The Meyerhoff Symphony Hall was a fat brown brick cylinder, with a curving drive full of stopped cars discharging passengers. The rain drizzled down listlessly, as if weary of falling, but too stubborn to quit. Michael parked the Corvette in the parking lot across the from the hall and we hurried quickly through the damp air, dodging puddles.

I bought two tickets, then we checked our overcoats. Several women—and a few men—gave Michael's skin-tight white turtleneck admiring glances, but he was oblivious. I smiled to myself, then ascended the steps to the balcony level, Michael's long legs keeping up easily with my brisk pace. I found our seats, close to the left wall, where we could overlook James' box while anyone in the box would have to crane his neck over his shoulder to see us. I pulled the tails of my tuxedo out of the way and sat down carefully, wishing I had worn the tailless tuxedo instead. Michael settled down beside me, denim-clad legs blocking the aisle. I noticed a number of other patrons in jeans along with the more numerous suits and gowns; I had been afraid they would not admit him in such casual dress. Chalk up one more change to the passing years.

The lights flashed, giving us the five minute warning, and I had just started to wonder if James was going to stand me up when a young man with wavy black hair and a black leather jacket entered the booth below us. He checked the numbers on the chairs, then settled in the middle seat of the first row. He slipped off his jacket, revealing bulging shoulders in a tight black tee shirt.

"I think my dinner has arrived," I said softly to Michael.

He scowled at me. "Don't go thinking with your eyeteeth, you'll only get into trouble."

I smiled. "Trouble is fun."

He glared at me.

"And I thought you weren't the jealous type!"

"I'm not the jealous type, I'm the smart type. If you go thinking with your hormones instead of your brain you'll end up in another one of your harebrained predicaments and I'll have to rescue you again."

"Doesn't sound so bad to me."

"I ought to wallop you up side the head!"

"I'm only teasing!"

He gave me another black look, but I could tell he was not really angry with me. I squeezed his hand. "I'm going to go down and see what's happening."

"You want me to come with you?"

I considered. "No. You can keep an eye on me from up here. I shouldn't be gone long."

"Well, okay." I settled into the seat next to the strange young man and smiled affably at him. He might be a random stranger, seated next to James' seat by accident. Not likely, but possible. He looked at me in surprise, and I showed him my ticket.

"Looks like we're going to be keeping each other company tonight."

He smiled invitingly. "Sounds good to me."

Bingo. I could not be getting this lucky all by myself. But I decided to play along as if I had no idea who might have sent him.

"Rafael Guitierrez, Junior," I said, offering my hand.

He took it limply, as if he was not sure what to do with it. "Kevin Siegel."

If the Semitic nose and swarthy complexion hadn't tipped me as to his ancestry, the name would have. I gave him a quick appraisal: Young, about twenty-one, and short, five-six at most. He had brown hair and a faint line of mustache across his upper lip, and a muscular, compact body. His pants were gray denim with factory supplied patches artfully arranged. He had nice legs, too.

"Pleased to meet you," I said, fulfilling the formalities.

He nodded nervously, suddenly tongue-tied. His eyes swept over my hand-tailored tuxedo and he knew he was badly outclassed.

"First time at the symphony?" I asked. He had the street hardened edge that spoke more of garage bands than classical music.

"Yes," he admitted.

"Mine too." He blinked and looked confused.

I smiled pleasantly. "First time at the Meyerhoff," I clarified. "I've been in plenty of other symphony halls. Occasionally as a performer."

"What instrument do you play?" he asked, and he actually seemed curious.

"Piano and harpsichord. I also coach voice, though it's been a while."

Voice teachers are like accountants: Least likely suspects for anything nefarious. I smiled engagingly, deliberately trying to subvert his connection to James. My smile seemed to work, for the pattering of his heart eased a bit. I let him mull things over while I surveyed the hall.

The boxes were irregular semicircles attached to the wall like fungus growing on a tree trunk. The walls and ceiling were white, except for the stage and its walls which were blonde wood. Large wooden discs were hung from the ceiling by wires over the central part of the audience. The ceiling itself was decorated with large, slotted hemispheres looking for all the world like giant screwheads. I looked at these features and swallowed disappointment.

"Too bad," I murmured.

"About what?" he asked, instantly nervous again.

I smiled. "The poor acoustics." I pointed to the discs. "Those redirect the sound from the stage to the audience. If you happen to be sitting under them, the sound is probably quite good. But not for the rest of the hall."

"Oh."

"I didn't expect Carnegie Hall where you can hear a pin drop in the last row, but still, I had hoped for a competent design."

He regarded me dubiously as if acoustics were the last thing he expected to be discussing on an assignation James had set up. Just then the house lights dimmed.

"When will James be joining us?" I asked quietly while he was blinking his eyes.

Caught by surprise he said, "A little later. He was delayed at the office."

Mixed in with Kevin's clean male scent was a faint whiff of pipe tobacco. Kevin had seen James in person recently, because the smell was not yet stale. Perhaps he had stopped by the office before coming to the hall, but then again, perhaps James was somewhere out of sight, watching me. Hairs stood up on the back of my neck, and I felt very much like a target. I looked past Kevin's head, located Michael, and smiled, but I did not feel reassured.

"So how did you meet James?" I asked in a friendly way,

218 / Gary Bowen

both to disarm his suspicions and to learn anything that might be useful in beating James at his own game.

He looked abashed, then said, "I guess you could say it was business."

"Really? Are you in the law business?"

Two bright spots of color appeared on his cheeks. "No. I'm a prostitute." He would not meet my eyes.

I smiled gently. "I've had occasion to use the services of the Athanasian fellowship myself. It's a venerable profession, even if it isn't exactly respectable."

He smiled in relief. "The Athanasian Fellowship. I've never heard it put that way before. It sounds religious, almost."

I grinned. "It is religious. Athanasius was a bishop who promulgated a creed beginning , 'Whosoever wills.'"

He groaned. "Ain't it the truth!"

The random tuning noises of the orchestra hushed, and the conductor entered. We all clapped politely, and I settled down to enjoy the program. I was rather surprised: The orchestra had developed a lot in the last fifteen years. It was still not what you would call a world class symphony, but for a regional orchestra it gave a solid, if undramatic, performance.

Kevin sat quietly beside me, listening to the music, and stealing glances at me out of the corner of his eye. He neither fidgeted nor slept, which amazed me. When the lights came up for intermission I smiled genuinely at him, and he smiled shyly back at me.

"That was kind of nice," he said, drawing a cigarette from his left coat pocket.

"You can't smoke that here."

He held onto to it. "I was gonna take it outside."

"All right. I'll keep you company." I was not about to let him have time to concoct some scheme with James.

Michael rose when we rose, and I jerked my head towards the side of the building. He nodded as if he understood, and Kevin and I exited the box. We avoided the throng in the main hall by taking the emergency stair and stepping out through the brown metal fire door. Kevin zipped his jacket against the cold, and followed the curve of the building around back where the wind could not find us. I was cold too, but for me it was a matter of comfort, not health. He put his cigarette in his mouth, then cupped his hands around the lighter, as much for warmth as to get the cigarette going.

"I haven't had a cigarette in years," I said enviously.

He looked surprised.

"Want one?"

"Yes, please."

He offered me the crumpled pack and I withdrew one of the slim white cylinders. I put it in my mouth, leaning forward to accept a light from his lighter. I puffed several times until I got it going, noticing as I did that he was looking past me.

"I gave up smoking when I was in Budapest and couldn't get good cigarettes," I said, glancing around casually, alert for a perfectly timed arrival by James. I stood with my back to the wall blowing smoke rings, childishly delighted that I still remembered how.

"You're not really immune to AIDS, are you?"

He said it in a tone of voice that told me he was not sure what to believe, but he wanted to be able to say, "Ha ha. I knew you were pulling my leg."

"Is that what James told you?"

"Yes."

"I might be," I said meditatively. "I don't know."

"Have you been tested?" He was trying hard to appear calm, but his heart was racing. The subject was important to him.

"Not yet."

"If you were immune, that could be the key to saving millions of lives!"

"Including yours," I said quietly.

He recoiled, then his face fell. He nodded.

We stood in silence, the rain pattering down the only sound. Distantly the sounds of muted traffic came to us, along with the indistinguishable hum that was the natural sound of a big city. I drew fiercely upon my cigarette, then tossed the butt into the gutter where it sizzled and drowned. I could turn my back on a cause, I could turn my back on millions of people. But one face, up close, someone whose name I knew, someone who shared fears I feared and loves I loved, someone who wanted nothing more than to live life as I lived, that was impossible to ignore.

"You will cooperate with the lab, won't you?" he beseeched me.

I thought about AIDS, illness piling upon illness, the body's defenses slowly crumbling, then collapsing utterly. A long, slow death. I did not wish that on any man. Not even James. If a man is to die, let it be quick and clean.

But there were so many of them, and only one of me! It would take an army to tend the needs of the sick, an army of vampires. All beholden to James, all grateful to him for their lives, dependent upon him for their blood, obedient to his will.

That was what James wanted: To be King of the Vampires, arbiter of life and death itself.

"No."

"Why not?" he demanded, his face turning white and pinched.

"Because he's the wrong man to do it."

"He's the right man!" he interrupted fiercely. "The one

with the money and the vision and the ability to make it happen!"

"No," I said. "He's selfish—"

"You're selfish! You could save millions of people, but you won't!" He right hand dipped into his coat pocket and clenched on something small. Not a gun, much too small and light to be a gun.

"Give me that." I reached for it at the same time he took it out of his pocket. A sudden small pain pierced my flesh as the needle bit deep into my hand. Kevin backpedaled rapidly while I stared in shocked horror at the small hypodermic protruding from my palm, the pain evaporating as the drug ate at my nerves. I tore the thing loose and threw it away, but it was too late. Cold numbness flowed along my veins, deadening my arm, reaching toward my heart and brain.

Where was Michael? I staggered along the wall, heading back the way I had come, hoping to find him just around the curve of the building, arms reaching out to catch me as I fell... I was alone. I bounced against the wall, right leg twisting under me, left fingers biting into the brown bricks, holding me up, right arm useless. A few feet away was the fire door, my escape from the trap I had walked into, my salvation from whatever James had planned for me. I lurched forward, reaching numbly for the handle. My vision blurred, and I concentrated, forcing my fingers to close on the handle, shifting my balance so that my weight pulled on the handle of the door.

It did not yield. Hazily I realized that it was locked, and I closed my eyes and extended my power, trying to find the shape of the lock with my mind, but unable to trip the tumblers. My heart fluttered as tendrils of cold poison wrapped around it, and I gasped for breath, finding it hard to breathe as the insidious power of the drug touched my vital organs. Cold tentacles of oblivion reached up my throat to strangle me from the inside.

I cried out in panic, my partially paralyzed vocal cords giving out a distorted yelp. My spine began to buckle, my hips no longer secure in their upright position, my legs melting, knees hitting the pavement, until at last my fingernails lost their bite on the bricks, and I collapsed in a heap.

Kevin hovered near, waiting for oblivion to claim me. The street was deserted, nobody was coming to my rescue. My head spun, and blackness crowded around the edges of my sight.

"You don't know what he's doing," I croaked through Novocaine numb lips.

"He's looking for a cure for AIDS. That's good enough for me."

"—vampires." My words were badly slurred, and he ignored me, stepping down the alley to wave his arm in signal.

James was coming, and James wanted to use my body to make a billion dollars. I had to get up, I had to get help. I could not lie there and let them take me, I had to try. My fingers hooked into the spaces between bricks, clenching tightly. Now up. Lean on my arms, drag my feet underneath me, pull up. Good. Now reach for another brick, reset my fingers, and drag myself up a few more inches.

Kevin turned in astonishment.

"You're not human!"

And a good thing too.

Forcing my numb legs to move, I got my feet flat on the sidewalk, my face banging against the rough wall as I staggered through walking motions. I pulled myself along the wall, limbs flopping wildly, face collecting lacerations I could not feel as I crawled sideways along the wall like a spider. Somewhere up ahead were people were standing smoking and drinking under the marquee, and if I could reach them James would not dare lay a hand on me.

I paused to rest, panting for breath, wondering if I had gained any ground at all or if that was an illusion. I dared not look back, turning my head to look over my shoulder required an extra bit of energy I could not spare. Kevin approached warily, second hypodermic in his hand. He tossed the orange safety tip into the gutter, and pointed the gleaming needle at me. I was barely upright now, a second jolt of that stuff would put me out completely.

Michael! Help me!

Kevin darted forward, and I flung my arm up wildly, trying to knock it away from him. I thought I had succeeded, then I saw the needle embedded in my bicep, the plunger partially depressed. Kevin danced out of reach as I pawed for him, seeing but not feeling my movements. The needle dropped to the pavement. I tried to speak, but no words came, only a mewling sound like a wounded kitten.

My vision went gray and fuzzy, shapes more than a few feet away blurring into smears of color, and nothing more. My shoulder leaned against the wall, wooden legs straining to prop me up. I had to get away. James was coming. James would hurt me. I had to run, had to hide. How long had it been since Kevin waved? Seconds? Minutes? I had no idea. How much time did I have to escape? None.

At the sound of a car engine I turned my head and saw the out-of-focus image of a bronze Cadillac pull to the curb. A double image of James stepped from the driver's seat to the curb. He stood behind his door, hand in his trench coat pocket.

"Put him in the car," James ordered.

Kevin took my arm.

"Rafael!" Michael shouted.

I looked vainly for him, but my sight was too badly blurred for me to distinguish anything. I heard his boots clattering on the sidewalk as he ran towards us.

"Hurry up," James snapped.

"No," I mumbled.

James pulled a snub-nosed pistol from his pocket.

"Gun!" I croaked, not loud enough to carry.

Kevin stood frozen, staring in shocked horror at the gun. Michael continued running towards us, and I had the horrible feeling of being the only one who could see and understand, and I was incapable of movement.

If I don't move, they will kill Michael just like they killed Valentin.

I lurched forward, the gun cracking like a lightning strike, the smell of burnt sulfur tainting the autumn air. A sledgehammer hit me in the chest, and before I could fall two more bullets clawed through my body. A short and fiery hole tore through my left arm splattering a great deal of blood, and a streak of fire traced a line along my ribs, exiting through the back of my jacket. Worst of all was the pain in my chest, which felt as though I had been kicked by an elephant. My breastbone had cracked, but not broken under the impact.

Pain was the perfect antidote to the drug Kevin had used. I remained on my feet, operating my body with the same power I used to open locks. James' eyes met mine in disbelief. Two massive bloodstains blotted the front of my white waistcoat, either of them apparently lethal. I smiled a nasty death's head grin at him.

"I'm undead, or did you forget?"

He leaped into his Cadillac, and I leaped after him, my drugged and wounded body sprawling headlong on the pavement. I lifted my head, saw the car backing away.

"Die!" I cried at the fleeing shape.

The car swerved, backed over the opposite curb, the rear fender caught a lamppost, and the front end skewed around. The engine stalled and James slumped over the wheel. I had no idea if he was alive or dead; my power was exhausted. My head dropped to the pavement.

Michael knelt beside me, touched my shoulder, and asked, "Rafael? Can you hear me?" I turned my head but I could not see him very well.

"Help me," I whispered.

He eased me to a sitting position, leaning against his chest as he knelt behind me, my head lying back against his shoulder, my breath coming raggedly through my lips. His arms cradled me, and his warmth was a much needed balm to the icy cold that pervaded my flesh.

"Call an ambulance!" he snapped at Kevin. Kevin ran, soft soled shoes making little sound on the pavement.

The bullet through my arm had opened an artery and my blood was draining away, and with it my strength. My heart stumbled in its cadence, fluttering erratically as it tried to pump too little blood through cyanose veins. I had never been so cold in my life.

"I'm dying, Michael," I mumbled.

"No!" he cried, head bent close to mine, hot tears dropping from his face to mine. "I won't let you die, you can't die! Not you!" I had wailed over Valentin the same way, refusing to accept either his death or my own, and so I had given myself thirty-five years of hell.

"Let me go, Michael. Grieve, and go on." My voice was reduced to a papery whisper.

"Don't you love me? How can you leave me if you love me?"

How many times had I stood over Valentin's grave, asking the same question? But Valentin had been a man of ordinary capabilities, and he had come to an ordinary end.

Yet in Michael I saw a spirit like my own. We were children of the same blood, and each of us had inherited the stubborn, intransigent spirit that balked against the rule of Death.

My fingers fumbled into my pocket and pulled out the small brown box. I snapped it open to reveal two gold bands nestled together in the velvet. The diamonds glittered in the light from the street lamps, cold and hard.

"I love you forever," I whispered.

"Not even death can part us!" he swore in reply.

I almost laughed to see how he reminded me of myself, but the sound turned to a cough and Michael had to catch the rings before I lost them.

"Promise me you won't let them bury me, or autopsy me..." I coughed again, dark blood splattering from my lips. Darkness crowded the edges of my vision. I did not have long.

He slid the ring with the initial M onto my ring finger. "I promise." Then he slipped the R onto his own finger.

"I'll come back, Michael. No matter what."

"I believe you. I'll be waiting."

Then Death laid his velvet cloak over me, suffocating with its soft darkness.

Chapter Twelve
EPILOGUE

I have labored sore and suffered death,
And now I rest and draw my breath;
But I shall come and call right soon
Heaven and death and hell to doom;
And then shall know both devil and man
What I was and what I am.

—Anonymous, 15th Century

Baltimore, 16 October 1991

Zoæ called on us while I was convalescing. Michael ushered her into the living room, where I was sitting on the sofa, dressed in a navy blue cardigan over a white oxford shirt with the collar open, blue jeans, and my stocking feet propped on the butler's table. My wounds were still bandaged, stiff and sore, but healing cleanly and rapidly. She sat down in the wing chair where I had sat the last time she called. This time she had apparently come straight from work, because she was wearing a gray suit of skirt and jacket, with a small maroon bow tie. Ties never look right on women.

"How are you feeling?" she asked, her voice carefully neutral.

I shrugged my right hand, as moving any other part of my body hurt.

"Recovering."

"You should have stayed at the hospital."

"After they put three pints of blood in me, stitched up my wounds, and taped everything back together again, there wasn't anything else for them to do. So I came home. Michael takes care of me as well as any nurse."

Michael was sitting on the floor beside me, dressed in his usual ratty blue jeans and a red cotton sweater. My hand fell on his shoulder.

After a short silence, Zoæ spoke again. "In related matters, Violeta Duran denies ever signing an affidavit. She says she did speak to James briefly by telephone, but was unaware of any 'disappearance.' Bertolo Guitierrez, your father's brother in Spain, says the same thing. Neither of them was ever notified about your father's death. I took the liberty of doing so; it was necessary to explain why I was asking about affidavits and disappearances. They want to meet you."

"I'll bet they do."

She did not ask me what I meant by that. Instead she said, "I've notified the insurance company of the fraud. They'll be investigating too. I'm optimistic that we'll be able to prove our case, but don't expect it immediately. It could take months to satisfy them and get them to pay your claim."

"And?"

She sighed. "Dad is in jail and under psychiatric care. I'm wondering if it would be acceptable to you for him be committed to a mental hospital instead of prosecuting him."

"Are you asking as my lawyer, or as the daughter of the man in question?"

She sighed deeply. "I'm still your lawyer, until you choose to discharge me. Considering the conflict of interest, discharging me would probably be wise."

I nodded in understanding. "I've been happy with your services so far. I see no reason to discontinue them."

I mulled over her question. An asylum would be a lot harsher than a prison, but there was always the possibility that he could be released far earlier than a prison would. On the other hand, it would mean the police would no longer have any reason to show up on my doorstep and ask me questions about my personal life.

"I'd be willing to accept those terms if I am notified whenever they consider releasing him. I want to be able to testify on my own behalf, and I want them to convince me he won't try to harm me."

"If they thought he was going to harm you, they would certainly not release him."

"I need to be sure of that."

"But the concept of hospitalization rather than imprisonment is acceptable to you?"

I debated with myself. The man I used to be wanted him dead, wanted the threat to Michael and me permanently obliterated from the face of the earth.

"If he's committed, will you be his guardian?"

"Yes."

Knowing James, being in the custody of his child would gall him far more than the faceless, impersonal custody of the state.

"All right. An asylum, with the conditions I have outlined. When the arrangements are made, I'll withdraw the charges against him."

She made notes on her legal pad.

"Anything else?"

I shook my head.

"It seems cruel," Michael said gravely. "Perhaps prison would be better. He's done wrong, let him pay for his crimes. I don't see the need for anything beyond that."

"He's ill," she said. "None of this would have happened if he were well."

Michael gave me a hard look.

"I think it would have. He committed forgery and fraud

and embezzlement years ago, when his mind was sound. If he came unhinged, it was confrontation with his own guilt that did it."

Zoæ shifted uncomfortably. "We don't know that. The delusions he's suffering don't develop in a matters of days or weeks. It takes time. Recent events simply revealed his illness."

Michael gave me another hard look, waiting for me to speak.

When I did not, he said, "Suppose everything James said was true. What would you do then?"

Zoæ's regarded Michael thoughtfully, then transferred her pensive gaze to me. I sat quietly, hoping she would not be able to overcome her own innate rationality and seriously consider what Michael was suggesting.

"If there was only one Rafael Guitierrez, and you were him, it would be fraud to try to collect the life insurance. As to what Dad did, it's still embezzlement and attempted kidnapping and murder."

We three sat in silence for a long time.

At last she said, "You are Rafael Guitierrez, aren't you? In spite of this masquerade, in spite your papers and everything, you are who Dad says you are."

I let out my breath in a long sigh. I did not realize I had been holding it.

"Yes."

Michael relaxed, and took my pale hand in his, the ring gleaming against his tan skin. Zoæ studied our hands, then searched my face.

"He says you're a vampire."

My grip tightened upon Michael's hand. "Yes, I am a vampire. But I am also a man."

"Dad isn't crazy," she said softly.

"Not that particular way, no." A little silence fell.

"Did you bite him?"

"In self defense, yes."

"He says he drank your blood."

I shook my head. "No. Never. I wouldn't allow it. That's why he had to resort to violence."

"Dad says your blood can be used to cure all the ills of humanity."

"I doubt it. Maybe some things, but at the price of turning people into vampires."

"There ought to be a way around it."

"Michael thinks so. He's persuaded me to take myself to the university hospital."

"I have?" Michael asked in surprise.

"You and Kevin and James and the press of recent events. Yes."

His eyes shone. "Good."

To see him looking at me with such approval made me a little giddy. I would do just about anything for that look.

Zoë gathered her things and rose. "You're fortunate to have a second chance at life. Some are not granted that grace."

"Everybody has a second chance. It's just that most people don't realize it."

She smiled wanly. "Don't screw up, Rafael. Whatever you turn out to be, for God's sake, be worth this agony."

There was nothing I could answer to that, so I sat silently while Michael showed her to the front door. I listened to her high heels clacking down the steps and across the walk, and the car door slam. The car pulled away, then Michael closed the front door and came and settled on the sofa next to me, lacing his arm gently around my shoulders.

"Thank you for telling her the truth."

"I don't see that it's any better for her to think her father is a criminal instead of a lunatic," I grumbled.

"Doesn't matter. She deserves the truth."

"Hmph. I don't see why."

He laughed and mussed my hair. "I love you, even if you are a grouch."

I smiled in spite of myself. "I love you, even if you are reforming me."

"No," he corrected. "You love me because I'm reforming you. If you really liked the way you used to be, you never would have spent fifteen years locked in a dark hole."

How could I argue with the man? I loved him. And besides, he was right. "Stop making sense," I ordered. "Kiss me instead." And he did.

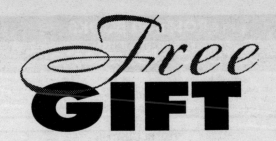

ROSEBUD BOOKS

THE ROSEBUD READER

Rosebud Books—the hottest-selling line of lesbian erotica available—here collects the very best of the best. Rosebud has contributed greatly to the burgeoning genre of lesbian erotica—to the point that authors like Lindsay Welsh, Aarona Griffin and Valentina Cilescu are among the hottest and most closely watched names in lesbian and gay publishing. Here are the finest moments from Rosebud's contemporary classics. $5.95/319-8

ALISON TYLER

THE BLUE ROSE

The tale of a modern sorority—fashioned after a Victorian girls' school. Ignited to the heights of passion by erotic tales of the Victorian age, a group of lusty young women are encouraged to act out their forbidden fantasies—all under the tutelage of Mistresses Emily and Justine, two avid practitioners of hard-core discipline! $5.95/335-X

ELIZABETH OLIVER

PAGAN DREAMS

Cassidy and Samantha plan a vacation at a secluded bed-and-breakfast, hoping for a little personal time alone. Their hostess, however, has different plans. The lovers are plunged into a world of dungeons and pagan rites, as the merciless Anastasia steals Samantha for her own. B&B—B&D-style! $5.95/295-7

SUSAN ANDERS

PINK CHAMPAGNE

Tasty, torrid tales of butch/femme couplings—from a writer more than capable of describing the special fire ignited when opposites collide. Tough as nails or soft as silk, these women seek out their antitheses, intent on working out the details of their own personal theory of difference. $5.95/282-5

LAVENDER ROSE

Anonymous

A classic collection of lesbian literature: From the writings of Sappho, Queen of the island Lesbos, to the turn-of-the-century *Black Book of Lesbianism*; from *Tips to Maidens* to *Crimson Hairs*, a recent lesbian saga—here are the great but little-known lesbian writings and revelations. $4.95/208-6

EDITED BY LAURA ANTONIOU

LEATHERWOMEN II

A follow-up volume to the popular and controversial *Leatherwomen*. Laura Antoniou turns an editor's discerning eye to the writing of women on the edge—resulting in a collection sure to ignite libidinal flames. Leave taboos behind—because these Leatherwomen know no limits.... $4.95/229-9

LEATHERWOMEN

These fantasies, from the pens of new or emerging authors, break every rule imposed on women's fantasies. The hottest stories from some of today's newest and most outrageous writers make this an unforgettable exploration of the female libido. $4.95/3095-4

LESLIE CAMERON

THE WHISPER OF FANS

"Just looking into her eyes, she felt that she knew a lot about this woman. She could see strength, boldness, a fresh sense of aliveness that rocked her to the core. In turn she felt open, revealed under the woman's gaze—all her secrets already told. No need of shame or artifice...." $5.95/259-0

ROSEBUD BOOKS

AARONA GRIFFIN

PASSAGE AND OTHER STORIES

An S/M romance. Lovely Nina is frightened by her lesbian passions until she finds herself infatuated with a woman she spots at a local café. One night Nina follows her and finds herself enmeshed in an endless maze leading to a mysterious world where women test the edges of sexuality and power. $4.95/3057-1

VALENTINA CILESCU

THE ROSEBUD SUTRA

"Women are hardly ever known in their true light, though they may love others, or become indifferent towards them, may give them delight, or abandon them, or may extract from them all the wealth that they possess." So says *The Rosebud Sutra*—a volume promising women's inner secrets. One woman learns to use these secrets in a quest for pleasure with a succession of lady loves.... $4.95/242-6

THE HAVEN

The shocking story of a dangerous woman on the run—and the innocents she takes with her on a trip to Hell. J craves domination, and her perverse appetites lead her to the Haven: the isolated sanctuary Ros and Annie call home. Soon J forces her way into the couple's world, bringing unspeakable lust and cruelty into their lives. The Dominatrix Who Came to Dinner! $4.95/165-9

MISTRESS MINE

Sophia Cranleigh sits in prison, accused of authoring the "obscene" *Mistress Mine*. For Sophia has led no ordinary life, but has slaved and suffered—deliciously—under the hand of the notorious Mistress Malin. How long had she languished under the dominance of this incredible beauty? $4.95/109-8

LINDSAY WELSH

PROVINCETOWN SUMMER

This completely original collection is devoted exclusively to white-hot desire between women. From the casual encounters of women on the prowl to the enduring erotic bonds between old lovers, the women of *Provincetown Summer* will set your senses on fire! A nationally best-selling title.$5.95/362-7

NECESSARY EVIL

What's a girl to do? When her Mistress proves too systematic, too by-the-book, one lovely submissive takes the ultimate chance—choosing and creating a Mistress who'll fulfill her heart's desire. Little did she know how difficult it would be—and, in the end, rewarding.... $5.95/277-9

A VICTORIAN ROMANCE

Lust-letters from the road. A young Englishwoman realizes her dream—a trip abroad under the guidance of her eccentric maiden aunt. Soon the young but blossoming Elaine comes to discover her own sexual talents, as a hot-blooded Parisian named Madelaine takes her Sapphic education in hand. $5.95/365-1

A CIRCLE OF FRIENDS

The author of the nationally best-selling *Provincetown Summer* returns with the story of a remarkable group of women. Slowly, the women pair off to explore all the possibilities of lesbian passion, until finally it seems that there is nothing—and no one—they have not dabbled in. $4.95/250-7

PRIVATE LESSONS

A high voltage tale of life at The Whitfield Academy for Young Women—where cruel headmistress Devon Whitfield presides over the in-depth education of only the most talented and delicious of maidens. Elizabeth Dunn arrives at the Academy, where it becomes clear that she has much to learn—to the delight of Devon Whitfield and her randy staff of Mistresses! $4.95/116-0

ROSEBUD BOOKS

BAD HABITS

What does one do with a poorly trained slave? Break her of her bad habits, of course! The story of te ultimate finishing school, *Bad Habits* was an immediate favorite with women nationwide. "Talk about passing the wet test!... If you like hot, lesbian erotica, run—don't walk...and pick up a copy of *Bad Habits*."—*Lambda Book Report* $4.95/3068-7

ANNABELLE BARKER

MOROCCO

A luscious young woman stands to inherit a fortune—if she can only withstand the ministrations of her cruel guardian until her twentieth birthday. With two months left, Lila makes a bold bid for freedom, only to find that liberty has its own excruciating and delicious price.... $4.95/148-9

A.L. REINE

DISTANT LOVE & OTHER STORIES

A book of seductive tales. In the title story, Leah Michaels and her lover Ranelle have had four years of blissful, smoldering passion together. One night, when Ranelle is out of town, Leah records an audio "Valentine," a cassette filled with erotic reminiscences.... $4.95/3056-3

RHINOCEROS BOOKS

EDITED BY AMARANTHA KNIGHT

FLESH FANTASTIC

A volume dedicated to the wildest fantasies. Humans have long toyed with the idea of "playing God": creating life from nothingness, bringing Life to the inanimate. Now Amarantha Knight, author of the phenomenal "Darker Passions" series of erotic horror novels, collects the best stories exploring not only the allure of Creation, but the lust that may well follow.... $6.96/352-X

GARY BOWEN

DIARY OF A VAMPIRE

"Gifted with a darkly sensual vision and a fresh voice, [Bowen] is a writer to watch out for." —*Cecilia Tan*

The chilling, arousing, and ultimately moving memoirs of an undead—but all too human—soul. Bowen's Rafael, a red-blooded male with an insatiable hunger for same, is the perfect antidote to the effete malcontents haunting bookstores today. *Diary of a Vampire* marks the emergence of a bold and brilliant vision, firmly rooted in past *and* present. $6.95/331-7

RENE MAIZEROY

FLESHLY ATTRACTIONS

Lucien Hardanges was the son of the wantonly beautiful actress, Marie-Rose Hardanges. When she decides to let a "friend" introduce her son to the pleasures of love, Marie-Rose could not have foretold the erotic excesses that would lead to her own ruin and that of her cherished son. $6.95/299-X

EDITED BY LAURA ANTONIOU

SOME WOMEN

Over forty essays written by women actively involved in consensual dominance and submission. Professional mistresses, lifestyle leatherdykes, whipmakers, titleholders—women from every conceivable walk of life lay bare their true feelings about about issues as explosive as feminism, abuse, pleasures and public image. $6.95/300-7

RHINOCEROS BOOKS

BY HER SUBDUED

Stories of women who get what they want. The tales in this collection all involve women in control—of their lives, their loves, their men. So much in control, in fact, that they can remorselessly break rules to become the powerful goddesses of the men who sacrifice all to worship at their feet. $6.95/281-7

JEAN STINE

SEASON OF THE WITCH

"A future in which it is technically possible to transfer the total mind... of a rapist killer into the brain dead but physically living body of his female victim. Remarkable for intense psychological technique. There is eroticism but it is necessary to mark the differences between the sexes and the subtle altering of a man into a woman." —*The Science Fiction Critic* $6.95/268-X

JOHN WARREN

THE LOVING DOMINANT

Everything you need to know about an infamous sexual variation—and an unspoken type of love. Mentor—a longtime player in the dominance/submission scene—guides readers through this world and reveals the too-often hidden basis of the D/S relationship: care, trust and love. $6.95/218-3

GRANT ANTREWS

SUBMISSIONS

Once again, Antrews portrays the very special elements of the dominant/submissive relationship...with restraint—this time with the story of a lonely man, a winning lottery ticket, and a demanding dominatrix. One of erotica's most discerning writers. $6.95/207-8

MY DARLING DOMINATRIX

When a man and a woman fall in love it's supposed to be simple, uncomplicated, easy—unless that woman happens to be a dominatrix. Curiosity gives way to unblushing desire in this story of one man's awakening to the joys to be experienced as the willing slave of a powerful woman. A touching volume, devoid of sleaze or shame. $6.95/3055-5

LAURA ANTONIOU WRITING AS "SARA ADAMSON"

THE TRAINER

The long-awaited conclusion of Adamson's stunning Marketplace Trilogy! The ultimate underground sexual realm includes not only willing slaves, but the exquisite trainers who take submissives firmly in hand. And it is now the time for these mentors to divulge their own secrets—the desires that led them to become the ultimate figures of authority. Only Sara Adamson could conjure so bewitching a portrait of punishing pleasure. $6.95/249-3

THE SLAVE

The second volume in the "Marketplace" trilogy. *The Slave* covers the experience of one exceptionally talented submissive who longs to join the ranks of those who have proven themselves worthy of entry into the Marketplace. But the price, while delicious, is staggeringly high.... Adamson's plot thickens, as her trilogy moves to a conclusion in the forthcoming *The Trainer*. $6.95/173-X

THE MARKETPLACE

"Merchandise does not come easily to the Marketplace.... They haunt the clubs and the organizations.... Some of them are so ripe that they intimidate the poseurs, the weekend sadists and the furtive dilettantes who are so endemic to that world. And they never stop asking where we may be found...." $6.95/3096-2

THE
WET FOREVER

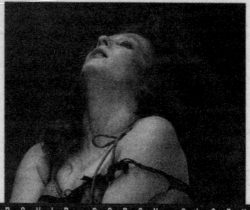

DAVID AARON CLARK

"Evocative and poetic."
Terence Sellers, author of *The Correct Sadist*

$6.95 • RHINOCEROS BOOKS

RHINOCEROS BOOKS

THE CATALYST

After viewing a controversial, explicitly kinky film full of images of bondage and submission, several audience members find themselves deeply moved by the erotic suggestions they've seen on the screen. "Sara Adamson"'s sensational debut volume! $5.95/328-7

DAVID AARON CLARK

SISTER RADIANCE

From the author of the acclaimed *The Wet Forever*, comes a chronicle of obsession, rife with Clark's trademark vivisections of contemporary desires, sacred and profane. The vicissitudes of lust and romance are examined against a backdrop of urban decay and shallow fashionability in this testament to the allure—and inevitability—of the forbidden. $6.95/215-9

THE WET FOREVER

The story of Janus and Madchen, a small-time hood and a beautiful sex worker, *The Wet Forever* examines themes of loyalty, sacrifice, redemption and obsession amidst Manhattan's sex parlors and underground S/M clubs. Its combination of sex and suspense led Terence Sellers to proclaim it "evocative and poetic." $6.95/117-9

ALICE JOANOU

BLACK TONGUE

"Joanou has created a series of sumptuous, brooding, dark visions of sexual obsession and is undoubtedly a name to look out for in the future." —*Redeemer*

Another seductive book of dreams from the author of the acclaimed *Tourniquet*. Exploring lust at its most florid and unsparing, *Black Tongue* is a trove of baroque fantasies—each redolent of the forbidden and inexpressible. Joanou creates some of erotica's most unforgettable characters. $6.95/258-2

TOURNIQUET

A heady collection of stories and effusions from the pen of one our most dazzling young writers. Strange tales abound, from the story of the mysterious and cruel Cybele, to an encounter with the sadistic entertainment of a bizarre after-hours cafe. A sumptuous feast for all the senses.. $6.95/3060-1

CANNIBAL FLOWER

"She is waiting in her darkened bedroom, as she has waited throughout history, to seduce the men who are foolish enough to be blinded by her irresistible charms....She is the goddess of sexuality, and *Cannibal Flower* is her haunting siren song."—Michael Perkins $4.95/72-6

MICHAEL PERKINS

EVIL COMPANIONS

Set in New York City during the tumultuous waning years of the Sixties, *Evil Companions* has been hailed as "a frightening classic." A young couple explores the nether reaches of the erotic unconscious in a shocking confrontation with the extremes of passion. With a new introduction by science fiction legend Samuel R. Delany. $6.95/3067-9

AN ANTHOLOGY OF CLASSIC ANONYMOUS EROTIC WRITING

Michael Perkins, acclaimed authority on erotic literature, has collected the very best passages from the world's erotic writing—especially for Rhino*ceros* readers. "Anonymous" is one of the most infamous bylines in publishing history—and these steamy excerpts show why! Dozens of examples of the best erotica. $6.95/140-3

RHINOCEROS BOOKS

THE SECRET RECORD: Modern Erotic Literature

Michael Perkins, a renowned author and critic of sexually explicit fiction, surveys the field with authority and unique insight. Updated and revised to include the latest trends, tastes, and developments in this misunderstood and maligned genre. An important volume for every erotic reader and fan of high quality adult fiction. $6.95/3039-3

HELEN HENLEY

ENTER WITH TRUMPETS

Helen Henley was told that woman just don't write about sex—much less the taboos she was so interested in exploring. So Henley did it alone, flying in the face of "tradition" by producing *Enter With Trumpets*, a touching tale of arousal and devotion in one couple's kinky relationship. $6.95/197-7

PHILIP JOSE FARMER

FLESH

Space Commander Stagg explored the galaxies for 800 years, and could only hope that he would be welcomed home by an adoring—or at least *appreciative*—public. Upon his return, the hero Stagg is made the centerpiece of an incredible public ritual—one that will repeatedly take him to the heights of ecstasy, and inexorably drag him toward the depths of hell. $6.95/303-1

A FEAST UNKNOWN

"Sprawling, brawling, shocking, suspenseful, hilarious…"—Theodore Sturgeon Farmer's supreme anti-hero returns. *A Feast Unknown* begins in 1968, with Lord Grandrith's stunning statement: "I was conceived and born in 1888." Slowly, Lord Grandrith—armed with the belief that he is the son of Jack the Ripper—tells the story of his remarkable and unbridled life. Beginning with his discovery of the secret of immortality, Grandrith's tale proves him no raving lunatic—but something far more bizarre…. $6.95/276-0

THE IMAGE OF THE BEAST

Herald Childe has seen Hell, glimpsed its horror in an act of sexual mutilation. Childe must now find and destroy an inhuman predator through the streets of a polluted and decadent Los Angeles of the future. One clue after another leads Childe to an inescapable realization about the nature of sex and evil…. $6.95/166-7

SAMUEL R. DELANY

EQUINOX

The *Scorpion* has sailed the seas in a quest for every possible pleasure. Her crew is a collection of the young, the twisted, the insatiable. A drifter comes into their midst, and is taken on a fantastic journey to the darkest, most dangerous sexual extremes—until he is finally a victim to their boundless appetites. $6.95/157-8

ANDREI CODRESCU

THE REPENTANCE OF LORRAINE

"One of our most prodigiously talented and magical writers."
—NYT **Book Review**

An aspiring writer, a professor's wife, a secretary, gold anklets, Maoists, Roman harlots—and more—swirl through this spicy tale of a harried quest for a mythic artifact. Written when the author was a young man, this lusty yarn was inspired by the heady—and hot—days and nights of the Sixties. Includes a special Introduction by the author, painting a vivid portrait of *Lorraine*'s creation. $6.95/329-5

RHINOCEROS BOOKS

DAVID MELTZER
ORF
He is the ultimate musician-hero—the idol of thousands, the fevered dream of many more. And like many musicians before him, he is misunderstood, misused—and totally out of control. Every last drop of feeling is squeezed from a modern-day troubadour and his lady love. $6.95/**110-1**

LEOPOLD VON SACHER-MASOCH
VENUS IN FURS
This classic 19th century novel is the first uncompromising exploration of the dominant/submissive relationship in literature. The alliance of Severin and Wanda epitomizes Sacher-Masoch's dark obsession with a cruel, controlling goddess and the urges that drive the man held in her thrall. The letters exchanged between Sacher-Masoch and an aspiring writer he sought as the avatar of his forbidden desires—are also included. $6.95/**3089-X**

SOPHIE GALLEYMORE BIRD
MANEATER
Through a bizarre act of creation, a man attains the "perfect" lover—by all appearances a beautiful, sensuous woman but in reality something far darker. Once brought to life she will accept no mate, seeking instead the prey that will sate her hunger for vengeance. A biting take on the war of the sexes, this debut goes for the jugular of the "perfect woman" myth. $6.95/**103-9**

TUPPY OWENS
SENSATIONS
A piece of porn history. Tuppy Owens tells the unexpurgated story of the making of *Sensations*—the first big-budget sex flick. Originally commissioned to appear in book form after the release of the film in 1975, *Sensations* is finally released under Masquerade's stylish Rhino*ceros* imprint. $6.95/**3081-4**

DANIEL VIAN
ILLUSIONS
Two disturbing tales of danger and desire in Berlin on the eve of WWII. From private homes to lurid cafés to decaying streets, passion is explored, exposed, and placed in stark contrast to the brutal violence of the time. A singularly arousing volume. $6.95/**3074-1**

PERSUASIONS
"The stockings are drawn tight by the suspender belt, tight enough to be stretched to the limit just above the middle part of her thighs..." A double novel, including the classics *Adagio* and *Gabriela and the General*, this volume traces desire around the globe. International lust! $6.95/**183-7**

LIESEL KULIG
LOVE IN WARTIME
An uncompromising look at the politics, perils and pleasures of sexual power. Madeleine knew that the handsome SS officer was a dangerous man. But she was just a cabaret singer in Nazi-occupied Paris, trying to survive in a perilous time. When Josef fell in love with her, he discovered that a beautiful and amoral woman can sometimes be wildly dangerous. $6.95/**3044-X**

MASQUERADE BOOKS

BEAUTY OF THE BEAST   *Carole Remy*
A shocking tell-all, written from the point-of-view of a prize-winning reporter.
And what reporting she does! All the secrets of an uninhibited life are
revealed, and each lusty tableau is painted in glowing colors. Join in on her
scandalous adventures—and reap the rewards of her extensive background in
Erotic Affairs! $5.95/332-5

NAUGHTY MESSAGE   *Stanley Carten*
Wesley Arthur, a withdrawn computer engineer, discovers a lascivious message on his answering machine. Aroused beyond his wildest dreams by the
unmentionable acts described, Wesley becomes obsessed with tracking down
the woman behind the seductive voice. His search takes him through strip
clubs and no-tell motels—and finally to his randy reward.... $5.95/333-3

The Marquis de Sade's JULIETTE   *David Aaron Clark*
The Marquis de Sade's infamous Juliette returns—and at the hand of David
Aaron Clark, she emerges as the most powerful, perverse and destructive
nightstalker modern New York will ever know. Under this domina's tutelage,
two women come to know torture's bizarre attractions, as they grapple with
the price of Juliette's promise of immortality.
Praise for Dave Clark:
"David Aaron Clark has delved into one of the most sensationalistically taboo
aspects of eros, sadomasochism, and produced a novel of unmistakable literary
imagination and artistic value."   —Carlo McCormick, *Paper* $5.95/240-X

THE PARLOR   *N.T. Morley*
Lovely Kathryn gives in to the ultimate temptation. The mysterious John and
Sarah ask her to be their slave—an idea that turns Kathryn on so much that
she can't refuse! But who are these two mysterious strangers? Little by little,
Kathryn comes to know the inner secrets of her stunning keepers.$5.95/291-4

NADIA   *Anonymous*
"Nadia married General the Count Gregorio Stenoff—a gentleman of noble
pedigree it is true, but one of the most reckless dissipated rascals in Russia…"
Follow the delicious but neglected Nadia as she works to wring every drop of
pleasure out of life—despite an unhappy marriage. A classic title providing a
peek into the secret sexual lives of another time and place. $5.95/267-1

THE STORY OF A VICTORIAN MAID   *Nigel McParr*
What were the Victorians really like? Chances are, no one believes they were
as stuffy as their Queen, but who would have imagined such unbridled lib-
ertines! One maid is followed from exploit to smutty exploit! $5.95/241-8

CARRIE'S STORY   *Molly Weatherfield*
"I had been Jonathan's slave for about a year when he told me he wanted to
sell me at an auction. I wasn't in any condition to respond when he told me
this…" Desire and depravity run rampant in this story of uncompromising
mastery and irrevocable submission. $5.95/228-0

CHARLY'S GAME   *Bren Flemming*
Charly's a no-nonsense private detective facing the fight of her life. A rich
woman's gullible daughter has run off with one of the toughest leather dykes
in town—and Charly's hired to lure the girl back. One by one, wise and
wicked women ensnare one another in their lusty nets! $4.95/221-3

ANDREA AT THE CENTER   *J.P. Kansas*
Kidnapped! Lithe and lovely young Andrea is, without warning, whisked
away to a distant retreat. Gradually, she is introduced to the ways of the
Center, and soon becomes quite friendly with its other inhabitants—all of
whom are learning to abandon all restraint in their pursuit of the deepest sexual satisfaction. $5.95/324-4

MASQUERADE BOOKS

ASK ISADORA
Isadora Alman

An essential volume, collecting six years' worth of Isadora Alman's syndicated columns on sex and relationships. Alman's been called a "hip Dr. Ruth," and a "sexy Dear Abby," based upon the wit and pertinence of her advice. Today's world is more perplexing than ever—and Isadora Alman is just the expert to help untangle the most personal of knots. $4.95/61-0

THE SLAVES OF SHOANNA
Mercedes Kelly

Shoanna, the cruel and magnificent, takes four maidens under her wing—and teaches them the ins and outs of pleasure and discipline. Trained in every imaginable perversion, from simple fleshly joys to advanced techniques, these students go to the head of the class! $4.95/164-0

LOVE & SURRENDER
Marlene Darcy

"Madeline saw Harry looking at her legs and she blushed as she remembered what he wanted to do.... She casually pulled the skirt of her dress back to uncover her knees and the lower part of her thighs. What did he want now? Did he want more? She tugged at her skirt again, pulled it back far enough so almost all of her thighs were exposed...." $4.95/3082-2

THE COMPLETE *PLAYGIRL* FANTASIES
Editors of Playgirl

The best women's fantasies are collected here, fresh from the pages of *Playgirl*. These knockouts from the infamous "Reader's Fantasy Forum" prove, once again, that truth can indeed be hotter, wilder, and *better* than fiction. $4.95/3075-X

STASI SLUT
Anthony Bobarzynski

Need we say more? Adina lives in East Germany, far from the sexually liberated, uninhibited debauchery of the West. She meets a group of ruthless and corrupt STASI agents who use her as a pawn in their political chess game as well as for their own perverse gratification— until she uses her talents and attractions in a final bid for total freedom! $4.95/3050-4

BLUE TANGO
Hilary Manning

Ripe and tempting Julie is haunted by the sounds of extraordinary passion beyond her bedroom wall. Alone, she fantasizes about taking part in the amorous dramas of her hosts, Claire and Edward. When she finds a way to watch the nightly debauch, her curiosity turns to full-blown lust! $4.95/3037-7

LOUISE BELHAVEL

FRAGRANT ABUSES

The saga of Clara and Iris continues as the now-experienced girls enjoy themselves with a new circle of worldly friends whose imaginations match their own. Perversity follows the lusty ladies around the globe! $4.95/88-2

DEPRAVED ANGELS

The final installment in the incredible adventures of Clara and Iris. Together with their friends, lovers, and worldly acquaintances, Clara and Iris explore the frontiers of depravity at home and abroad. $4.95/92-0

TITIAN BERESFORD

CINDERELLA

Beresford triumphs again with this intoxicating tale, filled with castle dungeons and tightly corseted ladies-in-waiting, naughty viscounts and impossibly cruel masturbatrixes—nearly every conceivable method of erotic torture is explored and described in lush, vivid detail. $4.95/305-8

JUDITH BOSTON

Young Edward would have been lucky to get the stodgy old companion he thought his parents had hired for him. Instead, an exquisite woman arrives at his door, and Edward finds his compulsively lewd behavior never goes unpunished by the unflinchingly severe Judith Boston! $4.95/273-6

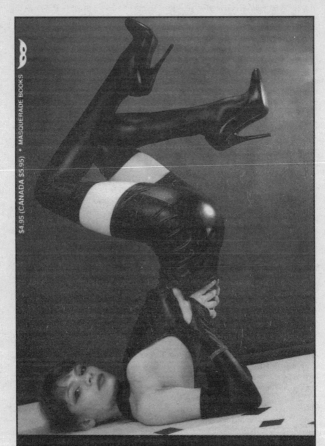

$4.95 (CANADA $5.95) • MASQUERADE BOOKS

NINA FOXTON

A N O N Y M O U S

MASQUERADE BOOKS

NINA FOXTON

An aristocrat finds herself bored by amusements for "ladies of good breeding." Instead of taking tea with proper gentlemen, Nina invents a contraption to "milk" them of their most private essences. Her frisky plan guarantees that no man ever says "No" to Nina! $4.95/145-4

A TITIAN BERESFORD READER

A captivating collection! Beresford's fanciful settings and outrageous fetishism have established his reputation as one of modern erotica's most imaginative and spirited writers. Wild dominatrixes, deliciously perverse masochists, and mesmerizing detail are the hallmarks of the Beresford tale—and can be encountered her in abundance. $4.95/114-4

CHINA BLUE

KUNG FU NUNS

"When I could stand the pleasure no longer, she lifted me out of the chair and sat me down on top of the table. She then lifted her skirt. The sight of her perfect legs clad in white stockings and a petite garter belt further mesmerized me. I lean particularly towards white garter belts." The infamous China Blue returns!
                                                                $4.95/3031-8

HARRIET DAIMLER

DARLING • INNOCENCE

In *Darling*, a virgin is raped by a mugger. Driven by her urge for revenge, she searches New York in a furious sexual hunt that leads to rape and murder. In *Innocence*, a young invalid determines to experience sex through her voluptuous nurse. Two critically acclaimed novels explode in one quality volume!
                                                                $4.95/3047-4

AKBAR DEL PIOMBO

SKIRTS

Randy Mr. Edward Champdick enters high society—and a whole lot more—in his quest for ultimate satisfaction. For it seems that once Mr. Champdick rises to the occasion, nothing can bring him down. Rampant ravishment follows this libertine wherever he goes! $4.95/115-2

DUKE COSIMO

A kinky romp played out against the boudoirs, bathrooms and ballrooms of the European nobility, who seem to do nothing all day except each other. The lifestyles of the rich and licentious are revealed in all their glory. Lust-styles of the rich and infamous! $4.95/3052-0

A CRUMBLING FAÇADE

The return of that incorrigible rogue, Henry Pike,who continues his pursuit of sex, fair or otherwise, in the most elegant homes of the most debauched aristocrats. No one can resist the irrepressible Pike! $4.95/3043-1

PAULA

"How bad do you want me?" she asked, her voice husky, breathy. I shrank back, for my desire for her was swelling to unspeakable proportions. "Turn around," she said, and I obeyed....This canny seductress tests the mettle of every man who comes under her spell—and every man does! $4.95/3036-9

ROBERT DESMOND

PROFESSIONAL CHARMER

A gigolo lives a parasitical life of luxury by providing his sexual services to the rich and bored. Traveling in the most exclusive circles, this gun-for-hire will gratify the lewdest and most vulgar sexual cravings! This dedicated pro leaves no one unsatisfied. $4.95/3003-2

MASQUERADE BOOKS

RETURN TO TIMBERLAND

It's time for a trip back to Timberland, the world's most frenzied sexual resort! Prepare for a vacation filled with delicious decadence, as each and every visitor is serviced by unimaginably talented submissives. These nubile maidens are determined to make this the raunchiest camp-out ever! $5.95/257-4

SARAH JACKSON

SANCTUARY

Tales from the Middle Ages. *Sanctuary* explores both the unspeakable debauchery of court life and the unimaginable privations of monastic solitude, leading the voracious and the virtuous on a collision course that brings history to throbbing life. $5.95/318-X

HELOISE

A panoply of sensual tales harkening back to the golden age of Victorian erotica. Desire is examined in all its intricacy, as fantasies are explored and urges explode. Innocence meets experience time and again. $4.95/3073-3

JOYCELYN JOYCE

PRIVATE LIVES

The illicit affairs and lecherous habits of the illustrious make for a sizzling tale of French erotic life. A wealthy widow has a craving for a young busboy; he's sleeping with a rich businessman's wife; her husband is minding his sex business elsewhere! $4.95/309-0

CANDY LIPS

The world of publishing serves as the backdrop for one woman's pursuit of sexual satisfaction. From a fiery femme fatale to a voracious Valentino, she takes her pleasure where she can find it. Luckily for her, it's most often found between the legs of the most licentious lovers! $4.95/182-9

KIM'S PASSION

The life of a beautiful English seductress. Kim leaves India for London, where she quickly takes upon herself the task of bedding every woman in sight! One by one, the lovely Kim's conquests accumulate, until she finds herself in the arms of gentry and commoners alike. $4.95/162-4

CAROUSEL

A young American woman leaves her husband when she discovers he is having an affair with their maid. She then becomes the sexual plaything of various Parisian voluptuaries. Wild sex, low morals, and ultimate decadence in the flamboyant years before the European collapse. $4.95/3051-2

SABINE

There is no one who can refuse her once she casts her spell; no lover can do anything less than give up his whole life for her. Great men and empires fall at her feet; but she is haughty, distracted, impervious. It is the eve of WW II, and Sabine must find a new lover equal to her talents. $4.95/3046-6

THE WILD HEART

A luxury hotel is the setting for this artful web of sex, desire, and love. A newlywed sees sex as a duty, while her hungry husband tries to awaken her to its tender joys. A Parisian entertains wealthy guests for the love of money. Each episode provides a new variation in this lusty Grand Hotel! $4.95/3007-5

JADE EAST

Laura, passive and passionate, follows her husband Emilio to Hong Kong. He gives her to Wu Li, a connoisseur of sexual perversions, who passes her on to Madeleine, a flamboyant lesbian. Madeleine's friends make Laura the centerpiece in Hong Kong's infamous underground orgies. $4.95/60-2

MASQUERADE BOOKS

RAWHIDE LUST

Diana Beaumont, the young wife of a U.S. Marshal, is kidnapped as an act of vengeance against her husband. Jack Beaumont sets out on a long journey to get his wife back, but finally catches up with her trail only to learn that she's been sold into white slavery in Mexico. $4.95/55-6

THE JAZZ AGE

The time: the Roaring Twenties. A young attorney becomes suspicious of his mistress while his wife has an fling with a lesbian lover. *The Jazz Age* is a romp of erotic realism from the heyday of the speakeasy. $4.95/48-3

AMARANTHA KNIGHT

THE DARKER PASSIONS:
THE FALL OF THE HOUSE OF USHER

The Master and Mistress of the house of Usher indulge in every form of decadence, and are intent on initiating their guests into the many pleasures to be found in utter submission. But something is not quite right in the House of Usher, and the foundation of its dynasty begins to crack.... $5.95/313-9

THE DARKER PASSIONS: *FRANKENSTEIN*

What if you could create a living, breathing human? What shocking acts could it be taught to perform, to desire, to love? Find out what pleasures await those who play God.... $5.95/248-5

THE DARKER PASSIONS: *DR. JEKYLL AND MR. HYDE*

It is an old story, one of incredible, frightening transformations achieved through mysterious experiments. Now, Amarantha Knight explores the steamy possibilities of a tale where no one is quite who—or what—they seem. Victorian bedrooms explode with hidden demons. $4.95/227-2

THE DARKER PASSIONS: *DRACULA*

"Well-written and imaginative, Amarantha Knight gives fresh impetus to this myth, taking us through the sexual and sadistic scenes with details that keep us reading.... This author shows superb control. A classic in itself has been added to the shelves." —Divinity $5.95/326-0

ALIZARIN LAKE

THE EROTIC ADVENTURES OF HARRY TEMPLE

Harry Temple's memoirs chronicle his amorous adventures from his initiation at the hands of insatiable sirens, through his stay at a house of hot repute, to his encounters with a chastity-belted nympho—and many other exuberant and over-stimulated partners. $4.95/127-6

EROTOMANIA

The bible of female sexual perversion! It's all here, everything you ever wanted to know about kinky women past and present. From simple nymphomania to the most outrageous fetishism, all secrets are revealed in this look into the forbidden rooms of feminine desire. $4.95/128-4

AN ALIZARIN LAKE READER

A selection of wicked musings from the pen of Masquerade's perennially popular author. It's all here: *Business as Usual, The Erotic Adventures of Harry Temple, Festival of Venus,* the mysterious *Instruments of the Passion,* the devilish *Miss High Heels*—and more. $4.95/106-3

MISS HIGH HEELS

It was a delightful punishment few men dared to dream of. Who could have predicted how far it would go? Forced by his sisters to dress and behave like a proper lady, Dennis finds he enjoys life as Denise much more! Crossdressed fetishism run amuck! $4.95/3066-0

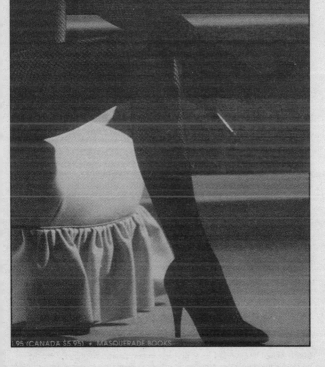

THE COMPLETE
Erotic
Reader

MASQUERADE BOOKS

ALL THE WAY

Two excruciating novels from Paul Little in one hot volume! *Going All the Way* features an unhappy man who tries to purge himself of the memory of his lover with a series of quirky and uninhibited women. *Pushover* tells the story of a serial spanker and his celebrated exploits in California. Two over-the-top sex marathons! $4.95/3023-7

CAPTIVE MAIDENS

Three beautiful young women find themselves powerless against the wealthy, debauched landowners of 1824 England. They are banished to a sexual slave colony where they are corrupted into participation in every imaginable perversion. $4.95/3014-8

SLAVE ISLAND

A leisure cruise is waylaid, finding itself in the domain of Lord Henry Philbrock, a sadistic genius, who has built a hidden paradise where captive females are forced into slavery. The ship's passengers are kidnapped and spirited to his island prison, where the women are trained to accommodate the most bizarre sexual cravings of the rich, the famous, the pampered and the perverted. Slutty slaves degraded! $4.95/3006-7

MARY LOVE

THE BEST OF MARY LOVE

Mary Love leaves no coupling untried and no extreme unexplored in these scandalous selections from *Mastering Mary Sue, Ecstasy on Fire, Vice Park Place, Wanda,* and *Naughtier at Night.* $4.95/3099-7

ECSTASY ON FIRE

The inexperienced young Steven is initiated into the intense, throbbing pleasures of manhood by the worldly Melissa Staunton, a well-qualified teacher of the sensual arts. Soon he's in a position—or two—to give lessons of his own! Innocence and experience in an erotic explosion! $4.95/3080-6

NAUGHTIER AT NIGHT

"He wanted to seize her. Her buttocks under the tight suede material were absolutely succulent—carved and molded. What on earth had he done to deserve a morsel of a girl like this?" $4.95/3030-X

RACHEL PEREZ

ODD WOMEN

These women are lots of things: sexy, smart, innocent, tough—some even say odd. But who cares, when their combined ass-ettes are so sweet! There's not a moral in sight as an assortment of Sapphic sirens proves once and for all that comely ladies come best in pairs. $4.95/123-3

AFFINITIES

"Kelsy had a liking for cool upper-class blondes, the long-legged girls from Lake Forest and Winnetka who came into the city to cruise the lesbian bars on Halsted, looking for breathless ecstasies. Kelsy thought of them as icebergs that needed melting, these girls with a quiet demeanor and so much under the surface...." A scorching tale of lesbian libidos unleashed, from an uncommonly vivid writer. $4.95/113-6

CHARLOTTE ROSE

A DANGEROUS DAY

A new volume from the best-selling author who brought you the sensational *Women at Work* and *The Doctor Is In*. And if you thought the high-powered entanglements of her previous books were risky, wait until Rose takes you on a journey through the thrills of one dangerous day! $5.95/293-0

MASQUERADE BOOKS

THE DOCTOR IS IN

"Finally, a book of erotic writing by a woman who isn't afraid to get down—and with deliciously lavish details that open out floodgates of lust and desire. Read it alone ... or with somebody you really like!"

—*Candida Royalle*

From the author of the acclaimed *Women at Work* comes a delectable trio of fantasies inspired by one of life's most intimate relationships. Charlotte Rose once again writes about women's forbidden desires, this time from the patient's point of view. $4.95/195-0

WOMEN AT WORK

Hot, uninhibited stories devoted to the working woman! From a lonesome cowgirl to a supercharged public relations exec, these women know how to let off steam after a tough day on the job. Includes "A Cowgirl's Passion," ranked #1 on Dr. Ruth's list of favorite erotic stories for women! $4.95/3088-1

SYDNEY ST. JAMES

RIVE GAUCHE

Decadence and debauchery among the doomed artists in the Latin Quarter, Paris circa 1920. Expatriate bohemians couple with abandon—before eventually abandoning their ambitions amidst the intoxicating temptations waiting to be indulged in every bedroom. Finally, "creative impulse" takes on a whole new meaning—with the creation of wild sexual heat! $5.95/317-1

THE HIGHWAYWOMAN

A young filmmaker making a documentary about the life of the notorious English highwaywoman, Bess Ambrose, becomes obsessed with her mysterious subject. It seems that Bess touched more than hearts—and plundered the treasures of every man and maiden she met on the way. $4.95/174-8

GARDEN OF DELIGHT

A vivid account of sexual awakening that follows an innocent but insatiably curious young woman's journey from the furtive, forbidden joys of dormitory life to the unabashed carnality of the wild world. Pretty Pauline blossoms with each new experiment in the sensual arts. $4.95/3058-X

ALEXANDER TROCCHI

THONGS

"...In Spain, life is cheap, from that glittering tragedy in the bullring to the quick thrust of the stiletto in a narrow street in a Barcelona slum. No, this death would not have called for further comment had it not been for one striking fact. The naked woman had met her end in a way he had never seen before—a way that had enormous sexual significance. My God, she had been..." $4.95/217-5

HELEN AND DESIRE

Helen Seferis' flight from the oppressive village of her birth became a sexual tour of a harsh world. From brothels in Sydney to harems in Algiers, Helen chronicles her adventures fully in her diary. Each encounter is examined in the scorching and uncensored diary of the sensual Helen! $4.95/3093-8

THE CARNAL DAYS OF HELEN SEFERIS

Private Investigator Anthony Harvest is assigned to save Helen Seferis, a beautiful Australian who has been abducted. Following clues in Helen's explicit diary of adventures, he Helen, the ultimate sexual prize. $4.95/3086-5

WHITE THIGHS

A fantasy of obsession from a modern erotic master. This is the story of Saul and his sexual fixation on the beautiful, tormented Anna. Their scorching passion leads to murder and madness every time they submit to their lusty needs. Saul must possess Anna again and again. $4.95/3009-1

MASQUERADE BOOKS

SCHOOL FOR SIN

When Peggy leaves her country home behind for the bright lights of Dublin, her sensuous nature leads to her seduction by a stranger. He recruits her into a training school where no one knows what awaits them at graduation, but each student is sure to be well schooled in sex! $4.95/ **89-0**

MY LIFE AND LOVES (THE 'LOST' VOLUME)

What happens when you try to fake a sequel to the most scandalous autobiography of the 20th century? If the "forgers" are two of the most important figures in modern erotica, you get a masterpiece, and THIS IS IT! One of the most thrilling forgeries in literature. $4.95/ **52-1**

MARCUS VAN HELLER

TERROR

Another shocking exploration of lust by the author of the ever-popular *Adam & Eve*. Set in Paris during the Algerian War, *Terror* explores the place of sexual passion in a world drunk on violence. *Terror* reveals the legendary Van Heller at the top of his game. $5.95/ **247-7**

KIDNAP

Private Investigator Harding is called in to investigate a mysterious kidnapping case involving the rich and powerful. Along the way he has the pleasure of "interrogating" an exotic dancer named Jeanne and a beautiful English reporter, as he finds himself enmeshed in the crime underworld. $4.95/ **90-4**

LUSCIDIA WALLACE

KATY'S AWAKENING

Katy thinks she's been rescued after a terrible car wreck. Little does she suspect that she's been ensnared by a ring of swingers whose tastes run to domination and unimaginably depraved sex parties. With no means of escape, Katy becomes the newest initiate into this sick private club—much to her pleasure! $4.95/ **308-2**

FOR SALE BY OWNER

Susie was overwhelmed by the lavishness of the yacht, the glamour of the guests. But she didn't know the plans they had for her. Sexual torture, training and sale into slavery! $4.95/ **3064-4**

THE ICE MAIDEN

Edward Canton has ruthlessly seized everything he wants in life, with one exception: Rebecca Esterbrook. Frustrated by his inability to seduce her with money, he kidnaps her and whisks her away to his remote island compound, where she emerges as a writhing, red-hot love slave! $4.95/ **3001-6**

DON WINSLOW

THE MANY PLEASURES OF IRONWOOD

Seven lovely young women are employed by The Ironwoood Sportsmen's club for the entertainment of gentlemen. A small and exclusive club with seven carefully selected sexual connoisseurs, Ironwood is dedicated to the relentless pursuit of sensual pleasure. $5.95/ **310-4**

CLAIRE'S GIRLS

You knew when she walked by that she was something special. She was one of Claire's girls, a woman carefully dressed and groomed to fill a role, to capture a look, to fit an image crafted by the sophisticated proprietress of an exclusive escort agency. High-class whores blow the roof off! $4.95/ **108-X**

GLORIA'S INDISCRETION

"He looked up at her. Gloria stood passively, her hands loosely at her sides, her eyes still closed, a dreamy expression on her face ... She sensed his hungry eyes on her, could almost feel his burning gaze on her body...." $4.95/ **3094-6**

Initiation Rites

A N O N Y M O U S

MASQUERADE BOOKS

THE MASQUERADE READERS

THE COMPLETE EROTIC READER

The very best in erotic writing together in a wicked collection sure to stimulate even the most jaded and "sophisticated" palates. $4.95/3063-6

THE VELVET TONGUE

An orgy of oral gratification! *The Velvet Tongue* celebrates the most mouthwatering, lip-smacking, tongue-twisting action. A feast of fellatio and *soixante-neuf* awaits readers of excellent taste at this steamy suck-fest. $4.95/3029-6

A MASQUERADE READER

Strict lessons are learned at the hand of *The English Governess*. Scandalous confessions are found in *The Diary of an Angel*, and the story of a woman whose desires drove her to the ultimate sacrifice in *Thongs* completes the collection. $4.95/84-X

THE CLASSIC COLLECTION

SCHOOL DAYS IN PARIS

A delicious duo of erotic awakenings. The rapturous chronicles of a well-spent youth! Few Universities provide the profound and pleasurable lessons one learns in after-hours study—particularly if one is young and bursting with promise, and lucky enough to have Paris as a playground. A stimulating look at the breathless pursuits of young adulthood. $5.95/325-2

MAN WITH A MAID

The adventures of Jack and Alice have delighted readers for eight decades! A classic of its genre, *Man with a Maid* tells an outrageous tale of desire, revenge, and submission. Over 200,000 copies in print! $4.95/307-4

MAN WITH A MAID II

Jack's back! With the assistance of the perverse Alice, he embarks again on a trip through every erotic extreme. Jack leaves no one unsatisfied—least of all, himself, and Alice is always certain to outdo herself in her capacity to corrupt and control. An incendiary sequel! $4.95/3071-7

MAN WITH A MAID: The Conclusion

The final chapter in the epic saga of lust that has thrilled readers for decades. The adulterous woman who is corrected with enthusiasm and the maid who receives grueling guidance are just two who benefit from these lessons! The can't-miss conclusion to one of erotica's most famous tales. $4.95/3013-X

Confessions of a Concubine II: HAREM SLAVE

The concubinage continues, as the true pleasures and privileges of the harem are revealed. For the first time, readers are invited behind the veils that hide uninhibited, unimaginable pleasures from the world.... $4.95/226-4

CONFESSIONS OF A CONCUBINE

What *really* happens behind the plush walls of the harem? An inexperienced woman, captured and sentenced to service the royal pleasure, tells all in an outrageously unrestrained memoir. No affairs of state could match the passions of a young woman learning to relish a life of ceaseless sexual servitude. $4.95/154-3

INITIATION RITES

Every naughty detail of a young woman's breaking in! Under the thorough tutelage of the perverse Miss Clara Birchem, Julia learns her wicked lessons well. During the course of her amorous studies, the resourceful young lady is joined by an assortment of lewd characters. $4.95/120-9

TABLEAUX VIVANTS

Fifteen breathtaking tales of erotic passion. Upstanding ladies and gents soon adopt more comfortable positions, as wicked thoughts explode into sinfully scrumptious acts. Carnal extremes and explorations abound in this tribute to the spirit of Eros—the lustiest common denominator! $4.95/121-7

MASQUERADE BOOKS

LADY F.

An uncensored tale of Victorian passions. Master Kidrodstock suffers deliciously at the hands of the stunningly cruel and sensuous Lady Flayskin—the only woman capable of taming his wayward impulses. $4.95/102-0

SACRED PASSIONS

Young Augustus comes into the heavenly sanctuary seeking protection from the enemies of his debt-ridden father. Within these walls he learns lessons he could never have imagined and soon concludes that the joys of the body far surpass those of the spirit. $4.95/21-1

CLASSIC EROTIC BIOGRAPHIES

JENNIFER III

The further adventures of erotica's most daring heroine. Jennifer, the quintessential beautiful blonde, has a photographer's eye for detail—particularly details of the masculine variety! A raging nymphomaniac! $5.95/292-2

JENNIFER AGAIN

One of contemporary erotica's hottest characters returns, in a sequel sure to blow you away. Once again, the insatiable Jennifer seizes the day—and extracts from it every last drop of sensual pleasure! $4.95/220-5

JENNIFER

From the bedroom of an internationally famous—and notoriously insatiable—dancer to an uninhibited ashram, *Jennifer* traces the exploits of one thoroughly modern woman. $4.95/107-1

ROSEMARY LANE *J.D. Hall*

The ups, downs, ins and outs of Rosemary Lane. Raised as the ward of Lord and Lady D'Arcy, after coming of age she discovers that her guardians' generosity is boundless—as they contribute to her carnal education! $4.95/3078-4

THE ROMANCES OF BLANCHE LA MARE

When Blanche loses her husband, it becomes clear she'll need a job. She sets her sights on the stage—and soon encounters a cast of lecherous characters intent on making her path to sucksess as hot and hard as possible! $4.95/101-2

KATE PERCIVAL

Kate, the "Belle of Delaware," divulges the secrets of her scandalous life, from her earliest sexual experiments to the deviations she learns to love. Nothing is secret, and no holes barred in this titillating tell-all. $4.95/3072-5

THE AMERICAN COLLECTION

LUST *Palmiro Vicarion*

A wealthy and powerful man of leisure recounts his rise up the corporate ladder and his corresponding descent into debauchery. A tale of a classic scoundrel with an uncurbed appetite for sexual power! $4.95/82-3

WAYWARD *Peter Jason*

A mysterious countess hires a tour bus for an unusual vacation. Traveling through Europe's most notorious cities, she picks up friends, lovers, and acquaintances from every walk of life in pursuit of pleasure. $4.95/3004-0

LOVE'S ILLUSION

Elizabeth Renard yearned for the body of Dan Harrington. Then she discovers Harrington's secret weakness: a need to be humiliated and punished. She makes him her slave, and together they commence a journey into depravity that leaves nothing to the imagination—*nothing!* $4.95/100-4

THE RELUCTANT CAPTIVE

Kidnapped by ruthless outlaws who kill her husband and burn their prosperous ranch, Sarah's journey takes her from the bordellos of the Wild West to the bedrooms of Boston, where she's bought by a stranger from her past. $4.95/3022-9

RICHARD KASAK BOOKS

EURYDICE

F/32

F/32 has been called "the most controversial and dangerous novel ever written by a woman." With the story of Ela (whose name is a pseudonym for orgasm), Eurydice won the National Fiction competition sponsored by Fiction Collective Two and Illinois State University. A funny, disturbing quest for unity, *F/32* prompted Frederic Tuten to proclaim "almost any page ... redeems us from the anemic writing and banalities we have endured in the past decade of bloodless fiction." $10.95/350-3

LARRY TOWNSEND

ASK LARRY

Twelve years of Masterful advice from Larry Townsend (*Run, Little Leatherboy, Chains*), the leatherman's long-time confidant and adviser. Starting just before the onslaught of AIDS, Townsend wrote the "Leather Notebook" column for *Drummer* magazine, tackling subjects from sexual technique to safer sex, whips to welts, Daddies to dog collars. Now, with *Ask Larry*, readers can avail themselves of Townsend's collected wisdom as well as the author's contemporary commentary—a careful consideration of the way life has changed in the AIDS era, and the specific ways in which the disease has altered perceptions of once-simple problems. $12.95/289-2

RUSS KICK

OUTPOSTS:
A Catalog of Rare and Disturbing Alternative Information

A huge, authoritative guide to some of the most offbeat and bizarre publications available today! Rather than simply summarize the plethora of controversial opinions crowding the American scene, Russ Kick has tracked down the real McCoy and compiled over five hundred reviews of work penned by political extremists, conspiracy theorists, hallucinogenic pathfinders, sexual explorers, religious iconoclasts and social malcontents. Better yet, each review is followed by ordering information for the many readers sure to want these remarkable publications for themselves. $18.95/0202-8

WILLIAM CARNEY

THE REAL THING

Carney gives us a good look at the mores and lifestyle of the first generation of gay leathermen. A chilling mystery/romance novel as well. —Pat Califia

With a new Introduction by Michael Bronski. Out of print for years, *The Real Thing* has long served as a touchstone to any consideration of gay "edge fiction." First published in 1968, this uncompromising story of New York leathermen received instant acclaim.. Out of print for years, *The Real Thing* returns from exile, ready to thrill a new generation—and reacquaint itself with its original audience. $10.95/280-9

MICHAEL LASSELL

THE HARD WAY

Lassell is a master of the necessary word. In an age of tepid and whining verse, his bawdy and bittersweet songs are like a plunge in cold champagne. —Paul Monette

The first collection of renowned gay writer Michael Lassell's poetry, fiction and essays. Widely anthologized and a staple of gay literary and entertainment publications nationwide, Lassell is regarded as one of the most distinctive talents of his generation. As much a chronicle of post-Stonewall gay life as a compendium of a remarkable writer's work. $12.95/231-0

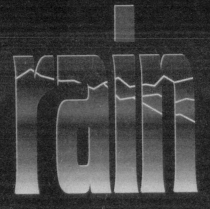

GUILLERMO BOSCH

rain

An Adult Fairy Tale

"This book will sear the flesh off your fingers."
—Peter Lefcourt, author of *Di and I*

RICHARD KASAK BOOKS

LOOKING FOR MR. PRESTON

Edited by Laura Antoniou, *Looking for Mr. Preston* includes work by **Lars Eighner**, Pat Califia, Michael Bronski, Felice Picano, Joan Nestle, Larry Townsend, Sasha Alyson, Andrew Holleran, Michael Lowenthal, and others who contributed interviews, essays and personal reminiscences of John Preston—a man whose career spanned the industry from the early pages of the *Advocate* to various national bestseller lists. Preston was the author of over twenty books, including *Franny, the Queen of Provincetown*, and *Mr. Benson*. He also edited the noted *Flesh and the Word* erotic anthologies, *Personal Dispatches: Writers Confront AIDS*, and *Hometowns*,. More importantly, Preston became a personal inspiration, friend and mentor to many of today's gay and lesbian authors and editors. Ten percent of the proceeds from sale of the book will go to the AIDS Project of Southern Maine, for which Preston had served as President of the Board. $23.95/288-4

AMARANTHA KNIGHT, EDITOR
LOVE BITES

A volume of tales dedicated to legend's sexiest demon—the Vampire. Amarantha Knight, herself an author who has delved into vampire lore, has gathered the very best writers in the field to produce a collection of uncommon, and chilling, allure. Including such names as Ron Dee, Nancy A. Collins, Nancy Kilpatrick, Lois Tilton and David Aaron Clark, *Love Bites* is not only the finest collection of erotic horror available—but a virtual who's who of promising new talent. $12.95/234-5

MICHAEL LOWENTHAL, EDITOR
THE BEST OF THE BADBOYS

A collection of the best of Masquerade Books' phenomenally popular Badboy line of gay erotic writing. Badboy 's sizable roster includes many names that are legendary in gay circles. The very best of the leading Badboys is collected here, in this testament to the artistry that has catapulted these "outlaw" authors to bestselling status. John Preston, Aaron Travis, Larry Townsend, John Rowberry, Clay Caldwell and Lars Eighner are here represented by their most provocative writing. Michael Lowenthal both edited this remarkable collection and provides the Introduction. $12.95/233-7

GUILLERMO BOSCH
RAIN

An adult fairy tale, *Rain* takes place in a time when the mysteries of Eros are played out against a background of uncommon deprivation. The tale begins on the 1,537th day of drought—when one man comes to know the true depths of thirst. In a quest to sate his hunger for some knowledge of the wide world, he is taken through a series of extraordinary, unearthly encounters that promise to change not only his life, but the course of civilization around him. A remarkable debut novel. $12.95/232-9

LUCY TAYLOR
UNNATURAL ACTS

"A topnotch collection..." —*Science Fiction Chronicle*

A remarkable debut volume from a provocative writer. *Unnatural Acts* plunges deep into the dark side of the psyche, far past all pleasantries and prohibitions, and brings to life a disturbing vision of erotic horror. Unrelenting angels and hungry gods play with souls and bodies in Taylor's murky cosmos: where heaven and hell are merely differences of perspective; where redemption and damnation lie behind the same shocking acts. $12.95/181-0

RICHARD KASAK BOOKS

SAMUEL R. DELANY

THE MOTION OF LIGHT IN WATER

"A very moving, intensely fascinating literary biography from an extraordinary writer. Thoroughly admirable candor and luminous stylistic precision; the artist as a young man and a memorable picture of an age." —William Gibson

The first unexpurgated American edition of award-winning author Samuel R. Delany's riveting autobiography covers the early years of one of science fiction's most important voices. Delany paints a vivid and compelling picture of New York's East Village in the early '60s—a time of unprecedented social transformation. Startling and revealing, ***The Motion of Light in Water*** traces the roots of one of America's most innovative writers. $12.95/133-0

THE MAD MAN

For his thesis, graduate student John Marr researches the life and work of the brilliant Timothy Hasler: a philosopher whose career was cut tragically short over a decade earlier. Marr encounters numerous obstacles, as other researchers turn up evidence of Hasler's personal life that is deemed simply too unpleasant. Marr soon begins to believe that Hasler's death might hold some key to his own life as a gay man in the age of AIDS.

This new novel by Samuel R. Delany not only expands the parameters of what he has given us in the past, but fuses together two seemingly disparate genres of writing and comes up with something which is not comparable to any existing text of which I am aware.... What Delany has done here is take the ideas of Marquis de Sade one step further, by filtering extreme and obsessive sexual behavior through the sieve of post-modern experience.... —Lambda Book Report

Reads like a pornographic reflection of Peter Ackroyd's Chatterton or A.S. Byatt's Possession.... Delany develops an insightful dichotomy between [his protagonist]'s two worlds: the one of cerebral philosophy and dry academia, the other of heedless, 'impersonal' obsessive sexual extremism. When these worlds finally collide ... the novel achieves a surprisingly satisfying resolution.... —Publishers Weekly $23.95/193-4

KATHLEEN K.

SWEET TALKERS

Here, for the first time, is the story behind the provocative advertisements and 970 prefixes. Kathleen K. opens up her diary for a rare peek at the day-to-day life of a phone sex operator—and reveals a number of secrets and surprises. Because far from being a sleazy, underground scam, the service Kathleen provides often speaks to the lives of its customers with a directness and compassion they receive nowhere else. $12.95/192-6

ROBERT PATRICK

TEMPLE SLAVE

...you must read this book. It draws such a tragic, and, in a way, noble portrait of Mr. Buono: It leads the reader, almost against his will, into a deep sympathy with this strange man who tried to comfort, to encourage and to feed both the worthy and the worthless... It is impossible not to mourn for this man—impossible not to praise this book.

—Quentin Crisp

*This is nothing less than the secret history of the most theatrical of theaters, the most bohemian of Americans and the most knowing of queens. Patrick writes with a lush and witty abandon, as if this departure from the crafting of plays has energized him. **Temple Slave** is also one of the best ways to learn what it was like to be fabulous, gay, theatrical and loved in a time at once more and less dangerous to gay life than our own.* —Genre

Temple Slave tells the story of the Espresso Buono—the archetypal alternative performance space—and the talents who called it home. $12.95/191-8

SWEET TALKERS

WORDS FROM THE MOUTH OF A "PAY TO SAY" GIRL

KATHLEEN K.

RICHARD KASAK BOOKS

DAVID MELTZER

THE AGENCY TRILOGY

...'*The Agency*' is clearly Meltzer's paradigm of society; a mindless machine of which we are all 'agents' including those whom the machine supposedly serves.... —Norman Spinrad

With the Essex House edition of *The Agency* in 1968, the highly regarded poet David Meltzer took America on a trip into a hell of unbridled sexuality. The story of a supersecret, Orwellian sexual network, *The Agency* explored issues of erotic dominance and submission with an immediacy and frankness previously unheard of in American literature, as well as presented a vision of an America consumed and dehumanized by a lust for power. $12.95/216-7

SKIN TWO

THE BEST OF *SKIN TWO* Edited by Tim Woodward

For over a decade, *Skin Two* has served the international fetish community as a groundbreaking journal from the crossroads of sexuality, fashion, and art, *Skin Two* specializes in provocative, challenging essays by the finest writers working in the "radical sex" scene. Collected here are the articles and interviews that established the magazine's reputation. Including interviews with cult figures Tim Burton, Clive Barker and Jean Paul Gaultier. $12.95/130-6

CARO SOLES

MELTDOWN!

An Anthology of Erotic Science Fiction and Dark Fantasy for Gay Men

Editor Caro Soles has put together one of the most explosive, mind-bending collections of gay erotic writing ever published. *Meltdown!* contains the very best examples of this increasingly popular sub-genre: stories meant to shock and delight, to send a shiver down the spine and start a fire down below. An extraordinary volume, *Meltdown!* presents both new voices and provocative pieces by world-famous writers Edmund White and Samuel R. Delany.
$12.95/203-5

BIZARRE SEX

BIZARRE SEX AND OTHER CRIMES OF PASSION
Edited by Stan Tal

Stan Tal, editor of *Bizarre Sex*, Canada's boldest fiction publication, has culled the very best stories that have crossed his desk—and now unleashes them on the reading public in *Bizarre Sex and Other Crimes of Passion*. Over twenty small masterpieces of erotic shock make this one of the year's most unexpectedly alluring anthologies. Including such masters of erotic horror and fantasy as Edward Lee, Lucy Taylor and Nancy Kilpatrick, *Bizarre Sex and Other Crimes of Passion*, is a treasure-trove of arousing chills. $12.95/213-2

PAT CALIFIA

SENSUOUS MAGIC

A new classic, destined to grace the shelves of anyone interested in contemporary sexuality.
Sensuous Magic is clear, succinct and engaging even for the reader for whom S/M isn't the sexual behavior of choice.... Califia's prose is soothing, informative and non-judgmental—she both instructs her reader and explores the territory for them.... When she is writing about the dynamics of sex and the technical aspects of it, Califia is the Dr. Ruth of the alternative sexuality set.... —Lambda Book Report

Don't take a dangerous trip into the unknown—buy this book and know where you're going!—SKIN TWO $12.95/131-4

RICHARD KASAK BOOKS

GAUNTLET

THE BEST OF *GAUNTLET* Edited by Barry Hoffman

No material, no opinion is taboo enough to violate Gauntlet's *purpose of 'exploring the limits of free expression'—airing all views in the name of the First Amendment.*
—Associated Press

Gauntlet has, with its semi-annual issues, taken on such explosive topics as race, pornography, political correctness, and media manipulation—always publishing the widest possible range of opinions. Only in *Gauntlet* might one expect to encounter Phyllis Schlafley *and* Annie Sprinkle, Stephen King *and* Madonna—often within pages of one another. The most provocative articles have been gathered by editor-in-chief Barry Hoffman, to make *The Best of Gauntlet* a riveting exploration of American society's limits. $12.95/202-7

MICHAEL PERKINS

THE GOOD PARTS: An Uncensored Guide to Literary Sexuality

Michael Perkins, one of America's only critics to regularly scrutinize sexual literature, presents sex as seen in the pages of over 100 major volumes from the past twenty years. *The Good Parts* takes an uncensored look at the complex issues of sexuality investigated by so much modern literature. $12.95/186-1

JOHN PRESTON

HUSTLING:
A Gentleman's Guide to the Fine Art of Homosexual Prostitution

John Preston solicited the advice of "working boys" from across the country in his effort to produce the ultimate guide to the hustler's world.

...fun and highly literary. What more could you expect from such an accomplished activist, author and editor? —Drummer $12.95/137-3

MY LIFE AS A PORNOGRAPHER
And Other Indecent Acts

...essential and enlightening...His sex-positive stand on safer-sex education as the only truly effective AIDS-prevention strategy will certainly not win him any conservative converts, but AIDS activists will be shouting their assent.... [My Life as a Pornographer] *is a bridge from the sexually liberated 1970s to the more cautious 1990s, and Preston has walked much of that way as a standard-bearer to the cause for equal rights....*
—Library Journal

My Life as a Pornographer...*is not pornography, but rather reflections upon the writing and production of it. Preston ranges from really superb journalism of his interviews with denizens of the S/M demi-monde, particularly a superb portrait of a Colt model Preston calls "Joe" to a brilliant analysis of the "theater" of the New York sex club, The Mineshaft.... In a deeply sex-phobic world, Preston has never shied away from a vision of the redemptive potential of the erotic drive. Better than perhaps anyone in our community, Preston knows how physical joy can bridge differences and make us well.*
—Lambda Book Report
$12.95/135-7

LARS EIGHNER

ELEMENTS OF AROUSAL

Critically acclaimed gay writer Lars Eighner develops a guideline for success with one of publishing's best kept secrets: the novice-friendly field of gay erotic writing. In *Elements of Arousal*, Eighner details his craft, providing the reader with sure advice. Because *Elements of Arousal* is about the application and honing of the writer's craft, which brought Eighner fame with not only the steamy *Bayou Boy*, but the illuminating *Travels with Lizbeth*. $12.95/230-2

RICHARD KASAK BOOKS

MARCO VASSI

THE STONED APOCALYPSE

" *...Marco Vassi is our champion sexual energist.*"—VLS

During his lifetime, Marco Vassi was hailed as America's premier erotic writer and most worthy successor to Henry Miller. His work was praised by writers as diverse as Gore Vidal and Norman Mailer, and his reputation was worldwide. *The Stoned Apocalypse* is Vassi's autobiography, financed by his other ground-breaking erotic writing. $12.95/132-2

A DRIVING PASSION

While the late Marco Vassi was primarily known and respected as a novelist, he was also an effective and compelling speaker. *A Driving Passion* collects the wit and insight Vassi brought to his infamously revealing lectures, and distills the philosophy—including the concept of Metasex—that made him an underground sensation. An essential volume. $12.95/134-9

THE EROTIC COMEDIES

A collection of stories from America's premier erotic philosopher. Marco Vassi was a dedicated iconoclast, and *The Erotic Comedies* marked a high point in his literary career. Scathing and humorous, these stories reflect Vassi's belief in the power and primacy of Eros in American life, as well as his commitment to the elimination of personal repression through carnal indulgence. $12.95/136-5

THE SALINE SOLUTION

During the Sexual Revolution, Marco Vassi established himself as an intrepid explorer of an uncharted sexual landscape. During this time he also distinguished himself as a novelist, producing *The Saline Solution* to great acclaim. With the story of one couple's brief affair and the events that lead them to desperately reassess their lives, Vassi examines the dangers of intimacy in an age of freedom. $12.95/180-2

CHEA VILLANUEVA

JESSIE'S SONG

"*It conjures up the strobe-light confusion and excitement of urban dyke life, moving fast and all over the place, from NYC to Tucson to Miami to the Philippines; and from true love to wild orgies to swearing eternal celibacy and back. Told in letters, mainly about the wandering heart (and tongue) of writer and free spirit Pearly Does; written mainly by Mae-Mae Might, a sharp, down-to-earth but innocent-hearted Black Femme. Read about these dykes and you'll love them.*"
—Rebecca Ripley

A rich collection of lesbian writing from this uncompromising author. Based largely upon her own experience, Villanueva's work is remarkable for its frankness, and delightful in its iconoclasm. Widely published in the alternative press, Villanueva is a writer to watch. Toeing no line, *Jessie's Song* is certain to redefine all notions of "mainstream" lesbian writing, and provide a reading experience quite unlike any other this year. $9.95/235-3

SHAR REDNOUR, EDITOR

VIRGIN TERRITORY

An anthology of writing about the most important moments of life. Tales of first-time sensual experiences, from the pens of some of America's most uninhibited literary women. No taboo is unbroken as these women tell the whole truth and nothing but, about their lives as sexual women in modern times.

Included in this daring volume are such cult favorites as Susie Bright, Shannon Bell, Bayla Travis, Carol Queen, Lisa Palac and others. They leave no act undescribed, and prove once and for all that "beginner's luck" is the very best kind to have! $12.95/238-8

BADBOY BOOKS

THE JOY SPOT *Phil Andros*

"Andros gives to the gay mind what Tom of Finland gives the gay eye—this is archetypal stuff. There's none better."   —**John F. Karr, Manifest Reader**

A classic from one of the founding fathers of gay porn. *The Joy Spot* looks at some of Andros' favorite types—cops, servicemen, truck drivers—and the sleaze they love. Nothing's too rough, and these men are always ready. So get ready to give it up—or have it taken by force!   **$5.95/301-5**

THE ROPE ABOVE, THE BED BELOW *Jason Fury*

The irresistible Jason Fury returns! Once again, our built, blond hero finds himself in the oddest—and most compromising—positions imaginable. And his combination of heat and heart has made him one of gay erotica's most distinctive voices.   **$4.95/269-8**

SUBMISSION HOLDS *Key Lincoln*

A bright talent unleashes his first collection of gay erotica. From tough to tender, the men between these covers stop at nothing to get what they want. These sweat-soaked tales show just how bad boys can get....   **$4.95/266-3**

SKIN DEEP *Bob Vickery*

Skin Deep contains so many varied beauties no one will go away unsatisfied. From Daddy's Boys to horny go-go studs, no tantalizing morsel of manflesh is overlooked—or left unexplored! Beauty may be only skin deep, but a handful of beautiful skin is a tempting proposition.   **$4.95/265-5**

ANIMAL HANDLERS *Jay Shaffer*

Another volume from a master of scorching fiction. In Shaffer's world, each and every man finally succumbs to the animal urges deep inside. And if there's any creature that promises a wild time, it's a beast who's been caged for far too long....   **$4.95/264-7**

RAHM *Tom Bacchus*

A volume spanning the many ages of hardcore queer lust—from Creation to the modern day. The overheated imagination of Tom Bacchus brings to life an extraordinary assortment of characters, from the Father of Us All to the cowpoke next door, the early gay literati to rude, queercore mosh rats. No one is better than Bacchus at staking out sexual territory with a swagger and a sly grin.   **$5.95/315-5**

REVOLT OF THE NAKED *D. V. Sadero*

In a distant galaxy, there are two classes of humans: Freemen and Nakeds. Freemen are full citizens in this system, which allows for the buying and selling of Nakeds at whim. Nakeds live only to serve their Masters, and obey every sexual order with haste and devotion. Until the day of revolution—when an army of sex toys rises in anger.... By the author of *In the Alley.*   **$4.95/261-2**

WHiPs *Victor Terry*

Connoisseurs of gay writing have known Victor Terry's work for some time. With *WHiPs*, Terry joins Badboy's roster at last. Cruising for a hot man? You'd better be, because one way or another, these WHiPs—officers of the Wyoming Highway Patrol—are gonna pull you over for a little impromptu interrogation....   **$4.95/254-X**

PRISONERS OF TORQUEMADA *Torsten Barring*

The infamously unsparing Torsten Barring (*The Switch, Peter Thornwell, Shadowman*) weighs in with another volume sure to push you over the edge. How cruel *is* the "therapy" practiced at Casa Torquemada? Rest assured that Barring is just the writer to evoke such steamy malevolence.   **$4.95/252-3**

BADBOY BOOKS

SORRY I ASKED *Dave Kinnick*

Up close and very personal! Unexpurgated interviews with gay porn's rank and file. Haven't you wondered what it's like to be in porn pictures? Kinnick, video reviewer for *Advocate Men*, gets personal with the guys behind (and under) the "stars," and reveals the dirt and details of the porn business.

$4.95/3090-3

THE SEXPERT *Edited by Pat Califia*

For many years now, the sophisticated gay man has known that he can turn to one authority for answers to virtually any question on the subject of man-to-man intimacy and sexual performance. Straight from the pages of *Advocate Men* comes The Sexpert! From penis size to toy care, bar behavior to AIDS awareness, The Sexpert responds to real concerns with uncanny wisdom and a razor wit.

$4.95/3034-2

DEREK ADAMS

MY DOUBLE LIFE

Every man leads a double life, dividing his hours between the mundanities of the day and the outrageous pursuits of the night. In this, his second collection of stories, the author of *Boy Toy* and creator of sexy P.I. Miles Diamond shines a little light on what men do when no one's looking. Derek Adams proves, once again, that he's the ultimate chronicler of our wicked ways.

$5.95/314-7

BOY TOY

Poor Brendan Callan—sent to the Brentwood Academy against his will, he soon finds himself the guinea pig of a crazed geneticist. Brendan becomes irresistibly alluring—a talent designed for endless pleasure, but coveted by others with the most unsavory motives....

$4.95/260-4

CLAY CALDWELL

STUD SHORTS

"If anything, Caldwell's charm is more powerful, his nostalgia more poignant, the horniness he captures more sweetly, achingly acute than ever."
—*Aaron Travis*

A new collection of this legendary writer's latest sex-fiction. With his customary candor, Caldwell tells all about cops, cadets, truckers, farmboys (and many more) in these dirty jewels.

$5.95/320-1

QUEERS LIKE US

A very special delivery from one of gay erotica's premier talents. For years the name Clay Caldwell has been synonymous with the hottest, most finely crafted gay tales available. *Queers Like Us* is one of his best: the story of a randy mailman's trek through a landscape of willing, available studs.

$4.95/262-0

CLAY CALDWELL/LARS EIGHNER

QSFx2

A volume of the wickedest, wildest, other-worldliest yarns from two master storytellers. Caldwell and Eighner take a trip to the furthest reaches of the sexual imagination, sending back stories proving that as much as things change, one thing will always remain the same....

$5.95/278-7

LARS EIGHNER

WHISPERED IN THE DARK

Hailed by critics, Lars Eighner continues to produce gay fiction whose quality rivals the best in the genre. *Whispered in the Dark* demonstrates Eighner's unique combination of strengths: poetic descriptive power, an unfailing ear for dialogue, and a finely tuned feeling for the nuances of male passion.

$5.95/286-8

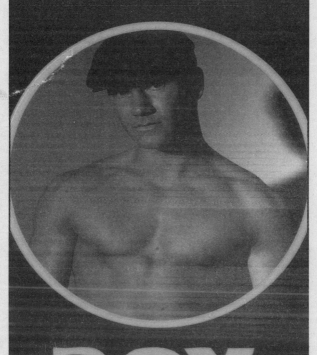

BOY
TOY

BADBOY BOOKS

AMERICAN PRELUDE

Praised by the *New York Times*, Eighner is widely recognized as one of our best, most exciting gay writers. What the *Times* won't admit, however, is that he is also one of gay erotica's true masters. Scalding heat blends with wry emotion in this red-blooded bedside volume. $4.95/170-5

LARRY TOWNSEND

BEWARE THE GOD WHO SMILES

A torrid time-travel tale from one of gay erotica's most notorious writers. Two lusty young Americans are transported to ancient Egypt—where they are embroiled in regional warfare and taken as slaves by marauding barbarians. The key to escape from this brutal bondage lies in their own rampant libidos, and urges as old as time itself. $5.95/321-X

RUN, LITTLE LEATHER BOY

The classic story of one man's sexual awakening. A chronic underachiever, Wayne seems to be going nowhere. When he is sent abroad, Wayne soon finds himself bored with the everyday and increasingly drawn to the masculine intensity of a dark sexual underground. Back in print to inspire a new generation, *Run, Little Leather Boy* is a favorite with gay readers. $4.95/143-8

SEXUAL ADV. OF SHERLOCK HOLMES

What Conan Doyle didn't know about the legendary sleuth. Holmes's most satisfying adventures, from the unexpurgated memoirs of the faithful Mr. Watson. "A Study in Scarlet" is transformed to expose Mrs. Hudson as a man in drag, the Diogenes Club as an S/M arena, and clues only Sherlock Holmes could piece together. $4.95/3097-0

AARON TRAVIS

BIG SHOTS

Two fierce tales in one electrifying volume. In *Beirut*, Travis tells the story of ultimate military power and erotic subjugation; *Kip*, Travis' hypersexed and sinister take on film noir, appears in unexpurgated form for the first time—including the final, overwhelming chapter. One of the rawest titles we've ever published. $4.95/112-8

SLAVES OF THE EMPIRE

"[A] wonderful mythic tale. Set against the backdrop of the exotic and powerful Roman Empire, this wonderfully written novel explores the timeless questions of light and dark in male sexuality. Travis has shown himself expert in manipulating the most primal themes and images. The locale may be the ancient world, but these are the slaves and masters of our time...." —John Preston $4.95/3054-7

JOHN PRESTON

TALES FROM THE DARK LORD

Twelve stunning works from the man called "the Dark Lord of gay erotica." The ritual of lust and surrender is explored in all its manifestations in this triumph of authority and vision from the Dark Lord! One of our most popular collections. $5.95/323-6

MR. BENSON

A classic novel from a time when there was no limit to what a man could dream of doing. Jamie is led down the path of erotic enlightenment by the magnificent Mr. Benson, learning to accept cruelty as love, anguish as affection, and this man as his master. $4.95/3041-5

HARD CANDY

SKYDIVING ON CHRISTOPHER STREET *Stan Leventhal*
"Positively addictive."   —Dennis Cooper

Aside from a hateful job, a hateful apartment, a hateful world and an increasingly hateful lover, life seems, well, *all right* for the protagonist of Stan Leventhal's latest novel, *Skydiving on Christopher Street*. Having already lost most of his friends to AIDS, how could things get any worse? But things soon do, and he's forced to endure much more....   **$6.95/287-6**

THE GAUDY IMAGE *William Talsman*

"To read *The Gaudy Image* now is not simply to enjoy a great novel or an artifact of gay history, it is to see first-hand the very issues of identity and positionality with which gay men and gay culture were struggling in the decades before Stonewall. For what Talsman is dealing with...is the very question of how we conceive ourselves gay."—from the Introduction by Michael Bronski
    $6.95/263-9

GAY COSMOS *Lars Eighner*

A thought-provoking volume from widely acclaimed author Lars Eighner. Eighner has distinguished himself as not only one of America's most accomplished new voices, but a solid-seller—his erotic titles alone have become bestsellers and classics of the genre. Eighner describes *Gay Cosmos* as being a volume of "essays on the place, meaning, and purpose of homosexuality in the Universe, and gay sexuality on human societies." A title sure to appeal not only to Eighner's gay fans, but the many converts who first encountered his moving nonfiction work.   **$6.95/236-1**

FELICE PICANO

AMBI*DEXTROUS*

The touching and funny memories of childhood—as only Felice Picano could tell them. **Ambi***dextrous* tells the story of Picano's youth in the suburbs of New York during the '50's. Beginning at age eleven, Picano's "memoir in the form of a novel" tells all: home life, school face-offs, the ingenuous sophistications of his first sexual steps. In three years' time, he's had his first gay fling—and is on his way to becoming the writer about whom the *L.A. Herald Examiner* said "[he] can run the length of experience from the lyrical to the lewd without missing a beat."   **$6.95/275-2**

MEN WHO LOVED ME

In 1966, at the tender-but-bored age of twenty-two, Felice Picano abandoned New York, determined to find true love in Europe. Almost immediately, he encounters Djanko—an exquisite prodigal who sweeps Felice off his feet with the endless string of extravagant parties, glamorous clubs and glittering premieres that made up Rome's *dolce vita*. When the older (slightly) and wiser (vastly) Picano returns to New York at last, he plunges into the city's thriving gay community—experiencing the frenzy and heartbreak that came to define Greenwich Village society in the 1970s. Lush and warm, *Men Who Loved Me* is a matchless portrait of an unforgettable decade.   **$6.95/274-4**

E-mail us:
Masq Bks @ aol.com

ORDERING IS EASY!

MC/VISA orders can be placed by calling our toll-free number

PHONE 800-375-2356 / FAX 212 986-7355

or mail this coupon to:

MASQUERADE BOOKS
DEPT. U54AT, 801 2ND AVE., NY, NY 10017

BUY ANY FOUR BOOKS AND CHOOSE ONE ADDITIONAL
BOOK, OF EQUAL OR LESSER VALUE, AS YOUR FREE GIFT.

QTY.	TITLE	NO.	PRICE
			FREE
			FREE

U54AT

	SUBTOTAL	
	POSTAGE and HANDLING	

We Never Sell, Give or Trade Any Customer's Name.   **TOTAL**

In the U.S., please add $1.50 for the first book and 75¢ for each additional book; in Canada, add $2.00 for the first book and $1.25 for each additional book. Foreign countries: add $4.00 for the first book and $2.00 for each additional book. No C.O.D. orders. Please make all checks payable to Masquerade Books. Payable in U.S. currency only. New York state residents add $8^{1/4}$% sales tax. Please allow 4-6 weeks delivery.

NAME _____

ADDRESS _____

CITY _____ STATE _____ ZIP _____

TEL ( ) _____

PAYMENT: ☐ CHECK ☐ MONEY ORDER ☐ VISA ☐ MC

CARD NO. _____ EXP. DATE _____